The Economics of Animal Health and Production

———————————

This book is dedicated to my boys Adam and Ben and my wife Rommy Evelyn,
who have sacrificed much during the book's preparation, and without their love and support
it would never have been possible.

The Economics of Animal Health and Production

By

Jonathan Rushton

With Guest Contributors

Foreword by

Peter R. Ellis OBE

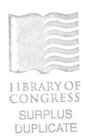
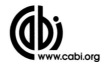

www.cabi.org

CABI is a trading name of CAB International

CABI Head Office
Nosworthy Way
Wallingford
Oxfordshire OX10 8DE
UK

Tel: +44 (0)1491 832111
Fax: +44 (0)1491 833508
Email: cabi@cabi.org
Web site: www.cabi.org

CABI North American Office
875 Massachusetts Avenue
7th Floor
Cambridge, MA 02139
USA

Tel: +1 617 395 4056
Fax: +1 617 354 6875
Email: cabi-nao@cabi.org

A catalogue record for this book is available from the British Library,
London, UK.

ISBN-13: 978-1-84593-194-0 (HB)

ISBN-13: 978-1-84593-875-8 (PB)

First published (HB) 2007
First paperback edition 2011

Printed and bound in the UK by MPG Books Group.

The paper used for the text pages of this book is FSC certified. The FSC
(Forest Stewardship Council) is an international network to promote responsible
management of the world's forests.

Contents

———————————————

Contributors

Principal author

Jonathan Rushton is an agricultural economist who specializes in livestock economics and development. He has experience of livestock development issues in Africa, Asia, Europe and Latin America through working with FAO, EU, DfID, IICA, ILRI, DANIDA, GTZ and USAID. His key interests are the role of livestock in the livelihoods of poor people worldwide, the impact of livestock diseases, the use of participatory methodologies in veterinary epidemiology and the marketing of agricultural products. He is a Senior Lecturer in animal health economics at the Royal Veterinary College, London.

Guest contributors

Vinod Ahuja is an Associate Professor at the Centre for Management in Agriculture, Indian Institute of Management, Ahmedabad. He has been involved in some of the ground-breaking research on service delivery for poor rural livestock producers and has published widely in this field. He currently combines his academic commitments with being the South Asian regional coordinator for FAO's Pro-Poor Livestock Policy Initiative.

Harvey Beck is an agricultural economist within the Department of Agriculture and Rural Development in Northern Ireland who is a specialist in the application of economic appraisal techniques. His doctorate from Reading University investigated the long-term benefits of agricultural research and the interaction between technical change in agriculture and agricultural policy. This, and a subsequent publication on the economics of mastitis control, laid the foundations for a continued interest in the economics of animal disease.

Pascal Bonnet is a veterinarian who specializes in epidemiology, animal health economics and health geography. He has worked in livestock research and development in Africa, Western and Central Asia, India, Western Europe and Latin America through working with the International Centre for Agricultural Research for Development (CIRAD), CGIAR (ILRI in Eastern Africa), various partners from civil society (NGOs, e.g. Action against Hunger), European Commission (EDF projects) and governmental agencies and ministries (i.e. Ministry of Agriculture, Ministry of Foreign Affairs and former Ministry of Cooperation, France). His key interests are livestock development approaches that combine geographical and economic analysis at micro or meso levels. He is currently working in Southern Africa as chief technical adviser for SADC, being posted by CIRAD.

C. Devendra is a specialist in animal nutrition and production systems. He has made significant contributions in these fields in Malaysia, in the Asian region and globally through assignments with the World Bank, UNDP, FAO, the Commonwealth Secretariat and USAID. He has also held the roles of Senior Program Officer for the Canadian International Development Research Center and Senior Associate for the International Livestock Research Institute in Kenya. Currently he is a consulting animal production systems specialist based in Malaysia.

Andrew James has worked in over 50 countries and is a regular contributor to FAO and OIE Expert consultations, particularly with reference to the control of transboundary diseases, disease surveillance and disease modelling. He is a member of the advisory committee for the FAO Emergency Programme for the Prevention of Transboundary Diseases (EMPRES), and was a member of the expert groups that developed epidemiological surveillance standards for declaring countries free of rinderpest, contagious bovine pleuropneumonia and foot-and-mouth disease. In recent years, he has managed the development of the InterAgri range of livestock information systems ranging from on-farm herd management systems through to national livestock databases.

David Leonard is a specialist in political science (BA from Haverford in 1963 and a PhD in Political Science from the University of Chicago in 1974). He has extensive experience of advising African governments in the field of animal health, and is a recognized global expert in the application of institutional economics for animal health service delivery. He was the Dean of International and Area Studies and Professor, Department of Political Science, University of California, Berkeley, USA, and is currently Professorial Fellow at the Institute of Development Studies, Brighton, UK.

Matthieu Lesnoff is a biometrician at the International Centre for Agricultural Research for Development (CIRAD). He has specialized in modelling demography of tropical livestock populations and disease dynamics. He has occupied various research positions in France, West Africa (CIRAD) and East Africa (ILRI: International Livestock Research Institute).

Joachim Otte is a graduate of the Veterinary College of Hanover with a specialization in veterinary epidemiology and economics. He has working experience in Latin America, Africa, Europe and Asia, where he primarily focused on the economic implications of animal health interventions. In 1998, he took up a post at FAO and currently occupies the position of coordinator of the Pro-Poor Livestock Policy Initiative.

Ugo Pica-Ciamarra is an agricultural economist with a specialization in institutional economics and economic development policies. His main areas of interest are pro-poor livestock policies, pro-poor institutional changes, and land policies in developing countries. He has worked for the University of Rome 'La Sapienza' and the Italian National Institute of Agricultural Economics (INEA), and currently works for the Pro-Poor Livestock Policy Initiative (PPLPI) at FAO Headquarters in Rome.

Liz Redmond is Director of Animal Health and Welfare Policy in the Department of Agriculture and Rural Development in Northern Ireland, and was formerly the Deputy Chief Veterinary Officer. She leads on the development of all aspects of animal health and welfare policy, and advises Ministers and the Northern Ireland Executives. She is a veterinary graduate from the University of Sydney, Australia, and she also holds a master's degree in agricultural economics from the University of Reading. She has previously worked for the Government of Botswana, for the FAO in Rome as part of a DfID-funded policy project to assist poor livestock farmers, and under contract to Defra on economic appraisal of disease control policy.

Hernán Rojas is a veterinary epidemiologist who has made significant contributions on animal health policy. He has a veterinary degree from the University of Chile, Santiago, and a Master's and PhD in veterinary epidemiology from the University of Reading, UK. Between 2001 and 2006, he was the Chief Veterinary Officer of Chile. Currently he is the Director of Chile's National Institute for Agriculture and Livestock Development (INDAP), which is part of the Ministry of Agriculture.

Alexandra Shaw is an economist, whose specialization is animal health. She began her working career in Nigeria, and later wrote her PhD on the economics of controlling tsetse and trypanosomiasis in West Africa. Most of her career has been focused on Africa, where she has worked in over twenty countries. She has also done some work in South America, for WHO on various zoonoses and worked on the economic aspects of animal health control programmes in the EU. She has taught veterinary economics in British, German, French and African universities. Currently, she divides her time between teaching and consultancy work. Her main research interests are trypanosomiasis and the economics of other zoonotic diseases.

Alistair Stott is head of the animal health economics team within the Research and Development Division of SAC. He graduated with a degree in agriculture in 1980, followed by a PhD in animal physiology and genetics. Alistair combines this strong scientific and agricultural background with nearly 15 years working in farm business management and animal health and welfare economics. His background is ideal for encouraging scientists and economists to work together to tackle problems facing agriculture. As well as animal health and welfare, he has worked on the development of selection indices for animal breeding.

Clem Tisdell has a broad range of research interests which include topics in agricultural and ecological economics, such as those involving livestock management, genetic diversity and animal health issues. He has been involved in consultancies or research projects for bodies such as ACIAR, FAO and ILRI. His applied research has focused mainly on Asia and the Pacific. He is currently Professor Emeritus in Economics at the University of Queensland (Australia) and is jointly investigating the adjustment of Vietnamese pig producers to changing market conditions.

Martin Upton has had a long career as an agricultural economist, first at the University of Ibadan, Nigeria, and subsequently at the University of Reading. Over the last 20 years he has specialized in the economics of livestock production, marketing and development policy, mostly in Africa and more recently in the UK. This has involved studies for ILCA and ILRAD (now ILRI), FAO, DfID and The Netherlands Government. For DEFRA, he led the Reading team conducting cost–benefit analysis of the 20-day standstill and continued as peer reviewer for further studies on FMD control. He is currently participating in a broad review of animal health and welfare policies for DEFRA.

Rommy Viscarra is a veterinary epidemiologist who specializes in animal health control and extension. She has experience in animal health issues in Bolivia and in the Americas through working with FAO, WHO, DANIDA and USAID. Her key interests are animal health education in schools to promote community development and sustainable livestock production. She is an independent consultant.

Preface

During the last 200 years, there has been massive socio-economic change through industrial and agricultural revolutions. This change has been associated with rapid increases in human and domestic livestock populations, and a movement of people from rural to urban areas. More than half the people in the world now live in urban environments where they have better access to work, but limited or no access to land and livestock to produce food. This implies that a majority of people are dependent on others for raw, semi-processed and processed food products. The efficient functioning of the livestock sector, encompassing all facets of input supply, production, processing and marketing, has become a critical issue for guaranteeing:

- that sufficient livestock products are available at affordable prices – food security; and
- that the livestock products are safe to eat – food safety.

Within the livestock sector, the livestock producers and business people involved in input supply and output processing and marketing need to be able to plan, make a profit and have a sustainable livelihood. The State also plays a critical role in facilitating how the livestock sector functions and develops in order to satisfy society's needs. Therefore, both the private and public sectors require economic theory and tools to understand the drivers of change for the livestock sector, and how to assess the impact of future actions and investments.

Background

The mid to late 18th century saw important advances in livestock production, in particular the recognition of more productive breeds. However, it was not until the middle of the following century that livestock production systems began to change. In Britain, the prices for meat began to rise in the 1840s, which stimulated an adoption of more intensive livestock production and a modification of housing systems. Around the same time livestock diseases became more problematic as livestock and livestock product movement increased and livestock value chains became longer and more complex. Of greatest note was the importance of economic diseases such as rinderpest, contagious bovine pleuropneumonia and foot-and-mouth disease (FMD). These diseases caused such problems that the State reacted and began to invest in veterinary services, education and research (Fisher, 1998). However, the response to diseases that cause less dramatic losses to production, yet have serious impacts on human health, was not addressed in many developed countries until much later (Fisher, 1998; Waddington, 2002; see also Alexandra P.M. Shaw, Chapter 14). At international level, concerns on the need to control rinderpest stimulated the creation of the international office of animal health in the 1920s.

These initial investments in animal health and production, mainly associated with developed countries, were stimulated by large changes in livestock production and their associated value chains, perhaps best described as the first livestock revolution. The changes in the livestock sector created new disease problems, and also amplified the impact of contagious diseases. The response over time has been a combined public and private effort to control animal diseases in order to minimize their socio-economic impact. In some cases this has led to the eradication of disease in a number of countries.

Through a process of investigation of livestock production systems (Steinfeld and Mäki-Hokkonen, 1995; Sere and Steinfeld, 1996), and followed by an analysis of the supply and demand of livestock products (Delgado et al., 1999), it was realized that a new livestock revolution had begun. Unlike the previous revolutions, this was based largely on monogastric production and, to some extent, on changes in milk production. Similar to the early changes in livestock production and supply chains, it was being driven on the demand side by rapid human population increases, growing urban populations and increasing incomes. On the supply side, production and processing technologies had improved; there was availability of cheap feed grains and a reduction in bulk transport costs. The production changes of this new livestock revolution have been concentrated in the developing countries. Some raised concerns that the changes may leave some poor people behind (Haan et al., 2001; Heffernan, 2002; FAO, 2005; Owen et al., 2005) and others focused on the environmental impacts of change (de Haan et al., 1997; Steinfeld et al., 2006). What was not anticipated were the growing problems with the control of transboundary animal diseases and, more specifically, the resurgence of zoonotic diseases (Greger, 2007).

Therefore, over a period of around 200 years, the world has moved from relatively simple livestock value chains to increasingly complex ones. In the simple livestock chains a high proportion of produce was either consumed in the farm household or sold in local and regional markets. In addition, much of this food was processed within the household (see Fig. 1).

In the complex food value chains that are now dominant in many parts of the world, primary production has complex relationships with consumers through processing and marketing companies. The links in the chain are maintained by middlemen, transport companies and finance groups. Where the value chains become integrated, i.e. owned and controlled by one company, the middlemen disappear. In addition, consumer demands have become more sophisticated for processed food and food with zero risk of food-borne diseases (see Fig. 2). These livestock value chains can also be global.

The adoption of more complex livestock value chains has not been gradual; rather it appears to have been in jumps. The first of these probably occurred in the mid 19th century in Europe and North America with linkages to Australia, New Zealand and probably Argentina, and the

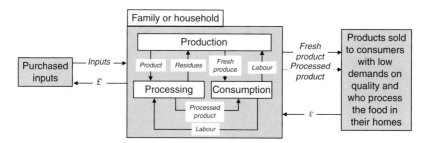

Fig. 1. Simple livestock value chains. (From Rushton and Viscarra, 2006.)

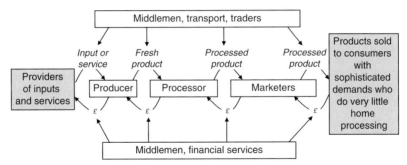

Fig. 2. A schematic diagram of the dominant complex livestock value chains. (From Rushton and Viscarra, 2006.)

second in the late 20th century mainly in Asia, but also in other developing countries. Both these jumps appear to be associated with societies in rapid transition from being largely rural to being urban and industrial. There is also an influence of the globalization of livestock and livestock product movement, associated with technological changes in transport and storage.

There has been a more gradual change in support of the new livestock value chains by animal health systems. The initial successes were with the control and eradication of rinderpest and contagious bovine pleuropneumonia in the late 1800s (Fisher, 1998). The distribution of livestock diseases began to change more rapidly in the 1960s and 1970s as European and North American countries and Japan began to make serious inroads into the control of a range of both transboundary and endemic diseases.[1] This was achieved through significant investments in human skills, building on previous investments in veterinary organizations, education and infrastructure from the mid 19th century onwards. The more recent investments, however, saw an intensified implementation of much more rigorous and organized programmes that used epidemiology and economics research to assist in decision making. Towards the end of the 1980s, many of these developed countries had become recognized as free from the major transboundary diseases and were beginning to make assessments of how to protect themselves from potential re-entries or re-emergence of disease. On a worldwide level, there were also successes that included the control and near eradication of rinderpest and the improved control of other transboundary diseases in developing countries with strong livestock export potential (Rushton, 2006). This would seem to indicate that methods of controlling disease, the production systems in which they are found and the methods used to assess their use are adequate.

However, there have been some major setbacks and large areas of the world have not been included in these advances (Rushton and Upton, 2006). The setbacks include:

- occasional introduction of transboundary diseases in developed countries such as FMD;
- emergence of new diseases such as bovine spongiform encephalopathy (BSE) and highly pathogenic avian influenza H5N1; and
- impact of food-borne pathogens such as *E. coli* O157 and *Salmonella*.

New problems relating to food-borne pathogens mean that the major impacts of livestock diseases are related to human health and welfare (see Alexandra P.M. Shaw, Chapter 14). In developed countries these impacts can be enormous, dwarfing the production losses due to disease. With other diseases there are large impacts due to food scares and trade restrictions, and implications in other larger aspects of the rural economy. This has raised questions

---

[1] It is recognized that some diseases were controlled well before this period (see Fisher, 1980); however major breakthroughs were mainly made in the period suggested.

about how to prevent the entry of exotic, contagious diseases and the most appropriate way to control such diseases if they occur. In particular, environmental and welfare concerns were raised about the large-scale slaughter and disposal of affected animals, and there were worries about the economic losses outside the livestock sector that were caused by animal disease control (Thompson *et al.*, 2002). In developed countries, there is also concern about endemic diseases, which are important in terms of production losses and control costs at farm level (Bennett, 2003), but remain largely uncontrolled. In developing countries investments in animal health are struggling to keep pace with the change in livestock sectors (Rushton *et al.*, 2006a), although countries with a strong interest in trade would appear to be responding more strongly (Rushton, 2006).

The increasing complexity of livestock production and their associated value chains had a background of changes in the political and institutional environment. From the late 1940s to the 1970s State action was accepted to be important in economic and agricultural development. However, during the 1980s, there was a change in thinking that stressed the market as a way to organize economic activity, supported by a small or even a minimal role for the State.

In this context, safeguarding animal health was until the 1980s regarded as an inherently public and therefore predominantly governmental service. At this point the provision of animal health services became more open to the use of market institutions, and there were evaluations of government services against those of the private sector. Market failures in animal health services remained, for which there is a role for the State in the correction of such failures through the provision of goods and services, the setting and enforcement of regulations and through taxes and subsidies. In addition, other policies such as education and infrastructure can have important impacts on livestock disease prevention, control and eradication. However, understanding which interventions require public support goes well beyond the traditional analysis of farm-level technical animal health interventions. Such analysis requires both the old and new methods and skills (see Hernán Rojas, Chapter 23, on the changes in cost–benefit analysis in Chile).

The major questions for the economics of animal health and production

Rushton *et al.* (2007) developed a list of the major questions that need to be addressed by the economics of animal health and production based on the recent experiences with transboundary, food-borne and endemic diseases. They identified the following:

- How can one guarantee not just reasonably priced livestock products (*food security*) but also food that has low or almost no risk in terms of spreading disease (*food safety*) and from farming and processing systems that guarantee that animals are treated humanely (*animal welfare*)?
  - Food safety and other quality attributes have become an overriding concern for many developed countries in recent times and in part this reflects not just the power of media, but also the fact that food-borne diseases cause losses that make production losses at farm level appear insignificant (Perry *et al.*, 2001, 2005; Rushton, 2002).
  - Animal welfare and ecologically 'sound' production practices are increasingly important and economically have become a selling point in many livestock product chains (Pritchard, 2004).
  - There is an increasing tendency to introduce food safety and welfare attributes into international law through the World Organization for Animal Health (OIE) and the World Trade Organization (WTO; Byron Nelson, 2005).
- What is the optimal level of resource allocation to the detection and prevention of exotic and emerging diseases?

- It is important to recognize that even if an optimum level is identified through data collection and modelling (see Alistair Stott, Chapter 9), it will change over time with changes in the livestock sector. In order to address this constant evolution a data collection, analysis and monitoring structure is critical to ensure that policy makers have up-to-date information at hand (see Andrew James, Chapter 8).
- With regard to the allocation of resources, there is a need to think about how to balance the allocation of resources between insurance that involves 'active' measures such as surveillance and vaccination versus more 'passive' measures such as the purchase of insurance policies and the establishment of contingency funds in the prevention, control and eradication of animal diseases (Rushton *et al.*, 2006b).
- Where livestock value chains are increasingly concentrated into large industrial integrated systems, who should insure against a contagious disease outbreak? Large industrial units have a much larger potential to contaminate and spread infectious agents in the surrounding environment than smaller units and the spillover costs are often borne by the State (Otte *et al.*, 2007). Striking a balance where some of the spillover costs are recognized by the private sector could have important and positive implications for production-level biosecurity measures.
- Is there a justification to allocate public resources for campaigns to control and eradicate endemic diseases?
- What methodologies can improve the implementation of animal disease control programmes that are assessed to be nationally economically profitable?
- In an animal health system what roles should the public veterinary services and the private sector play to improve the welfare benefits from animal disease control investments?
  - The improvements in animal disease status should take into account the needs of all socio-economic groups, poor and rich, producers and consumers.
  - It should be recognized that ideally each country would develop an animal health system according to its stage of development, cultural and social needs, rather than following models.
- At international level, where do responsibilities lie for the control of transboundary diseases? This is particularly relevant for countries that are poor and have the potential to export livestock products, but have difficulties in achieving OIE/WTO regulations to enter into attractive export markets.

It is difficult and in most cases impossible to separate science from economics in addressing animal health and disease problems. Epidemiology is so tightly mixed with economics that often one forgets to say epidemiological and economic analysis of a disease and its control. For example, costs and benefits of disease control influence the willingness to participate in surveillance programmes and disease control strategies, and trade influences the movement of livestock and livestock products, which in turn influences the spread and maintenance of diseases.

The Book Objective and Structure

The challenges and opportunities for the economics of animal health and production require a *holistic or systems perspective* which combines an analysis of the political economy, the economic incentives, the social acceptability and the technical feasibility of disease control measures and programmes. With this in mind, the book sets out to provide the theoretical and practical basis to assess livestock systems and animal disease control for farm, private enterprise and government policy through the provision of data collection and analysis methods and examples of their application in decision making.

Book structure

The book draws on an extensive review of the literature on animal health economics (Rushton, 2002) and experience in livestock issues in Europe, Asia, Africa and Latin America. It is the work of a number of authors who are well respected in their own fields of economics and have also made significant contributions to livestock and animal health economics. The book is divided into the following chapter and three major parts:

- History of livestock and animal health economics (Chapter 1);
- Theory and tools for the economics of animal health and production (Part I);
- A review of the application of economics to animal diseases and health problems (Part II);
- Economic analysis and policy making: examples from around the world (Part III).

Part I, on economic theory and tools, includes an explanation of production economics theory supported by a contribution by Professor Clem Tisdell. The following chapter provides an overview of data collection management and methods, which is supported by a contribution from Dr Rommy Viscarra. In Chapter 7, the main tools available for farm-level assessment are presented and the chapter is supported by Dr Alistair Stott's explanation of optimization methods and Dr Andrew James' contribution on models and data collection. Chapter 10 covers the main tools for the assessment of markets, the economy and value chains followed by Professor Martin Upton's review of the main economic assessment methods and Professor David Leonard's introduction to Institutional Economics. Chapter 13 presents the importance and influence of social and cultural issues with regard to livestock decision making, and Dr Alexandra Shaw presents a good framework to assessing the impacts of animal diseases in a wider society context that includes human health. Part I concludes with a chapter on the general analysis of livestock systems.

Part II, on the review of the literature of studies on the economics of animal health and diseases, has chapters that cover diseases which affect a range of livestock species followed by chapters on diseases that affect large ruminants, small ruminants, pigs and poultry. Part III has contributions from around the world on the applications of the economics of animal health and production to different problems, in research, production and policy.

It is not the intention of the author that this book be read from cover to cover; it is a reference text that will introduce readers to theories and methods which are required to assess change in the livestock sector and assist decision makers at all levels in making investments and deciding on future strategies and policies. The examples presented are largely from real situations and serve to illustrate that the economic analysis of animal health and production requires a multidisciplinary and systems approach. This reflects the reality that faces livestock producers, agrobusiness people and policy makers involved in the livestock sector.

Foreword

At a time when the world faces a period of major changes in animal production to meet rapidly accelerating demand for animal products, it is highly opportune that CABI should have commissioned this study of relevant economic techniques. It is appropriate too that Jonathan Rushton has been chosen to edit the study because at the start of his career – as I saw first-hand – he made a remarkable socio-economic study of the roles of livestock in Indian villages. This complemented a deep knowledge of modern dairy farming acquired during his childhood on the family farm in England, and later he has practised his abilities as a consultant on the small, medium and very large livestock systems of Latin America, Africa, Asia and Europe. The contributors too have been well chosen to focus their knowledge on particular aspects of the complex methodologies now available.

In the 1960s, when supplies of animal products frequently exceeded consumer purchasing power, studies on the value of disease losses attracted little attention. However, as livestock development schemes expanded, trade diversified and awareness of disease risks for both humans and animals built up, and the need for socio-economic appraisal techniques has become more and more urgent. The rapid evolution of recording and computing technology now enables fully integrated analyses which can reflect the social as well as the economic implications of changes in animal production and health for farmers, human communities, nations and whole regions of the world.

This book should prove extremely useful for everyone concerned with production and health policies and I feel sure it will gain the wide readership it deserves.

Peter Ellis OBE
Former director of VEERU

Acknowledgements

I would like to thank my life-long mentors, my parents Bessie and Trevor Rushton, for continuing to teach me that learning never stops. I would like to thank my father for his generosity in providing the drawings for the book. My professional mentors are Peter and Mary Ellis, who skilfully guided me through the early stages of my career and have given regular inputs ever since. There are many teachers, colleagues and friends who have given support, guidance and encouragement at various times; in no particular order, these include: Chris Gilligan, Ruth Henderson, Ed Miller, Tahir Rehman, Martin Upton, Steve Wiggins, T. Gopal, Chengappa, Andrew James, Andrew Paterson, Alexandra Shaw, Peter Spradbrow, Clare Heffernan, Festus Murithi, Susan Ngongi, Steve Angus, Madelon Meijer, Hernán Rojas, Armando Gonzalez, Vitor Piçao, Jaime Romero, Nick Taylor, Joachim Otte, Anni McLeod, James and Anna McGrane, Gabriel Ayala, Robyn Alders, Simon Anderson, Andrew Dorward, Elaine Marshall, Kate Schreckenberg, Karin Schwabenbauer and Jémi Domenech. The contributors are recognized and thanked for their time and energy in developing their chapters.

The CABI team of Gareth Richards, David Hemmings and Rachel Cutts has given assistance, encouragement and badgered me where appropriate. In general, their support has been crucial in getting me motivated to write this document.

My family on the Rushton side (Jane, Richard, Ruth, Paul, Philip, John) and the Viscarras (Charo, Cecilia, Enrique, Valita) have all given encouragement and help at important moments. Finally, my wife, Rommy Evelyn, has been a vital driving force behind the book being completed through her professional advice and her love.

1 History of Livestock and Animal Health Economics

Origins of the Subject

The study of the economics of livestock and their associated diseases is relatively young in relation to other economic disciplines and has really grown out of the movement of the epidemiology of diseases that began in the 1960s and early 1970s. While it is recognized that some interest has been shown in developing ideas of livestock economics (Brown, 1979; Crotty, 1980; Gittinger, 1982; Simpson, 1988), the much larger contributions to thinking on the economics of livestock production systems and their associated chains have come from the animal health angle. This interest was generated by governments who were beginning the final stages of eradication of major diseases and also becoming aware of the economic impact of less dramatic diseases such as infertility and parasitism. These animal health initiatives coincided with the interest in the economic analysis of the use of public funds. Prior to this period, veterinary services had kept records of the costs and benefits of disease control without any detailed analysis.

In the mid-1960s, Peter Ellis and Heinz Konigshofer documented the information available from the veterinary services in the Food and Agriculture Organization/World Health Organization/World Organization for Animal Health (FAO/WHO/OIE) Animal Health Yearbook. In the following years, Bill R. Macallon and associates at the United States Department of Agriculture (USDA) made more comprehensive assessments of a number of specific diseases. From this point onwards a number of important schools of thought began to emerge.

Main schools of thought and their contributions to its development

This section will briefly examine the schools of thought identified, listing some of their contributions to knowledge and reasons behind their existence. The reference lists provide the major articles written by people identified. The following schools are identified:

1. Ellis, Morris, Hugh-Jones, Putt, James and Shaw at the Veterinary Epidemiology and Economics Research Unit (VEERU), University of Reading, UK;
2. Carpenter at the Department of Medicine and Epidemiology, School of Veterinary Medicine, University of California, Davis, USA;
3. McInerney and Howe at the University of Exeter, UK;
4. Dijkhuizen at the Animal Health Economics, Farm Management Group, Department of Economics and Management, Wageningen Agricultural University, The Netherlands; and

5. Emerging schools Tisdell, Harrison and Ramsay at the University of Queensland, Australia; Perry at the International Livestock Research Institute (ILRI), Kenya; and Bennett at the University of Reading.

Reading: Veterinary Epidemiology and Economics Research Unit (VEERU)

Peter Ellis was the founder of the Veterinary Epidemiology and Economics Research Unit (VEERU) at the University of Reading and in many ways a pioneer in the subject of animal health economics. His interest in economics evolved from work on foot-and-mouth disease (FMD) in South America where he discovered that FMD epidemiology could not be separated from livestock prices and farm management systems. When Ellis returned to the UK, he worked at the Agricultural Economics Research Institute in Oxford and was introduced to benefit–cost analysis by Ian Little, the co-author of the *Manual of Industrial Project Analysis in Developing Countries* (Little and Mirlees, 1968).

In 1970, Ellis moved to the University of Reading where he began an analysis of classical swine fever (CSF) eradication in the UK with finance from the Wellcome Foundation and an agreement with the Ministry of Agriculture, Fisheries and Food (MAFF; Ellis, 1972a). This was the first study to apply cost–benefit analysis techniques to an animal disease appraisal. The success of this study led to the interest in carrying out a similar one for brucellosis eradication in England and Wales (Hugh-Jones *et al.*, 1975). At this point Martin Hugh-Jones went to Reading for 2 years to work on this project.

During these early works on animal health economics in the UK, Roger Morris had been working at the Veterinary School of the University of Melbourne on various aspects of economics with particular emphasis on the economics of production disease. Ellis and Morris met at a meeting convened by WHO in 1970 in Geneva to discuss approaches to evaluating the control of zoonoses. Morris went to Reading on a sabbatical in 1972 where Ellis and Morris consolidated their views, which were presented at a follow-up workshop for WHO in Reading, in which Macallon

also participated. This workshop produced a four- or five-page working document, which, though never formally published, was widely distributed as a guideline for international project evaluations.

Morris during his sabbatical also collaborated with UK-practising vets who were involved in Dick Esslemont's study of oestrus behaviour in dairy cows. Morris lent a computer program which was modified to become 'Melbread' and later the DAISY information system which provided the basis for assessing the loss from infertility.

Demand for help from the European Economic Council/European Union (EEC/EU) and support for research from the Overseas Development Administration of the British Government, now DfID, resulted in the development of an interdisciplinary team that was in 1975 designated as VEERU. The early contributors to this group were Andrew James (economist), Nick Putt (veterinarian), Alexandra Shaw (economist), Lindsay Tyler (veterinarian), Dick Esslemont (farm management), Tony Woods (statistician), Andrew Stephens (veterinarian), Richard Matthewman (animal production), Howard Pharo (veterinarian) and at a later stage James Hanks (animal production), Anni McLeod (economist) and Jackie Leslie (economist).

In 1975, an increasing number of research students encouraged VEERU to establish a formal training programme, which offered short courses in epidemiology and economics and could be combined with research leading to an MPhil or a PhD degree. Later a specific MSc was offered. Many students from all over the world have passed through these courses.

The VEERU policy was to develop teams through studies and collaborative projects in different countries and to build around them training schemes for middle management in veterinary and livestock services. These initiatives have been supported by ODA, German Aid, Danish Aid, the British Council, FAO, OIE and the World Bank and many other agencies and involved a continuing series of visits to countries in Latin America, Africa, the Middle East, the Indian subcontinent and Asia by various combinations of staff.

In 1976, Ellis invited all the professionals he knew who were interested in veterinary epidemiology and economics to come to Reading for an exchange of ideas. About 80 people attended the meeting and the proceedings provided a reference document, which was very widely distributed (Ellis *et al.*, 1978). The main result of that meeting was the creation of the International Society of Veterinary Epidemiology and Economics (ISVEE) and a plan to hold meetings every 3 years. Morris was elected Chairman and offered Australia as the venue for the next meeting. Shortly after this meeting, the Society for Veterinary Epidemiology and Preventive Medicine (SVEPM) was founded in the UK and similar societies were created in France and other countries.

Some of the key people in the work of VEERU apart from Ellis are described below:

- Martin Hugh-Jones, now at the Department of Epidemiology and Community Health, Louisiana State University, was seconded to the University of Reading to work on the study of the economics of brucellosis eradication in England and Wales. He has since specialized in geographic information systems (GIS), modelling diseases such as anthrax, anaplasmosis dermatophilis and trypanosomiasis (a list of his publications is available in the reference list). What stands out in the work of Hugh-Jones is the thoroughness of the research; the economic impact assessments he has been involved in are based on a deep knowledge of the production system and epidemiology of the disease.

- Roger Morris, now at Massey University, New Zealand, was working on the economics of livestock disease in Australia at the same time that Ellis began working on this subject in the UK. He went to Reading for a sabbatical year in 1972 where he completed his thesis for a Master's from the University of Melbourne. He did his PhD supervised by Ellis in which he explored complementary methodology including the applications of risk analysis and chaos theory. He is one of the leading veterinary economists in the world and was co-editor of a book on animal health economics (Dijkhuizen and Morris, 1997).

- Nick Putt was an important figure in the epidemiology and economics of trypanosomiasis in Nigeria and Zambia. He directed the study on trypanosomiasis in Nigeria and also coordinated and authored some sections of the International Livestock Centre for Africa (ILCA) manual on epidemiology and economics (see below). Unfortunately, he died in the prime of his career in 1995.

- Alexandra Shaw, now an independent consultant, specialized in the economics of trypanosomiasis and its control, using her experiences from western Africa to explore not just the impact of the disease at herd level, but also its impact on land use and the general economy. She was also the key economist in the ILCA manual, which was the first to detail livestock disease economics techniques in book form, and she has been an important figure in the training of veterinarians and livestock productionists in the use of economic techniques around the world. She has also used her extensive language skills to forge links with West African, French and German institutions working in the field of epidemiology and economics.

- Andrew James, currently Director of VEERU, worked on early assessment of FMD costs and their control, first in general terms and then with examples from India. His later work concentrated on east coast fever (ECF), tick and tick-borne disease economics, with a series of papers based on experimental work in Zambia, Zimbabwe and Kenya. This work was coordinated with Rupert Pegram and Bruno Minjauw. James has also given important inputs to discussions on rinderpest and animal recording systems. Finally, probably his major contribution has been to clarify the concepts of production and productivity. His pioneering modelling work looking at production systems and returns to feed use is the basis for much research in animal disease economics currently coming from the VEERU group. He also developed the database PANACEA.

Their major contributions were in the early use in scientific studies of:

- cost–benefit analysis techniques;
- herd models (CLIPPER and LPEC);
- herd monitoring systems (DAISY, EVA, MONTY, INTERHERD);
- promoting the use of economic techniques in planning processes; and
- examining economic impact across different levels of society.

Their approach was and remains in the much more practical field of the economic assessment of animal disease based on detailed knowledge of the production system and the epidemiology of diseases within the production system. This was not popular and remains unpopular with the pure economist (see a list of publications by McInerney in the reference list).

Tim Carpenter (Davis, California)

Tim Carpenter was another pioneer in the field of animal health economics during the 1970s. His early work was on *Mycoplasma gallisepticum* (Carpenter *et al.*, 1979) and *Mycoplasma meleagridis* in turkeys (Carpenter, 1980). Carpenter was probably the first to examine the use of different economic analysis techniques in the study of diseases and their control such as:

- decision tree analysis (Carpenter and Norman, 1983; Carpenter *et al.*, 1987; Ruegg and Carpenter, 1989; Rodrigues *et al.*, 1990);
- microeconomic analysis of disease (Carpenter, 1983);
- simulation models to assess animal disease (Carpenter and Thieme, 1980);
- dynamic programming (Carpenter and Howitt, 1988);
- dual estimation approach to derive shadow prices for diseases (Vagsholm *et al.*, 1991);
- estimation of consumer surplus (Mohammed *et al.*, 1987);
- willingness to pay for vaccination (Thorburn *et al.*, 1987);
- linear programming (Carpenter, 1978; Carpenter and Howitt, 1980; Christiansen and Carpenter, 1983);
- use of economic analysis to review subsidies to veterinary support institutions (Carpenter and Howitt, 1982); and
- the use of the cost–benefit analysis approach for selecting veterinary services (Zessin and Carpenter, 1985).

Carpenter has also been involved in economic analysis with more conventional economic tools such as financial and cost–benefit analysis (Carpenter *et al.*, 1981a,b, 1988; Davidson *et al.*, 1981; Kimsey *et al.*, 1985; Mousing *et al.*, 1988; Vagsholm *et al.*, 1988; Sischo *et al.*, 1990). He has contributed to the discussion on the difficulties and problems of veterinary economics (Carpenter, 1994) and has been an important figure in the teaching of animal health economics (Carpenter, 1979).

Carpenter's work has been based on very thorough knowledge of the production system and the epidemiology of the disease concerned. He has been involved in the study of a number of diseases. What sets his contribution to the subject apart from other economists and veterinarians has been his willingness to experiment with a wide range of techniques.

John McInerney and Keith Howe at Exeter University, UK

John McInerney, during his time at the University of Reading, had some contact with the VEERU group. However, as an economist he was unhappy with the more practical approach to animal health economics that this group presented. With Keith Howe at Exeter, McInerney began research on the more theoretical economics of livestock disease, developing largely conceptual models of farmer behaviour towards disease (Howe, 1985; McInerney, 1988, 1999; Howe *et al.*, 1989; McInerney *et al.*, 1992; Howe and Christiansen, 2004). They continued this approach and to some extent with Richard Bennett at the University of Reading, in trying to teach their veterinary colleagues what economists do and how they approach assessment of disease (Howe, 1992). However, their influence on the thinking of animal health economics has largely been limited to concepts and theory. Howe was involved in early assessments of overall disease losses in the UK (Beynon and Howe, 1975) and they have had some involvement in analyses of mastitis (McInerney and Turner, 1989), tuberculosis (McInerney, 1986, 1987; Bourne *et al.*, 2000; Morrison *et al.*, 2000) and Aujesky disease (Willeberg *et al.*, 1996). McInerney has also had some input into animal welfare economics (McInerney, 1991, 1994).

This group is credited as being the first to begin thinking about the conceptual framework behind the economic analysis of disease and its control. However, it should be noted that the conceptual framework that was developed by McInerney has recently been criticized by Harrison *et al.* (1999), a group of economists based at the University of Queensland, Australia (see below).

Alt Dijkhuizen (Wageningen, The Netherlands)

In the 1970s, Dijkhuizen began investigations into the costs of disease with Renkema, but particularly with an emphasis on mastitis (Dijkhuizen, 1977; Dijkhuizen and Renkema, 1977, 1983; Dijkhuizen and Stelwagen, 1981, 1982) and diseases that affect dairy cattle (Renkema and Dijkhuizen, 1979; Dijkhuizen, 1983a,b). He also investigated the economics of animal surgery (Breukink and Dijkhuizen, 1982; Rougoor *et al.*, 1994) and production problems (Dijkhuizen, 1983a,b; Dijkhuizen *et al.*, 1984, 1985; Sol *et al.*, 1984; Joosten *et al.*, 1988). He used these earlier studies to begin research on the use of economic analysis techniques for animal disease (Renkema *et al.*, 1981; Renkema and Dijkhuizen, 1985; Berentsen *et al.*, 1992b; Dijkhuizen *et al.*, 1994, 1996, 1998; Buijtels *et al.*, 1996; Horst *et al.*, 1996; Rougoor *et al.*, 1996; Jalvingh *et al.*, 1998). This work culminated in a co-edited book on animal health economics (Dijkhuizen and Morris, 1997), of which full details are provided in the following section.

In addition, Dijkhuizen and his team, in particular Jalvingh and Huirne, have worked on the following diseases and disease problems:

- Pig disease economics (Dijkhuizen, 1987, 1989a), economics of pig fertility (Houben *et al.*, 1990; Dijkhuizen *et al.*, 1997b) and culling management (Scholman and Dijkhuizen, 1989); the particular diseases this group has worked on are: CSF (Horst *et al.*, 1997a; Dijkhuizen, 1999; Meuwissen *et al.*, 1999; Nielen *et al.*, 1999; Mangen *et al.*, 2001), porcine reproductive and respiratory syndrome in The Netherlands (Klink *et al.*, 1991) and Porcilis APP (Dijkhuizen and Valks, 1997).
- Cattle problems and diseases they have particularly worked on:

- reproductive economics in cattle and buffalo (Shah *et al.*, 1991);
- the economics of cattle lameness (Enting *et al.*, 1997);
- bovine respiratory diseases (Fels-Klerx *et al.*, 1999);
- economics of mastitis (Schakenraad and Dijkhuizen, 1990; Schepers and Dijkhuizen, 1991; Houben *et al.*, 1993, 1994; Barkema *et al.*, 1995; Rougoor *et al.*, 1999);
- paratuberculosis, particularly in The Netherlands (Benedictus *et al.*, 1985, 1986, 1987; van Schaik *et al.*, 1996);
- leptospirosis (van der Kamp *et al.*, 1990);
- bovine diarrhoea virus (Wentink and Dijkhuizen, 1990; Pasman *et al.*, 1994; Stelwagen and Dijkhuizen, 1998);
- bovine spongiform encephalopathy (BSE; Geurts *et al.*, 1997);
- bovine herpes virus (Noordegraaf *et al.*, 1999; van Schaik *et al.*, 1999; Noordegraaf *et al.*, 2000).
- FMD disease economics particularly with reference to control strategies at a time when Europe was contemplating changing a policy of annual vaccination to no vaccination and a stamping out policy (Dijkhuizen, 1988, 1989b; Berentsen *et al.*, 1990a,b, 1992a,b); they also contributed to discussions on the veterinary regulation associated with FMD (Berentsen *et al.*, 1991).
- Risk of exotic disease (Horst *et al.*, 1997b) and the incorporation of risk analysis into economic analysis (Dijkhuizen *et al.*, 1997a); within this work they looked at the possible use of insurance against the occurrence of contagious diseases (Meuwissen *et al.*, 1997), risks of animal movements introducing contagious diseases (Vos *et al.*, 1999) and the modelling of virus introduction with examples of CSF and FMD (Horst *et al.*, 1999).
- Animal welfare, food safety and animal health economics (Dijkhuizen, 1998).

Dijkhuizen developed his work from using animal recording systems such as PORKCHOP and developing the use of decision support systems such as CHESS. The recording systems' work extended beyond the farm level with analysis of national recording systems.

His modelling inputs have been to develop models to assist decision makers at farm, national and region levels.

In summary, Dijkhuizen has concentrated on the intensive pig and dairy sectors of The Netherlands. His work has been mainly on the important contagious diseases such as CSF and FMD, production diseases such as mastitis and production problems such as fertility. This has largely been focused on the Dutch commercial sector. However, his experience has also been used to examine different techniques for the economic assessment of diseases and the use of economic and risk analysis tools to aid decision makers. His contributions in these areas have been important in directing animal health policies in his own country.

Emerging schools

TISDELL, HARRISON AND RAMSAY AT THE UNIVERSITY OF QUEENSLAND, BRISBANE, AUSTRALIA. During the 1990s, an animal health project in Thailand was supported by the economics department at the University of Queensland headed by Tisdell. This project provided material for research into the economics of livestock diseases and their control with a focus on FMD economics. Tisdell (1995) and Harrison (1996) examined the use of cost–benefit analysis for assessing animal disease programmes. It is the first school to have carefully examined and criticized the McInerney conceptual theory and was able to do so on the basis of practical experience and intellectual capacity. These economists also investigated how animal health programmes can help sustainable development (Harrison and Tisdell, 1997) with particular reference to Thailand. Ramsay, Tisdell and Harrison (1997a,b,c) also looked at how better information for animal health could improve decision making and how this affected the benefits from these improved decisions. This work was based on analysis of the FMD programme in Thailand (Harrison and Tisdell, 1999) and research work on control of *Babesia bovis* in Australia (Ramsay, 1997). The economists involved in this research published many of their ideas on animal health economics in the Australian Centre for International

Agricultural Research (ACIAR) publication titled *Advances in the Collection, Management and Use of Animal Health Information* (Harrison and Sharma, 1999; Harrison *et al.*, 1999; Ramsay *et al.*, 1999a,b), and one of their main contributions has been to critically assess the conceptual models developed by McInerney on animal disease control. Their conclusions suggest that endemic diseases have two options: do nothing or eradication (Harrison *et al.*, 1999; Tisdell *et al.*, 1999). This view is based on the need for large fixed costs at the beginning of a programme, which initially have no benefits in terms of reducing disease losses, but are needed to lead to eradication of disease. If these initial fixed costs cannot be met, then there is no point in investing small amounts in the control of disease.

BENNETT AT THE UNIVERSITY OF READING, UK. Richard Bennett at the University of Reading has made contributions to the subject of animal health economics, initially with work on how to use information on animal health decisions (Bennett, 1991) and decision making for leptospirosis in cattle (Bennett, 1993). The main contribution of his work so far has been in the field of animal welfare economics (Bennett, 1995, 1998; Bennett and Larson, 1996; Blaney and Bennett, 1997; Anderson *et al.*, 1999) and assessing the losses from endemic diseases in the UK (Bennett *et al.*, 1997, 1999a,b; Bennett, 2000). His work on endemic diseases in the UK touches on the economics of impact and control of most of the diseases across a range of livestock.

PERRY, MUKHEBI, YOUNG, RANDOLPH, MCDERMOTT AND RICH AT THE INTERNATIONAL LIVESTOCK RESEARCH INSTITUTE (ILRI), NAIROBI, KENYA. The epidemiology and disease control unit at ILRI in Kenya was led by Brian Perry. Perry is one of the world's most prominent epidemiologist with a depth of experience in a range of diseases. In the early 1990s, Perry worked on the economic impact of ticks and tick-borne diseases (Perry *et al.*, 1990). This work was with Adrian Mukhebi and concerned the economic assessments of ECF (Mukhebi *et al.*, 1989, 1990) and theileriosis (Mukhebi *et al.*, 1992). He also wrote a paper with Young on the epidemiology and economics of tick-borne disease (Perry and Young, 1995).

Recently, Perry has made other important contributions to the field of animal health economics. He coordinated the first book to bring together a number of important themes in animal health economics: farm-level economic assessments; trade implications of sanitary requirements; and veterinary service delivery (Perry, 1999). In addition Perry, with Tom Randolph and John McDermott, has written papers on epidemiology and economics (Perry et al., 2001), economics of parasitic diseases (Perry and Randolph, 1999) and has carried out major research into FMD economics (Perry et al., 1999). He was also involved in the economic assessment of heartwater (Mukhebi et al., 1999). More recently Karl Rich has joined the ILRI team and has made contributions on animal health economics, particularly in the area of complex modelling to capture the impacts of animal diseases and their control (Rich et al., 2005).

In addition to the list presented, the following people should be added, and groups or focuses are also identified:

1. Alistair Stott at Scottish Agricultural College (Stott, 2005) has pioneered the use of optimization methods in animal health decision making and the book includes a contribution from Dr Stott.
2. There have been investigations into veterinary service delivery and the use of New Institutional Economics by World Bank economists (Umali et al., 1992). David Leonard and Vinod Ahuja have taken this early work to new levels with fieldwork and analysis in Africa and India, respectively (Leonard, 2000, 2004; Ahuja, 2004). Some interesting work in Africa on this subject area has been carried out by Cheik Ly (Ly, 2003). David Leonard makes a contribution in the applications section of the book.
3. FAO pioneered early classification systems to detail how the livestock production units were developing and where they were concentrating (Steinfeld and Mäki-Hokkonen, 1995; Sere and Steinfeld, 1996). Building on these approaches, it was recognized that a livestock revolution was ongoing, responding to the growing demands of urban populations in developing countries (Delgado et al., 1999). It was documented at an early stage that much of the growth in the livestock sector

was coming from the intensive monogastric systems and to some extent from a growth in milk production. For many reasons, these dramatic changes in livestock production were celebrated, some concerns were raised about poorer livestock producers being left behind (Haan et al., 2001; Heffernan, 2002; FAO, 2005; Owen et al., 2005) and issues on the potential negative impacts on the environment have been well investigated (de Haan et al., 1997; Steinfeld et al., 2006).
4. In FAO, there has also been the Pro-Poor Livestock Policy Initiative led by Joachim Otte investigating the use of a variety of economic methods. They have challenged the strong technical focus of animal health decision making and raised the need to see animal health problems as a mixture of policy, social and economic issues (FAO, 2007).[1]

Important references and books

With regard to the economics of livestock diseases some important books and papers are provided below:

- Putt, S.N.H., Shaw, A.P.M., Woods, A.J., Tyler, L. and James, A.D. (1988) *Veterinary Epidemiology and Economics in Africa. A manual for use in the design and appraisal of livestock health policy.* ILCA Manual No. 3, International Livestock Centre for Africa (now International Livestock Research Institute), Addis Ababa, Ethiopia.
  - This is the first book published on this subject and contains sections on 'The use of economics in the planning and evaluation of disease control programmes'; 'Estimating the costs of diseases and the benefits of their control'; and 'Economics and decision-making in disease control policy'. It also includes discussions of modelling techniques with an early example of the James' static herd model.
- McInerney, J.P., Howe, K.S. and Schepers, J.A. (1992) A framework for the economic

[1]http://www.fao.org/ag/againfo/projects/en/pplpi/

analysis of disease in farm livestock. *Preventive Veterinary Medicine* 13, 137–154.

- First outline of conceptual ideas for animal health economics, which introduces the need for thoughts on costs of disease control not just losses caused by disease. This is the basis for improving decisions on diseases.

- Dijkhuizen, A.A. and Morris, R.S. (eds) (1997) *Animal Health Economics: Principles and Applications*. University of Sydney, Postgraduate Foundation in Veterinary Science, Sydney, Australia.

  - The book brings together much of the modelling work of the Dijkhuizen group with contributions from other world leaders in animal health economics. The book contains the following sections:

    1. Framework and basic methods of economic analysis:
       (a) 'How economically important is animal disease and why?' (Morris, pp. 1–11);
       (b) 'Economic decision making in animal health management' (Dijkhuizen; R.B.M. Huirne; Morris, pp. 13–23);
       (c) 'Basic methods of economic analysis' (Huirne; Dijkhuizen, pp. 25–39); and
       (d) 'Economic impact of common health and fertility problems' (Dijkhuizen; Huirne; A.W. Jalvingh; J. Stelwagen, pp. 41–58).

    2. Advanced methods of economic analysis:
       (a) 'Critical steps in systems simulation' (Dijkhuizen; A.W. Jalvingh; R.B.M. Huirne, pp. 59–67);
       (b) 'Linear programming to meet management targets and restrictions' (Jalvingh; Dijkhuizen; J.A. Renkema, pp. 69–84);
       (c) 'Dynamic programming to optimise treatment and replacement decisions' (Huirne; Dijkhuizen; P. van Beek; Renkema, pp. 85–97);
       (d) 'Markov chain simulation to evaluate user-defined management strategies' (Jalvingh; Dijkhuizen; J.A.M. van Arendonk, pp. 99–113); and

       (e) 'Monte Carlo simulation to model spread in management outcomes' (W.E. Marsh; Morris, pp. 115–133).

    3. Risky choice in animal health management:
       (a) 'Scope and concepts of risky decision making' (R.B.M. Huirne; J.B. Hardaker, pp. 135–147);
       (b) 'Application of portfolio theory for the optimal choice of on-farm veterinary management programs' (D.T. Galligan; W.E. Marsh, pp. 149–157);
       (c) 'Modelling the economics of risky decision making in highly contagious disease control' (Dijkhuizen; A.W. Jalvingh; P.B.M. Berentsen; A.J. Oskam, pp. 159–170);
       (d) 'Risk analysis and the international trade in animals and their products' (S.C. MacDiarmid, pp. 171–185).

    4. Decision support in animal health management:
       (a) 'Examples of integrated information systems for decision making at farm and national level' (Morris; W.E. Marsh; R.L. Sanson; J.S. McKenzie, pp. 187–199);
       (b) 'Profitability of herd health control and management information systems under field conditions' (Dijkhuizen; J.A.A.M. Verstegen; R.B.M. Huirne; A. Brand, pp. 201–207);
       (c) 'Disease control programs in developing countries: prospects and constraints' (B.D. Perry); and
       (d) 'How do we integrate economics into the policy development and implementation process?' (A.D. James).

    5. Use of spreadsheets in animal health economics:
       (a) 'Building a spreadsheet model' (Morris; C.W. Rougoor; R.B.M. Huirne, pp. 233–245); and
       (b) 'Computer exercises on animal health economics' (Rougoor; A.W. Jalvingh; Dijkhuizen; Morris; Huirne, pp. 247–305).

- In 1998 OIE commissioned an edition of their journal titled 'The economics of animal disease control' (Perry, 1999).
  - This edition of *Scientifique et Technique* contains information on economic analysis techniques from farm level through to consumer surplus analysis. In addition, it looks at the importance of veterinary service delivery and trade implications with greater global movement of livestock and livestock products. Finally the edition has case studies on: FMD; rinderpest; rabies control; BVD.
- Animal health work supported and funded by ACIAR during the 1990s was published in a monograph titled *Understanding Animal Health in South-East Asia – Advances in the Collection, Management and Use of Animal Health Information* (Sharma and Baldock, 1999).
  - This ACIAR publication contains important ideas developed by Tisdell, Harrison and Ramsay on animal health economics, benefits from animal health projects, integrating economics with GIS systems for animal health decisions and improving animal health decisions through better information.

The above publications provide the reader with a very good basis for beginning economic assessment of livestock diseases, covering the conceptual aspects of disease losses and control of diseases (McInerney *et al.*, 1992; Harrison *et al.*, 1999) and information on the methodologies and techniques for the analysis of diseases and their control (Putt *et al.*, 1988; Dijkhuizen and Morris, 1997; Perry, 1999). In addition to these animal health economics texts, the papers by Upton (1989, 1993) and James and Carles (1996) on livestock productivity assessments are a very useful introduction to assessing livestock interventions and systems changes. Other overviews of the subject of animal health economics have been written by Rushton *et al.* (2007) and Howe and Christiansen (2004). The basis of the paper by Rushton *et al.* (2007) comes from the material presented in this section.

Summary

In summary, this chapter on the history of the economics of animal health and production demonstrates that it is a dynamic area of work and research. Doubts have been expressed whether this subject is a discipline (Howe and Christiansen, 2004), but it is clear that a small group of academics, consultants and other professionals are dedicated to investigating the economics of livestock systems and animal health problems associated with these systems. It is a relatively specialized area of economics in the sense that the underlying technical issues for livestock systems are very specific (Rushton *et al.*, 1999; Part I). However, in contrast to the well-documented social and economic importance of crop diseases (Apple, 1978), the economic implications of animal diseases have been comparatively understudied (Rushton *et al.*, 1999). McInerney (1996) urged that much more work be done in applying 'old economics' to the 'new problem' of livestock disease. In one sense, it seems extraordinary that livestock disease has still not been thoroughly explored within the analytical framework of production economics.

Rushton *et al.* (2007) also posed the question of whether the subject of animal health economics is moving and changing to meet the environment and challenges set by the livestock sector and society as a whole. In partial answer to this question, Part I will provide an overview of the theoretical basis for making assessments of animal health and production and introduce important data collection methods and practical tools. The intention is to provide the reader with an analytical framework to respond to the changing demands of society.

Part I

Theory and Tools for the Economics of Animal Health and Production

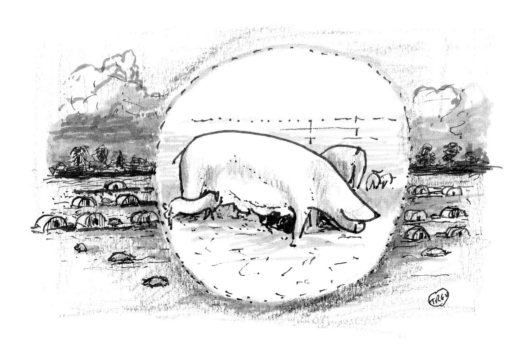

Introduction

In order to make economic assessments of animal health and production, it is important to have some understanding of the socio-economic setting of which the livestock system is part. In particular, animal diseases are often closely linked to socio-economic activities of the people who own and look after them and the consumers who eat livestock products.

Markets for livestock products drive animal and livestock product movement, which for many diseases are critical aspects of disease-agent maintenance and spread. These markets also influence the general development of livestock production methods. Markets, both input and output, can be modified by State policies on subsidies, research and general infrastructure development. In turn, animal diseases affect livestock systems with direct impacts and rather subtle implications that are much less obvious (Morris, 1997).

The linkages between government policy, markets, livestock systems and animal diseases create complexity in the study of the economics of animal health and production. In addition, livestock systems differ from other agricultural systems in the following ways:

- Most livestock systems take longer than a year to complete a full cycle.
- Livestock are mobile.
- In comparison with crop systems there are relatively few livestock, which makes collecting a representative sample more difficult.
- Livestock can reproduce.
- Livestock have an inherent capital value.

Farmers also keep livestock as a means of transforming resources into a wide range of outputs such as milk, meat, traction power, dung for fertilizer, fuel or buildings, hides, wool, fibre and/or animals. These outputs may be used for home consumption or they may be sold. In many societies, the ownership of livestock is important in terms of social status, and in countries with chronic inflation problems livestock are one of the few relatively safe investment options. Where owners have a social objective to increase the number of their animals and thus their wealth, the output can be viewed as a process of reinvestment. At a sector or national level, society has an interest in having livestock that can provide food in the most efficient manner. This system needs to be balanced against the possibility of being able to import similar products at competitive prices.

Therefore, livestock systems are relatively complex and serve various monetary and non-monetary purposes at individual, household, local and national levels. Added to this is that animal diseases are themselves complex. Such complexity requires a systems approach rather than a focus on individual units or linear relationships. However, a systems approach requires a good grounding in aspects of production economics, farm management tools, investment appraisal and modelling. No single aspect provides all the necessary information for a complete analysis of animal health and production,

but combined they become a powerful tool. The wide range of subjects that will be covered in Part I have required it to be split into the following chapters:

- A brief *introduction* on what is economics and how it can be useful for planning and policy processes is provided.
- A short explanation is given of some of the most important aspects of *production economics*, in part to provide a theoretical basis for the farm management tools described. For those interested, *Professor Clem Tisdell's* contribution gives an explanation of how this theoretical thinking can be applied to animal health.
- Analysis cannot be performed without data. Therefore, a chapter has been included that covers the different *data collection* methods. *Dr Rommy Viscarra* and *Dr Jonathan Rushton* provide a discussion of formal and informal data collection methods. A summary of the management of data collection exercises is provided as there is little point in having strong planning and analysis processes for the data if the collection is badly done.
- However, data are not useful until they have been analysed and turned into information. Analytical structures range from farm management tools to livestock and household models and through to sector or economy-wide models. This chapter focuses on *economic tools for livestock production* with practical examples and descriptions of tools at a local or national level. This part is supported by contributions from *Dr Andrew James* on modelling, *Dr Alistair Stott* on the use of optimization methods, *Professor Martin Upton* on the general strengths and weaknesses of a variety of policy tools, *Professor David Leonard* on institutional economics and animal health and *Dr Alexandra Shaw* on the economics of zoonoses.
- A final chapter has been included on the *general analysis of livestock systems*. This is supported by papers by *Dr Jonathan Rushton* and *Dr Rommy Viscarra* on the analysis of livestock systems in South America and a local analysis of livestock systems in southern Bolivia.

2 What Is Economics and How Is It Useful?

Introduction

Economics and the term economist were first used in the context of efficient management of agricultural estates by the Greek Xenophon between 394 and 365 BC (Backhouse, 2002). Lionel Robbins defines economics as 'the science which studies human behaviour as a relationship between ends and scarce means which have alternative uses' (cited by Backhouse, 2002, p. 3). While this definition captures many ideas such as prices, money, production, markets, bargaining, it does not capture policy issues. Marshall's (1920) definition that economics is 'the study of mankind in the ordinary business of life' is another good description but rather imprecise for the nature of the current book. Dijkuizen (1993) wrote that 'Non-economists often qualify economics as the discipline that simply measures things in monetary units, while other disciplines use physical units. This view is simplistic and inappropriate.' For the purposes of this book and Part I on theory and tools for the economics of animal health and production, economics is not concerned principally with money but with *making rational choices/decisions in the allocation of scarce resources for the achievement of competing goals.* Monetary units are simply used as a yardstick to compare the different resources and goals involved in the decision. The underlying theme is that economics helps us deal with problems of scarcity (Sloman, 1991).

Where this book sits in providing information for rational decision making is that understanding problems at farm, national or international level requires good information on objectives and constraints of the *people* implementing the actions of greatest interest in improving disease control and livestock production in general. In past times, this has focused at the farm level, but as described above the livestock sector now involves components of input industries, farm-level production and processing. All these components can have influences on the spread of diseases and also the nature of the impact of those diseases on society. This is particularly the case where diseases also affect humans, zoonoses and food-borne pathogens.

At the production level, economic theory and tools are particularly important in planning in order to assess the implications of allocating resources in a particular way before deciding whether to act. As Upton (1996) states, this is 'an essential part of rational decision making'. Formal procedures such as budgeting are used by large commercial units use for guiding agricultural and production practices, as they have closer control of the system and interaction with service providers (Upton, 1996). Smaller-scale farmers and agrobusiness people may not use these formal methods frequently, either through lack of knowledge or time. It must be recognized that the data collection and the use of economic tools for analysis themselves have a cost which in a small-scale operation may outstrip the benefits of their use in decision making. The implication is that economic theory and tools become more and more useful where the scale and complexity of the problem being dealt with increases. In this they provide a manageable framework that does not just rely on what can be remembered and assessed by one person.

In this sense, Upton (1996) also identified that planning tools are used in two different ways: to *prescribe* what farmers or agrobusiness people ought to do in order to advise on how systems can be improved; and to *predict* how farmers and agrobusiness people will respond to changes in prices, institutions or technology. The former is important in guiding the people actually involved in making decisions on a livestock situation and the latter in guiding policy makers in decisions on how to facilitate the livestock sector.

Important Economic Concepts

There are some underlying economic concepts that are important to clarify with regard to the allocation of scarce resources. These are choice and opportunity cost, rational decisions and the marginal costs and benefits.

Choice and opportunity cost

When making a choice or decision, there must be some sacrifice. In very simple terms if farmers have two livestock markets in their area that are run on the same day, they must decide which market will provide the best inputs or livestock for their farm. This requires sacrificing being able to buy the inputs and livestock that will be available at the market that they do not go to. At a livestock enterprise level, farmers may be advised that the fertility management of their animals can be improved if they spend more time making checks of the animals in the late evening.

However, this requires sacrificing time with their friends and family or perhaps reducing the amount of sleep they get. Similarly, people involved in agrobusiness make choices in the type of agricultural products they will focus on to process and sell. A company that has specialized in the slaughter and processing of pigs will have to sacrifice the possibility of using the slaughterhouse, human resources and finance for poultry. For governments, whether at local or national level, there are also decisions in how State money is spent. Decisions on whether to invest in a livestock research project may depend on whether this money could be better invested in an infrastructure project that generates electricity. At a consumer level, people with a limited budget may be able to afford a small beef steak per week, but with the same money could buy a chicken and three eggs.

The sacrifices involved in making decisions on how time or resources are used create costs. In other words, the production or consumption of one thing involves the sacrifice of alternatives. This sacrifice of alternatives in production (or consumption) of a good is known as its *opportunity cost*.

Rational choices

When making decisions of how to allocate scarce resources, farmers, agrobusiness people, government officials and consumers of livestock products need to assess the costs and benefits of their actions. Where a person makes a decision that generates *the greatest benefit relative to cost* an economist would say that a *rational choice* has been made. Therefore, the decision is not made on cost alone, but also comparing this cost with the benefit that is derived from spending the money and using the item purchased. People making rational decisions know the cost, but also understand the value of the decision. People making poor decisions might well know the cost of everything and the value of nothing!

At a personal level, consumers of ham have a wide range of products available at different prices. The purchase of the best hams may allow a person to buy only a little of that ham, but the memory and satisfaction of eating a little of this product may be much greater than eating a lot more of an inferior ham.

Similarly, firms that make feed inputs for livestock production will want to assess the investment and running costs required for a new feed mill versus the income that this mill will generate. A more complex decision-making process is carried out by governments when deciding which projects to fund and how big they should be. The government must weigh up the relative costs and benefits of each project to produce a mixture of projects that give the best chance for economic growth and encourage poorer groups in society. Therefore, a decision to run a dairy development project may be affected by a project to build a road, because the road is thought to benefit the country and its people more. A government has limited amount of funds, and therefore it requires a mechanism to ration this funding. One of the main mechanisms for allocating government funding is the use of the technique known as cost–benefit analysis.

Marginal costs and benefits

The above description of rational choices focuses on the comparison of total costs versus total benefits. This assumes that the best level of an input is known, or that amount that a person might be able to consume and continue to get the same satisfaction is known. In reality, people will experiment with the levels of inputs until they reach a level where they can see the greatest benefit. Consumers will also recognize that livestock product consumption creates a high pleasure for small amounts, but additional amounts create less and less pleasure. Therefore, reaching a rational choice on how much of an input to use or how much of a product to consume

often involves assessing the *marginal costs* of extra inputs or products versus the *marginal benefits* they create.

For example, the consumption of strong-flavoured cheese can create strong pleasure in small amounts, but in extreme cases may make people feel ill, if they eat too much. Pig farmers making rational decisions on how much time they need to spend on oestrus detection will compare the incremental amounts of time versus the extra benefits they produce. In this decision, the value of the time will vary according to the hour it has to be provided. So a farmer may have to consider the costs of checking his sows during unsociable hours, in terms of overtime payments to staff or the need to sacrifice their time with their friends and family. The farmer will not be interested in the overall piglet production, but in the extra piglets produced by the intervention. They will compare the marginal benefit with the marginal cost of the extra time spent on oestrus detection.

Summary

Economics is the study of *making rational choices/decisions in the allocation of scarce resources for the achievement of competing goals.* The underlying issue is that there is scarcity and it is not possible to do every activity at all the levels that one wants. Making decisions on how to allocate resources requires sacrifices that generate opportunity costs. These decisions are rational if they compare the cost of the decision versus the benefit generated. In general, such a rational decision-making process will compare the marginal costs of a decision versus the marginal benefits. These concepts are important for Part II, which covers production economics and applies these principles to animal health and production.

3 Livestock Production Economics

The conceptual basis of the livestock and farm production-level analysis tools that will be described in Chapter 4 is production economics. Doll and Orazem (1984) describe in detail all aspects of production economics, and its relationship to farm production-level analysis tools is described by Boehlje and Eidman (1984, pp. 86–127). The current chapter will present the basic principles of production economics with examples applied to livestock production systems.

The principles of production economics clarify 'the concepts of costs, output response to inputs, and the use of resources to maximise profits and/or minimise costs' (Doll and Orazem, 1984). Therefore, for the production-level decision makers seeking to maximize profit, the principles of production economics are very useful.

A farm environment is a complex mix of production activities; livestock, crops, household activities and non-agricultural activities and consumption activities; rest time, eating, purchase of goods. To achieve maximum returns from production activities requires knowledge of:

1. Agricultural practices – technical and husbandry.
2. How to allocate resources, available on and off the farm, and react to economic forces that have origins far from the farm.

The latter requires analysis tools to indicate the best use of resources and how to react to external changes. The logic of production economics provides a framework for decision making at the livestock unit, farm and agrobusiness levels. Based on the theory of the firm, the study of the principles of production economics should clarify the concepts of cost, output response to inputs, and the use of resources to maximize profits and/or minimize costs. Therefore, the principles of production economics should be extremely useful to the farm unit seeking profit and efficiency.

In addition to assisting in decision making, the general principles of production economics are useful for understanding the decision-making process. These principles can be applied to studying how different components of the livestock sector will react to changing prices and policy measures taken by a government, including disease control policies. However, such analyses will be realistic only if the analyst has a clear perception of the technical production problems facing the components of the livestock sector. By nature, then, production economics is a combination of the technical relationship between inputs and outputs and the costs and prices of these goods. It is therefore an interdisciplinary subject, looking beyond the biology and purely technical aspects of production.

Studying Production Processes

Production economics will help to answer the following types of question within the livestock sector:

1. What is efficient production? By examining the different stages of production.
2. How is the most profitable amount of an input determined? By assessing the relationship between input (factor) and product.
3. What is the best combination of a number of inputs? By examining the relationship between inputs called a factor/factor relationship.
4. What enterprise combination will maximize farm profits? By determining what is called a product/product relationship.
5. How will farm production respond to a change in the price of an output, e.g. milk or meat?
6. How much can a livestock farmer pay for a durable input, such as a bullock cart?
7. What should a manager do if they are uncertain about livestock production levels? For example, livestock production will be uncertain if a farmer is in a region with animal diseases. This requires risk analysis tools.
8. How will technical change affect output?

Answering these questions is not straightforward due to the complexities of livestock processes. Production is affected by inputs, some of which can be controlled by the farm unit, while others are random such as rainfall. Time is important, particularly as livestock cycles often take a number of years to complete. Even in livestock systems with short cycles such as poultry and pigs, there will be investments that will take years for repayment. Dealing with this complexity requires a framework, which production economics provides.

Biological scientists would establish experimental plots to determine the importance of the factors that affect production. For example, growth of pigs can be tested by varying the amount of essential amino acids in their diet. However, it is not possible to set up trials of this sort to test changes in the livestock markets. For example, introducing a bonus for milk produced based on milk quality and antibiotic residues may influence the level of veterinary product use and the quantity of milk produced. Establishing a similar trial to that described for the pig feeding trial, where only a small group of farmers are involved and milk quality prices are varied, will be difficult if not impossible. The farmers in the trial would probably demand a stable quality premium so that they can plan their production and if the trial is perceived to be beneficial farmers outside the trial will demand to be part of it.

Therefore, economists have developed a logical reasoning process that in every sense parallels the experiment of the animal production scientist. This process, embodied in the theory of the firm, predicts how the profit maximizing components of the livestock sector will respond to a change in price policy for livestock products and inputs, given that other variables do not change. One important difference is that while the experiment can be observed and measured, the reasoning of the economist is abstract. This abstraction makes the discipline appear more difficult than it actually is.

To study the livestock production process a distinction is made between inputs with the following different categories identified:

- *Variable inputs* can be controlled by the livestock system and vary with the level of livestock product produced. A good example would be feed, or veterinary care. This concept will be used again when farm management methods such as gross margin analysis are presented in Chapter 4.
- *Fixed inputs* do not change over the analysis period. They are the inputs in terms of infrastructure such as a building and can also include the investment in the animals themselves.
- *Random inputs* are associated with inputs that cannot be influenced by the livestock producer such as the weather, and in the market the prices of inputs and outputs. To simplify this, an economic analysis often assumes that these random inputs are constant. To generalize, the result would require further work on the robustness of the result with changes in important parameters.

The problem of random inputs will be dealt with later, but it is first necessary to have a starting point for building an economic analysis framework. The following is a brief description of the important initial assumptions of production economics:

1. The first set of assumptions is designed to make the production process stable during the period of study.
- Technology is assumed constant; the livestock system selects the most efficient known technology and does not change it during the production period.
- Institutional factors such as land ownership and government policies do not change.

2. A second set of assumptions is required to make the analysis of the production process easy to conceptualize.
- Production functions are drawn as smooth, well-behaved curves.
- Inputs are taken as being indivisible and mobile. Such assumptions are quite reasonable for some inputs, such as commercial fertilizer, but unrealistic for others, such as labour. The same assumptions of homogeneity and perfect divisibility are also applied to products.

3. A third category of assumptions is required to deal with the randomness of some inputs.
- Initially, the assumption of perfect certainty is made. This assumption is restrictive and implies that the farm unit has perfect knowledge of prices and the general environment and that the cost of obtaining this knowledge is zero. Because of this, price and livestock production uncertainties are removed. Clearly, the impact of random variables, particularly animal disease, on livestock production is important, but initially the production process will be presented without uncertainty in order to provide a basis for understanding decision-making processes.

4. A fourth category of assumptions is required to deal with time. Perfect certainty removes the random elements associated with time, but another problem remains. A dollar at farrowing time has a different value from a dollar at finishing time. This is called time discounting and is not initially considered. In the presence of perfect certainty and in the absence of time discounting, production can be abstracted from time and for practical purposes considered as instantaneous.

5. Finally goals of the livestock system must be considered:
- the initial assumption is that the livestock system is motivated by profits; and
- rationally seeking to maximize profits.

These assumptions allow the development of economic theory, and help to identify which facts are useful in examining problems such as:

1. Determining the best use of resources by livestock production, processing or production units, given the changing needs, values and goals of society.

2. Determining the consequences of alternative public and private policies[1] on output, profits and resource use within the livestock sector; these may include:
- evaluation of the effects of technical and institutional changes on production and resource use by the livestock sector or components of that sector;
- determination of the response of the livestock sector output in terms of livestock product supply and resource use to changes in prices.

3. Understanding the behaviour of the different components of the livestock sector as profit maximizing entities.

The Economic Setting for the Livestock Sector

Markets used by the livestock sector can be classified according to the:

- Number and size of the firms which sell their products to the markets.
- Number of buyers who purchase the livestock products and the amounts they purchase.
- Similarity or lack of similarity of animals and livestock products sold at the

---

[1]This recognizes that some livestock systems are private sector-led and private sector-regulated and their policies have a strong influence on livestock sector supply (see Henson, 2006, for more details).

markets. For example, cattle are kept for different purposes, and for dairy cattle there are different points in the production cycle such as heifers, in-calf cows and barren cows. For livestock products such as eggs, there are classifications based on species, breeds, size and type of production system. Different markets and traders often deal with different types of animals and livestock products.

- Ease with which firms may enter into, or cease, production of a livestock sector input, an animal or a livestock product; while not examined in any detail in this chapter, these transaction costs will be discussed more carefully in the contribution by David Leonard on institutional economics (see Chapter 12).

If we consider a livestock farm as a seller, livestock farmers all over a nation will produce beef, eggs, milk, etc. For any one product, beef for example, *so many sellers exist that the quantity sold by any one seller is infinitely small compared to the quantity sold by all other sellers.* The quantity of beef produced by one farm unit is minute compared to the beef produced annually by a nation.

Therefore, there are many sellers of livestock products, but that is not all. Agricultural products of a given type are similar in appearance and quality. *Livestock farmers sell a homogeneous product.* The beef raised by one farm unit may be of a higher quality than a neighbour's, but will be similar to the beef produced by a large number of other efficient farm units. In general, buyers do not prefer the products of one farmer to the products of a second. The result is that individual livestock farmers are generally unable to create a unique demand for their own particular products by special marketing methods such as advertising.

These two conditions, many sellers and homogeneous products, mean that *an individual livestock production system cannot influence the market price of their product.* The livestock production system can therefore be described as a *price taker*, meaning that it must take the market price as given.

Let us consider now the livestock production unit as a buyer. In general, it is one of many buyers, all of whom need the same or similar type of input. If the livestock production unit decides not to buy a veterinary input, the price will not be affected, as the individual livestock production unit's purchase represents an infinitesimal quantity relative to the total veterinary inputs sold. However, in general, most livestock producers *regard the price of inputs as given.*

Usually, farm units are only able to influence market prices themselves in a local market and not the general price level facing all farm units. There are also exceptions for specialty livestock products, but these tend to be for niche markets and have been established over long periods of time. These products are usually associated with regions. For livestock inputs where livestock production systems are very large, as is the trend in many developed countries and also in certain developing countries, there may be more bargaining power. Farmers may also form groups or cooperatives to have improved negotiation power for the purchase of inputs and the sale of outputs.

The type of market described above, with many buyers or sellers and a homogeneous product, is called a *purely competitive market.* Many of the markets in which livestock farmers buy and sell approximate pure competition. There are two more conditions for a purely competitive market:

1. Businesses must be free to enter into, or cease, production as they please. There should be no patents etc.

2. There should be no artificial restrictions placed on the supply of, or demand for, products. Thus, prices are free to vary, and equilibrium levels will be reached in the marketplace. In this way, increased production by the industry results in a lower market price and an increase in the quantity demanded and vice versa.

Pure competition is rarely found in the real world, but is considered worthy of study for the following reasons. First, it comes closer to approximating market conditions in agricultural production than any other type of market. Second, one of the characteristics of an industry selling in a purely competitive market is that profits are the result of natural rather than contrived scarcity. Profits made by livestock farms in India are due to them because they own milk animals that are naturally scarce. Profits from contrived scarcity would result if a farm purchased all milk animals in India and took them out of production. In an industry selling in a purely competitive market, however, no individual producer owns enough of any productive resource to be able to create artificial shortages.

In summary to this introduction and concepts for production economics, the key assumptions are the following:

- Inputs can be classified into variable, fixed and random inputs.
- Inputs are homogeneous and equivalent in quality and are *divisible* and *mobile*.
- There is perfect certainty.
- The production process is stable, i.e. during the analysis period there is *constant technology*.
- The goal of the livestock farmer or agribusiness person is *profit maximization*.
- The livestock farmer or agribusiness person is a price taker and cannot influence the price of either input or output.
- There are numerous producers, which implies there is *perfect competition*.

Relationship Between Inputs and Outputs

The management of a livestock production or processing enterprise, be it a large commercial company or a small subsistence farmer, requires decisions on the level of input use that is appropriate. This requires the use of information on the technical relationship between the inputs and the output and the prices of the inputs and output.

The underlying process of a livestock production system is biological with the level of output being directly related to the amount of input. Such a relationship can take on various forms of which the most common are the following:

Constant productivity is one where each unit of variable input added to the fixed inputs increases the livestock output by the same amount (see Fig. 3.1). Best examples of this type of relationship are bulky items such as the addition of new housing facilities for animals.

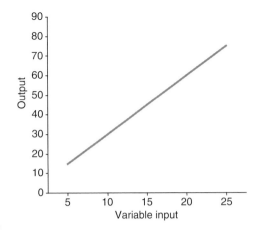

Fig. 3.1. Physical production function with constant productivity.

Diminishing productivity is one where each additional unit of the variable input adds less to the total livestock output than the previous unit (see Fig. 3.2). Many examples of this sort of response are seen in natural situations, an example would be additions of protein supplement to beef cattle.

Increasing productivity is one where each additional unit of the variable input adds more to total livestock output than the previous one (see Fig. 3.3). This sort of response will generally only be seen at very low levels of input use. Perhaps an example would be the period of compensatory growth seen in cattle that have been through the dry season.

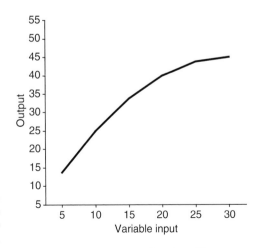

Fig. 3.2. Physical production function with diminishing productivity.

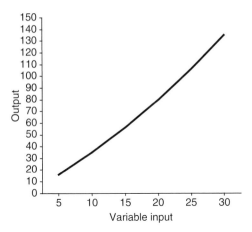

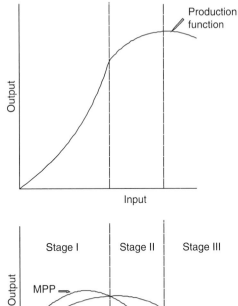

Fig. 3.3. Physical production function with increasing productivity.

Fig. 3.4. The classical production function and the three production phases.

The curve shown in the top graph of Fig. 3.4 represents an idealistic production function. It shows all aspects of productivity from increasing to diminishing. It is unlikely that a production function for an input to animal production system would look like this. One reason is that most production processes have some residual level of input. For example, in an experiment looking at the response to feeding concentrates the animal will be getting a certain level of nutrients from the forage. Therefore, the initial portion of the production function will not be displayed. The use of this idealistic function is to allow the building of a useful economic framework.

The input and output relationship is of interest, as it can be used to determine the efficient area of production and the optimum level of input use. However, the biological optimum level of input use is not necessarily the same as the economic optimum. To calculate, the latter requires input and output prices. Before introducing prices, it is necessary to look first at the relationships between inputs and outputs, which are represented by the production function.

Production Functions

Production is the process of using materials (inputs, factors, resources or productive services) to create goods or services (output or product). In a more practical context, the process of producing milk from cows requires inputs of land to produce fodder and feed, labour to care for the animals and capital to buy or hire the animals. These inputs are combined to produce milk. All livestock systems or agrobusiness enterprises are production activities.

Productivity is the relationship between output and input, and is used as an efficiency measure. In other words, it is the rate at which livestock output varies as additional equal units of variable input are used. In the curves presented above, productivity is the same throughout the increases in inputs for Fig. 3.1, i.e. constant productivity. For Fig. 3.2, each additional unit of input generates a smaller amount of output than the previous unit, i.e. decreasing productivity. Finally in Fig. 3.3, each additional unit of input generates a greater amount of output than the previous unit, i.e. increasing productivity.

To analyse livestock production processes, it is necessary to develop quantitative relationships between inputs and outputs, which is precisely what a *production function* does. A *production function* is a quantitative or mathematical description of various technical production possibilities facing a livestock farmer, livestock input supplier or livestock processing company. The production function gives the maximum output(s) in physical terms for each level of input(s) in physical terms. The production function can be expressed in three ways: tables, graphs or equations.

Tables

Tables are an obvious representation of a production function but are limited for analyses. They provide a useful starting point when looking at the relationship between inputs and outputs, but become increasingly complicated when expressing relationships between multiple inputs and an output.

- Tables represent a production function in a discrete or discontinuous manner.

Graphs

Graphs are a useful representation of production functions, but are limited by the number of inputs to output they can represent. It is easy to draw a graph of one input relating to one output, difficult to plot two inputs and one output and impossible to plot three and more inputs to one output. A graphical representation of an input to output can be seen in Figs 3.1–3.4. These are all single input and single output representations.

Figure 3.4 is a graph of a production function. This *line represents the frontier of technically feasible production* and is the most technically efficient region of production for the agricultural operation it represents. The area above the line is therefore a *technically infeasible* region with the present state of knowledge and the area below the line represents the *technically suboptimal points*. The graph contains no information on prices and is only related to the physical input and output levels.

- A graph can represent a production function either as a *discrete* or *discontinuous* relationship or a *continuous* relationship.
- A graph can be used to represent what happens with a technological change.

Equations

Equations provide the most analytically useful representation of the production function.

The generalized expression of a production function in equation form is as follows:

$$Y = f(X_1, X_2, X_3, \ldots X_{(n-1)}, X_n)$$

where Y = Output

X_1, X_2 = Inputs (resources)

f means function of and implies that a unique amount of output is derived from a given set of inputs.

In situations where some inputs do not change over the period of production (i.e. they are fixed costs or resources), the production function equation would be written in the following manner:

$$Y = f(X_1 \mid X_2, X_3, \ldots X_{(n-1)}, X_n)$$

When a production function is written in such a way it indicates that anything before the solid line is varied (i.e. variable costs or inputs), but after the solid line the inputs are kept constant (fixed cost or inputs).

Equations provide an easier method of expressing more complicated relationships on paper. More than one input can be introduced and still be expressed in a relatively simple form with an equation.

Summary

Tables, graphs and equations are the three theoretical methods of expressing a production function. All three methods provide a relationship between inputs and outputs, but equations are the most powerful for analytical work. It is noted that gross margins, enterprise budgets and farm budgets, which will be explained in Chapter 7, represent a point of a production function. They indicate the expected output levels for the inputs displayed, but provide no information on what would happen to the level of output with a change in any one of the inputs.

Terminology for Production Economics

The generalized equation for expressing the production function can be used to calculate the livestock output produced in a production process with any given level of input or combination of inputs. The total output produced is sometimes called the *total physical product* (TPP) and can be expressed in the following way:

Total physical product (TPP) =
$$Y = f(X_1 \mid X_2, \ldots, X_n)$$

There are two different measures of productivity used in production economics. Both are related to the production function and the TPP and are explained below.

The *average physical product (APP)* is the average livestock output per unit of variable input and can be calculated by dividing the total livestock output by the amount of variable input used. This is a measure of how efficiently input is converted to output. APP can be represented by the following equation:

Average physical product (APPx_1) =
$$\frac{Y}{X_1} = \frac{f(X_1 \mid X_2, \ldots, X_n)}{X_1}$$

The *marginal physical product (MPP)* is equal to the change in the amount of product produced over the change in the amount of input that is used. Therefore, if an extra amount of variable input, dx_i, produces dy of extra livestock output then the MPP$_{xi}$ is equal to dy/dx_i. MPP is equal to the slope of TPP and therefore represents the rate at which an input is transformed into an output. This can be represented by the following equation:

Marginal physical product (MPP$_{X_1}$) =
$$\frac{dY}{dX_1} = \frac{df(X_1 \mid X_2, \ldots, X_n)}{dX_1}$$

Elasticity of production (ε_p) is the percentage change of an output over the percentage change of an input. It is an indicator of the responsiveness of output to changes in input. It can either be represented as partial or factor elasticity (where only one input is varied, all others held constant) or function coefficient or total elasticity (where all inputs are varied by an equal amount). This can be represented by the following equation:

$$\varepsilon_p = \frac{\% \, change \, in \, output}{\% \, change \, in \, input} = \frac{\dfrac{dY}{Y}}{\dfrac{dX_1}{X_1}} = \frac{MPP_{X_1}}{APP}$$

Law of diminishing returns

In the production function drawn in Fig. 3.2, the relationship between the input and the output begins to show decreasing productivity. At this point, the increase in the level of input adds less and less output. This in its most basic form is the law of diminishing returns. A strict definition is as follows:

> The law of diminishing returns (also called the law of variable proportions) states that if increasing amounts of one input are added to a production process while all other inputs are held constant the amount of output added per unit of variable input will eventually decrease.

Note that the statement makes the allowance for a period of increasing as well as diminishing returns. Many people use the concept of marginal change, and often the law is referred to as the Law of Diminishing Returns.

Stages of production

APP, MPP and elasticity of production are all derived from the production function. They are useful in determining the region of rational production for an agricultural process. Figure 3.2 has a number of stages marked out on both graphs and these represent important areas with regard to economic decision making. These stages are described below.

Stage I

During this stage, the TPP is increasing at an increasing rate. Productivity is therefore increasing during this stage. In the bottom graph, it can be seen that during this stage APP is increasing and MPP is greater than APP. MPP also reaches a maximum during this stage. Elasticity of production is greater than one, which means that the response to increases in input levels is elastic.

End of stage I and beginning of stage II

MPP equals APP, elasticity of production is equal to one and APP reaches its maximum.

Stage II

During stage II, TPP is increasing at a diminishing rate and therefore productivity is decreasing. APP is greater than MPP. The efficiency of using a variable input is at its greatest where stage II begins; however, the efficiency of using the fixed inputs is greatest at the end of stage II. Optimal use of inputs lies somewhere in stage II and it depends upon the input costs and output prices. Throughout this stage elasticity of production is between one and zero and responsiveness of output to increases in input can be described as inelastic.

End of stage II and beginning of stage III

At the end of stage II, TPP reaches its maximum point and MPP equals zero. The elasticity of production also equals zero.

Stage III

During stage III, TPP declines, MPP is negative and APP is declining. It would be wasteful if producers were at this stage of the production function. Elasticity of production is less than zero.

The efficient usage of inputs: examination of the different stages of production

It would be irrational for a livestock farmer or agribusiness person to operate in stages I and III of production, regardless of the level of input and product prices. This is obvious for stage III where the addition of extra input is reducing the level of output. The logic of not producing in stage I of production is a little more difficult.

To understand why it is not sensible to produce in stage I of production, it is necessary to examine the full meaning of APP. APP measures the efficiency of resource use. The livestock farmer is interested in the most efficient use of his resources. During stage I, APP is increasing, implying that the level of efficiency with which a single input is being used is also increasing. The most efficient point of input usage is where the APP reaches its maximum. This is at the end of stage I and the beginning of stage II. Therefore, a livestock farmer would not be utilizing resources in the most efficient manner if they produced in stage I. This is illustrated by the following example.

Table 3.1 gives the offtake of sheep meat in kilograms with different levels of fertilizer application to a pasture. MPP and APP for the production function have been calculated, and indicate that Phase I runs from zero fertilizer use to the application of five units of fertilizer, and that Phase II runs from the application of five to ten units of fertilizer.

Figure 3.5 presents the graphical form of the production function and the associated productivity measures.

To demonstrate why a farmer would not produce in stage I, another constraint is added. The farmer has only 10 ha of land and ten units

Table 3.1. Relationship between fertilizer use and sheep meat production per hectare.

Quantity of fertilizer per hectare X_1	TPP (kg of meat/ha)	APP_{X1}	MPP_{X1}	Elasticity of production
0	0.0			
1	7.6	7.60	7.60	1.00
2	16.2	8.10	8.60	1.06
3	25.4	8.47	9.20	1.09
4	34.7	8.68	9.30	1.07
5	43.8	8.76	9.10	1.04
6	52.1	8.68	8.30	0.96
7	59.3	8.47	7.20	0.85
8	65.0	8.13	5.70	0.70
9	68.7	7.63	3.70	0.48
10	70.9	7.09	2.20	0.31
11	67.5	6.14	−3.40	−0.55

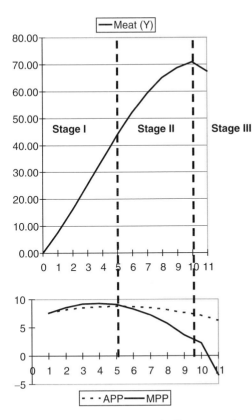

Table 3.2. Total sheep meat output with different combinations of fertilizer and land.

Units of fertilizer per hectare	Hectares of land used	Meat yield per hectare	Total meat production from ten units of fertilizer
1	10	7.6	76
2	5	16.2	81
3	3.33	25.4	84.582
4	2.5	34.7	86.75
5	2	43.8	87.6
6	**1.66**	**52.1**	**86.486**
7	1.43	59.3	84.799
8	1.25	65.0	81.25
9	1.11	68.7	76.257
10	1	70.0	70

Fig. 3.5. Relationship between fertilizer use and sheep meat production per hectare with measures of average and marginal physical products.

of fertilizer to spread on it. To obtain the best combination of the two inputs, all the units of fertilizer used and the amount of land used are varied. Table 3.2 shows that most sheep meat is produced if 1.66 ha land is used and that six units of fertilizer per hectare are applied to this land, i.e. within Phase II of the production function for fertilizer and meat production.

A comment on production functions and production economics

The ideal aim would be to produce an equation that would give us a precise method of calculating output from any given level of inputs. However, the difficulty in generating the production functions is a lack of data. As a consequence, researchers and livestock managers alike rely on few observations

and make large interpolations between data points. Therefore, equations are often good approximations, which take into account the cost of collecting data and their end use.

It will be noted here that the production function material from one area may not be applicable to other areas. The reason is relatively obvious in that important determinants not under the control of the manager and researcher play a large role in determining the level of production. Such items include climate and the quality of the soil.

What is often found with farmers is that they have reached an understanding of their own production functions through a long period of trial and error. They are therefore able to select the optimum use of an input from the knowledge that has been built up over many years. Problems tend to arise, however, when new inputs are introduced and farmers are unfamiliar with their use, or when there are fluctuations in the markets for inputs and outputs. Livestock research and dissemination of information on the use of new inputs are vital to assist livestock farmers in making optimum use of resources. Some elements of using research-guiding resources for animal health decision making are provided by Professor Clem Tisdell in Chapter 4 and Dr Alistair Stott when he examines how optimization methods can be used to look at farm-level data for disease control interventions (Chapter 9).

Necessary and sufficient conditions

The previous paragraphs defined a range of production where there is no possibility of producing the same amount of product with fewer inputs and no possibility of producing more product with the same amount of inputs. This is of course stage II of production when elasticity of production is greater than zero but less than one. This is a physical relationship and is universally applicable under any economic system. It is objective in nature and is a *necessary* condition of production.

The necessary condition produces a wide range of possibilities of input use for the livestock farmer, livestock input supplier or processor and some method is needed for narrowing it down. This can be done by adding choice indicators that reflect how a livestock farmer (the decision maker) chooses the level of inputs. In the idealistic situation, the livestock farmer is a profit maximizer, which implies that prices are the choice indicators to determine profit maximizing points for input use. This selection of choice indicators and determination of optimum points is our *sufficient* condition.

Production Economics: Profit Maximization Point for a Single Variable Input

The technical relationship between an input and livestock output has been examined and represented as a production function. This technical relationship has helped to make some recommendations about input use, with stage II of production defined as the rational region of production. If a product has any value at all, input should continue to be increased until at least stage II has been reached, the point of maximum physical efficiency. Even if the input is free it should not be used in stage III of production, as this will simply mean reducing the quantity of product produced.

The physical relationship is useful, but to determine the most profitable amount of variable input to be used, and hence the most profitable amount of product to be produced,

requires the prices of the input and output to be known. There are three methods of determining this profit maximization for a single input to single output relationship (factor/product):

1. Calculating the profit for different levels of input use and the resultant output;
2. Graphing the profit line to determine where it reaches a maximum;
3. Algebraically.

Before examining the use of these three methods, it is first necessary to provide some additional definitions.

Total value product (TVP) is the total monetary value of the production of an enterprise and can be written as:

$$TVP = P_Y * Y$$

where Y = the amount of output at any level of input; and P_Y = the price per unit of output.

Average value product (AVP) is APP times the price per unit of Y and can be written as:

$$AVP = APP * P_Y$$
$$= (Y / X) * P_Y$$
$$= TVP / X$$

Marginal value product (MVP or VMP) is MPP times the price per unit of Y. MVP is the slope of the TVP line. It can be written as:

$$MVP = MPP * P_Y$$
$$= (dY / dX) * P_Y$$
$$= d / dX(TVP)$$

Total variable costs (TVC) are the total monetary costs for a variable input used for production and can be written as:

$$TVC = P_x * X$$

where X = the amount of variable input used; and P_x = the price per unit of input.

Total fixed costs (TFC) are the total monetary value of fixed inputs used for production.

Total costs (TC) are the total monetary value of all costs of production and can be written as:

$$TC = TVC + TFC$$

Profit (π) is TVP minus TC. Profit is also called net returns or net revenue. It can be written as:

$$\text{Profit}(\pi) = \text{TVP} - \text{TC}$$
$$= \text{TVP} - \text{TVC} - \text{TFC}$$
$$= P_Y * Y - P_x * X - \text{TFC}$$

The production function is vital for calculating profit for the livestock enterprise. It relates TVP to the amount of input and TC to the amount of output: i.e. TVP is easily related to livestock output; it is price times quantity. In the same way, TC may be derived for various input amounts. However, only the production function can relate inputs to revenues and outputs to costs.

The following example will use two of the methods described above to determine the profit maximizing point for a single variable input to produce one output.

Table 3.3 provides data on the production function for milk yield of a cow with different levels of concentrate feeding. The following information is available on the prices of feed and milk:

Price per unit of milk (P_Y) = £2
Price per unit of feed (P_X) = £1
TFC = £10

Table 3.3 contains further information on technical and economic productivity measures and profit. The profit maximization point for the use of feed for milk production with the prices described is the use of 20 units of feed.

Figure 3.6 is a graphical representation of TVP from the varying levels of feed input.

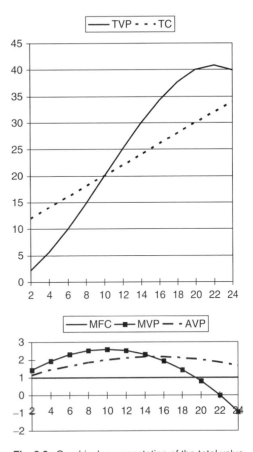

Fig. 3.6. Graphical representation of the total value product of milk production and varying levels of feed input use with the associated measures of economic productivity.

Table 3.3. Relationship between feed use for a dairy production with the associated value of output, costs, profitability and productivity measures.

Units of feed (X)	Milk output (Y)	APP	MPP	AVP	MVP	TVP	TFC	TVC	TC	Profit
2	1.14	0.57	0.72	1.14	1.45	2.28	10.00	2.00	12.00	−9.72
4	2.85	0.71	0.98	1.42	1.95	5.70	10.00	4.00	14.00	−8.30
6	5.00	0.83	1.16	1.66	2.31	10.00	10.00	6.00	16.00	−6.00
8	7.42	0.93	1.26	1.86	2.53	14.84	10.00	8.00	18.00	−3.16
10	10.00	1.00	1.30	2.00	2.60	20.00	10.00	10.00	20.00	0.00
12	12.58	1.05	1.26	2.10	2.53	25.16	10.00	12.00	22.00	3.16
14	15.01	1.07	1.16	2.14	2.31	30.02	10.00	14.00	24.00	6.02
16	17.15	1.07	0.98	2.14	1.95	34.30	10.00	16.00	26.00	8.30
18	18.87	1.05	0.72	2.10	1.45	37.74	10.00	18.00	28.00	9.74
20	**20.00**	**1.00**	**0.40**	**2.00**	**0.80**	**40.00**	**10.00**	**20.00**	**30.00**	**10.00**
22	20.42	0.93	0.00	1.86	0.01	40.84	10.00	22.00	32.00	8.84
24	19.97	0.83	−0.46	1.66	−0.93	39.94	10.00	24.00	34.00	5.94

It also shows the economic productivity measures and the cost lines. Where the cost line and TVP line cross, profit becomes positive, and where the slope of the cost line is equal to the slope of the TVP line, profit is maximized.

Algebraic solution to the profit maximization point for a single variable input

If profit is considered as a function of input, then the optimum amount of input is where profit is at a maximum. At the point where profit is at a maximum, the slope of the profit line is equal to zero. The slope of a line can be obtained by differentiating the equation of that line.

Therefore, consider the profit equation as a function of input:

$$\text{Profit} = P_Y f(X) - P_X X - \text{TFC}$$

If this function is differentiated with respect to X, the following equation is derived:

$$\frac{d\text{Profit}}{dX} = P_Y \frac{dY}{dX} - P_X$$

As this equation represents the slope of the profit line and the maximum point is reached where the slope equals zero, the following can be done to calculate the profit maximization point for a single variable input:

$$\frac{d\text{Profit}}{dX} = P_Y \frac{dY}{dX} - P_X = 0$$
$$= P_Y \text{MPP} - P_X = 0$$

or

$$P_Y \text{MPP} = P_X$$
$$\frac{\text{MVP}}{P_X} = 1$$

The profit maximization point solution to this generalized profit function implies:

> The use of an input should be increased until the point is reached whereby the last £ (or $, Kwacha, Rupee, Shilling, etc.) spent on the input returns exactly its incremental cost.

Therefore, if the MVP is greater than the price per unit of an input (or the marginal factor cost of an input), then profit can be increased by increasing input use. If MVP is less than price per unit of input, then profit can be increased by reducing input use. In the example above, the table and graphical solutions to identify profit maximization were imprecise, indicating that 20 units of feed should be used; in fact the profit maximization point can be calculated more accurately with an equation of the production and the prices at just under 20.

Production with Two Variable Inputs: Factor–Factor Relationship

The relationship between a single input and single output has been examined to determine a general profit maximizing point for that input. This point is reached where the MVP for the input is equal to the price per unit (or marginal factor cost) of that input. This principle will be useful for determining the best combination of two inputs and to develop a general theory on multiple input use.

In examining a livestock production system with two variable inputs and a single output, it is assumed that all other inputs are held constant, and that the livestock farmer can buy as much of either variable input without affecting the price of those inputs. The following generalized equation represents the production function facing the farmer:

$$Y = f(X_1, X_2 | X_3, X_4, ..., X_{(n-1)}, X_n)$$

Data for such a production function can also be represented in tabular form as Table 3.4 shows.

Alternatively it can be shown as a three-dimensional graph (see Fig. 3.7).

The production function is represented by a *production surface* in the graph. Any point on this surface represents the technically feasible level of production for a combination of the two variable inputs, soybean meal and fishmeal. Any point above this surface is technically infeasible and points below are technically suboptimal. Compare this with the production function for a single variable input and a single output.

It is possible using the profit maximizing point for a single variable input and data like those shown in Table 3.2 to find the profit

Table 3.4. Relationship between pig growth and the use of soybean meal and fishmeal.

Fishmeal (g)	Soybean meal (g)				
	60	80	100	120	140
	Growth (g)				
20	76	90	95	97	96
40	78	92	100	104	105
60	78	93	102	105	108
80	77	92	103	106	109

maximizing point for two variable inputs. For this, it is necessary to have some prices, which are given as:

Value of live weight gain = K 2.50/g
Price of soybean = K 0.2/g
Price of fishmeal = K 0.25/g

If the fishmeal is held constant at 20 g, then it is possible to determine the MVP of growth with increases of soybean meal (see Table 3.5).

From Table 3.5 it can be estimated that the profit maximizing point for pig growth with varying levels of soybean meal in the diet is 120 g of soybean meal. If the soybean meal is now held constant at 120 g, the fishmeal can be varied (see Table 3.6).

From Table 3.6, it can be estimated that the profit maximizing point for pig growth with varying levels of fishmeal is 40 g of fishmeal. There is one final check to examine if profit can be improved by further inputs and that is to increase both the fishmeal and the soybean meal at the same time (remember we are examining a production surface not a production line). Looking at the first table, increasing fishmeal by 20–60 g and soybean by 20–140 g will increase growth from 105 to 109 g. This will give a change in financial output of K 10 (4 * 2.5). The cost of the inputs to achieve this change

Table 3.5. The production function and measures of technical and economic productivity of soybean (variable input) and pig growth (output).

Soybean (g)	Growth (g)	MPP	MVP
60	76		
		0.7	1.75
80	90		
		0.25	0.625
100	95		
		0.1	0.25
120	**97**		
		−0.05	−0.125
140	96		

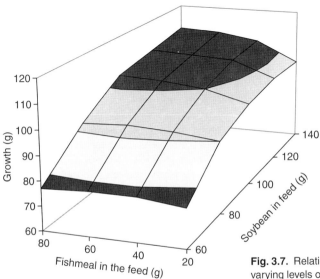

Fig. 3.7. Relationship between pig growth and varying levels of soybean and fishmeal.

Table 3.6. The production function and measures of technical and economic productivity of fishmeal (variable input) and pig growth (output).

Fishmeal (g)	Growth (g)	MPP	MVP
20	97		
		0.35	0.875
40	**104**		
		0.05	0.125
60	105		
		0.05	0.125
80	106		

Table 3.8. The profit from feeding varying levels of soybean meal and fishmeal and producing pig meat.

	Soybean meal (g)				
	60	80	100	120	140
Fishmeal (g)	Profit (Kwacha)				
20	173	204	212.5	213.5	207
40	173	204	220	226	224.5
60	168	201.5	220	223.5	**227**
80	160.5	194	217.5	221	224.5

in output is K 9 (((20 ∗ 0.25) + (20 ∗ 0.2)). This implies that the profit maximizing point, for this relationship at these prices, is 108 g of growth produced by feeding 140 g of soybean meal and 80 g of fishmeal.

Table 3.7 highlights the path that has been taken to seek the profit maximization point. If we had begun by holding the soybean meal constant at 60 g we would have reached the same profit maximization point (if you are not convinced try it yourself).

Finally, for those not convinced that this is the profit maximization point, examine the data presented in Table 3.8, which shows the profit of the production process as the value of the output (grams of growth multiplied by price per gram of growth) minus the cost of soybean and fishmeal. The highest profit is achieved with 60 g of fishmeal and 140 g of soybean meal. (Note: The addition of fixed costs to the calculation will make no difference to the profit maximization point, as these will always be constant.)

Table 3.7. Production function for pig growth (output) with varying levels of soybean and fishmeal (variable inputs) and the path to obtain the profit maximization point for the use of these two variable inputs.

	Soybean meal (g)				
	60	80	100	120	140
Fishmeal (g)	Growth (g)				
20	**76**	**90**	**95**	**97**	96
40	78	92	100	**104**	105
60	78	93	102	105	**108**
80	77	92	103	106	109

The above example shows that it is possible to determine a profit maximizing point for two inputs using the general theory developed for single input use. However, it is necessary to have some general theories for two inputs in order to determine:

1. The least cost combination of two inputs for any particular level of output;
2. The level of output that maximizes profit.

To ease the development of a general theory for the least cost combination, it is necessary to represent the relationship between an output and two inputs in a two-dimensional way. This is achieved by representing the different levels of output as lines known as *isoquants*. These lines:

1. Never cross;
2. Represent combinations of the two inputs that yield equal amounts of output;
3. Provide a substitution rate between the two inputs.

Isoquants are analogous to contour lines on a geography relief map. Figures 3.8 and 3.9 show a number of common sets of isoquant lines for two inputs.

The rate at which one input replaces another to maintain the same level of production is called the *marginal rate of technical substitution* (MRTS). MRTS is as important to the relationship between two variable inputs (factor–factor relationship) as the MPP is to the single variable input and output (factor–product) relationship. It is represented by the slope of the isoquant. The marginal rate of substitution of variable input X_2 for variable input X_1 (see Fig. 3.10) is defined as the amount by which X_1 must be decreased to

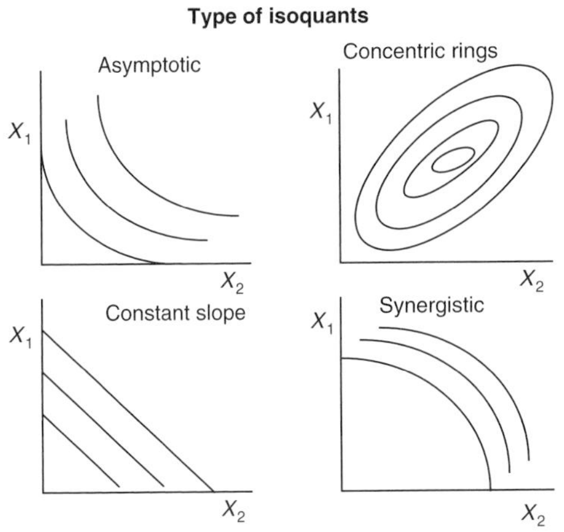

Type of isoquants

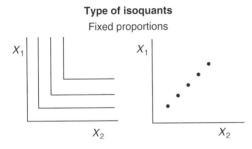

Fig. 3.8. Isoquants showing the relationship between two inputs and varying levels of output.

maintain output at a constant amount when X_2 is increased by one unit.

The MRTS of variable input X_2 for variable input X_1 can also be written as a formula:

$$\text{MRTS of } X_2 \text{ for } X_1 = dX_1 / dX_2$$

There are four basic rates of substitution:

1. *Decreasing rate of substitution* occurs when the input being increased substitutes for successively smaller amounts of the input being replaced. This type of substitution is shown by the asymptotic and concentric ring types of isoquants shown in Fig. 3.8. A real example of this type of situation would be the replacement of concentrate feed for forage in milk production.

2. *Constant rate of substitution* occurs when the amount of one input replaced by the other input does not change as the added

input increases in magnitude. In some literature, inputs that substitute at constant rates are termed 'perfect substitutes'. This type of substitution is shown by the constant slope type of isoquants demonstrated in Fig. 3.8. An example would be one type of concentrate feed for another.

3. *Complements* occur where inputs that increase output only when combined in fixed proportions are called technical complements. Examples would be labour and the introduction of a machine such as a tractor.

4. *Lumpy* occurs where both of the inputs are not completely divisible but exist only in discrete units; then the isoquants appear as dots which, when connected, appear as linear segments. Decision making with lumpy inputs, because of fewer alternatives, is less complex than when substitution relationships are continuous.

Factor–Factor Relationships: Least Cost Combinations and Profit Maximization Point

To develop the least cost and profit maximization points for two variable inputs and one output

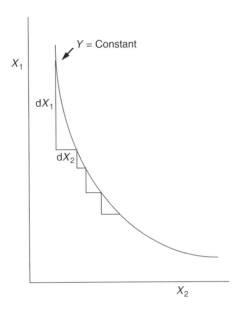

Fig. 3.10. The marginal rate of technical substitution for two variable inputs (X_1 and X_2) with constant level of output.

Type of isoquants

Fixed proportions

Fig. 3.9. Isoquants that show a fixed proportion relationship.

the concept of isocline will be introduced. An *isocline* is a line connecting points that have the same rate of technical substitution. The general equation for an isocline is as follows:

$$\text{MRTS of } X_2 \text{ for } X_1 = dX_1/dX_2 = \alpha$$

where α is an arbitrary constant.

Isoclines are of use in defining a rational region of production for two variable inputs and a single output. This can be done by deriving two special isoclines known as *ridge lines*. For one ridge line, the MRTS of variable input X_2 for variable input X_1 is equal to zero and for the other ridge line the MRTS of variable input X_2 for variable input X_1 is equal to ∞. Figure 3.11 presents this information graphically for variable inputs and outputs with asymptotic isoquants.

The area above the ridge line for variable input X_1 and to the right of the ridge line for variable input X_2 are irrational combinations of the variable inputs X_1 and X_2. In these regions, the MRTS is positive, indicating that instead of one input replacing another to maintain production at a certain level it will require extra amounts of both inputs to maintain that level of production.

How does the MPP of X_1 and X_2 relate to the MRTS? It is possible to examine this by carrying out some simple algebra.

To obtain a small change in output (Y) it is necessary to have a small change in variable input X_1 and a small change in variable input X_2. This can be written as a formula in the following way:

$$dY = (\text{small change in } X_1)*(\text{rate of transformation of } X_1 \text{ into } Y) + (\text{small change in } X_2)*(\text{rate of transformation of } X_2 \text{ into } Y)$$
$$= dX_1 * MPP_{X1} + dX_2 * MPP_{X2}$$

However, the definition of an isoquant implies that:

$$dY = 0$$

Therefore, $0 = dX_1 * MPP_{X1} + dX_2 * MPP_{X2}$

$$dX_1 * MPP_{X1} = -dX_2 * MPP_{X2}$$
$$dX_1/dX_2 = -MPP_{X2}/MPP_{X1}$$
$$\text{MRTS of } X_2 \text{ for } X_1 = -MPP_{X2}/MPP_{X1}$$

Least Cost Combination of Two Variable Inputs

To determine the least cost combination for two inputs, it is necessary to introduce a *budget/expenditure/isocost line*. This line represents a constant amount of money spent on the inputs and can be represented as the general equation:

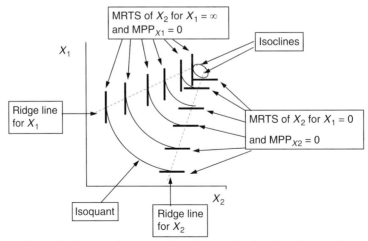

The region between the two isoclines is the rational region of production

Fig. 3.11. The rational region of production for two variable inputs and a single output.

$$C = P_{X1} * X_1 + P_{X2} * X_2$$

where C = Amount of capital (money)

P_{X1} = Price per unit of X_1

P_{X2} = Price per unit of X_2.

It can also be shown graphically as seen in Fig. 3.12.

Such an isocost line can be introduced into a graph with isoquant lines. The point of tangency of an isocost line and an isoquant line is the *least cost combination* for the two inputs (see Fig. 3.13). At this point of tangency the slopes of the isocost line and the isoquant line are equal.

The slope of an isoquant is represented by the MRTS of X_2 for X_1. By having a method to determine the slope of the isocost line, it will be possible to estimate the point where the slopes of the isoquant and isocost lines are equal. This of course is the least cost combination of two variable inputs for the production of a single output. The slope of a line is the *rise divided by the run*. For an isocost line, the rise is equal to zero minus the point where the isocost line crosses the X_1 axis. The point where the line crosses the X_1 axis is:

$$X_1 = C / P_{X1}$$

Therefore, the rise can be represented in the following way:

$$\text{Rise} = (0 - C / P_{X1})$$

Similarly, the run is equal to the point where the isocost line crosses the X_2 axis minus zero. The point where the line crosses the X_2 axis is:

$$X_2 = C / P_{X2}$$

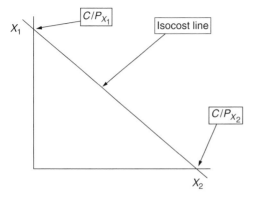

Fig. 3.12. Isocost line for two variable inputs.

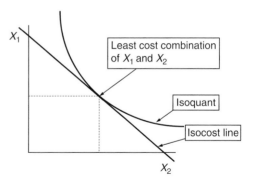

Fig. 3.13. Least cost line for two variable inputs and the isoquant for these two inputs, indicating the point of least cost combination of the inputs in the production of a single output.

Therefore, the run can be represented in the following way:

$$\text{Run} = (C / P_{X2} - 0)$$

The slope of the line is:

$$\text{Rise} / \text{Run} = (0 - C / P_{X1}) / (C / P_{X2} - 0)$$
$$= (-C / P_{X1}) * (P_{X2} / C)$$
$$= -P_{X2} / P_{X1}$$

This implies that the least cost combination of two inputs and a single output is reached where the MRTS of X_2 for X_1 will be equal to the price ratio of X_2 to X_1. The following can be expressed as a general formula:

$$\text{MRTS of } X_2 \text{ for } X_1 = -dX_1/dX_2 =$$
$$-\text{MPP}_{X2}/\text{MPP}_{X1} = -P_{X2}/P_{X1}$$

Figure 3.14 shows a family of isoquant curves and the least cost combination points for each isoquant. The isocline that joins these least cost combination points together is known as the *expansion path*. To reach the most profitable level of output for this two input single output scenario, it is necessary to move along to the end of this expansion path line.

Therefore, the most profitable level of production (output) must first satisfy the criterion of least cost combination of inputs. The general expression for an expansion path is given as:

$$\frac{\text{MPP}_{X2}}{\text{MPP}_{X1}} = \frac{P_{X2}}{P_{X1}}$$

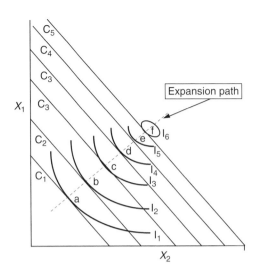

Fig. 3.14. The expansion path for two variable inputs and a single output.

Profit Maximization with Two Variable Inputs

If fixed costs are ignored, then a general relationship for two variable inputs can be derived. The following general equations can be written about the relationship:

$$\text{Output} = Y = f(X_1, X_2)$$
$$\text{TVP} = P_Y * Y = P_Y * f(X_1, X_2)$$
$$\text{TC} = P_{X1} * X_1 + P_{X2} * X_2$$

This implies that profit can be written as:

$$\text{Profit} = \text{TVP} - \text{TC}$$

$$\text{Profit} = P_Y * [f(X_1, X_2)] - [P_{X1} * X_1 + P_{X2} * X_2]$$
$$= P_Y * f(X_1, X_2) - P_{X1} * X_1 - P_{X2} * X_2$$

For profit to be at a maximum, the first condition that must be met is that the slope of the profit line equals zero for both variable inputs. Therefore, the following general equations can be written:

$$\frac{d\text{Profit}}{dX_1} = 0 \quad \text{Profit function for input } X_1$$

and

$$\frac{d\text{Profit}}{dX_2} = 0 \quad \text{Profit function for input } X_2$$

This implies that:

$$\frac{d\text{Profit}_{X1}}{dX_1} = \frac{P_Y * dY}{dX_1 - P_{X1}} = 0$$

and

$$\frac{d\text{Profit}_{X2}}{dX_2} = \frac{P_Y * dY}{dX_2 - P_{X2}} = 0$$

which can be simplified to:

$$\frac{P_Y * dY}{dX_1} = P_{X1}$$

and

$$\frac{P_Y * dY}{dX_2} = P_{X2}$$

or

$$\text{MVP}_{X1} = P_{X1}$$

and

$$\text{MVP}_{X2} = P_{X2}$$

This implies that, at the profit maximization point for two variable inputs, the ratio of MVP for input one to price per unit of input one should equal one and the ratio of MVP for input two to price per unit of input two should equal one:

$$\frac{\text{MPP}_{X2}}{P_{X2}} = \frac{\text{MPP}_{X1}}{P_{X1}} = 1$$

which means that, for a livestock production process with multiple inputs, the last pound (or kwacha, shilling, rupee, dollar) spent on each input must return exactly a pound (or kwacha, shilling, rupee, dollar).

Product–Product Relationships

The examination of the relationship between the production of two livestock products or the production of a livestock product and a crop product called the *product–product relationship* will help to answer the following question:

> What combination of enterprises should be produced from a given bundle of fixed and variable inputs?

The logic of product–product relationships is a formalization of the procedures used in budgeting and other planning techniques.

To answer the question it is necessary to look at something called a *production possibility curve*. This is analogous to an isoquant, but instead of output remaining constant it is the input levels that remain constant. The inputs can be switched between outputs. One question that will arise is how much input is available.

Unlimited inputs

If a livestock farmer, livestock input supplier or processor can buy as much of any input they require to maximize profit, it is not important to look at the allocation of resources between enterprises.

Limited inputs

With limited inputs available it is not certain that the optimum use for each livestock enterprise can be taken for granted. By definition, limited availability of inputs means that the total amount of input available is less than that amount needed to apply the optimum to each enterprise. Limited input situations are also referred to as *limited capital situations*.

When inputs are limited in quantity, livestock enterprises on the farm become uniquely related and can no longer be considered independently. The degree of interdependence among enterprises depends on their technical and economic relationships.

The concept of the production possibility curve is best demonstrated by an example. A livestock farmer has the opportunity to produce two outputs: sheep meat Y_1 and beef Y_2. We will assume that there is only one variable input feed X, all other inputs are fixed and specialized. This variable feed input can be used in both meat production processes. Table 3.9 gives the expected output with varying levels of input applied to sheep meat (Y_1) and beef enterprises (Y_2).

If the feed input is limited to seven units, then the relationship between sheep meat and beef is shown in Table 3.10.

The production possibility curve is a convenient device for depicting the two pro-

Table 3.9. Production functions for variable inputs of feed and outputs of sheep meat and beef.

Units of feed (X) used to produce sheep meat (Y_1)	Output of sheep meat (Y_1)	Units of feed (X) used to produce beef (Y_2)	Output of beef (Y_2)
0	0	0	0
1	7	1	12
2	13	2	22
3	18	3	30
4	22	4	36
5	25	5	40
6	27	6	42
7	28	7	43
8	27	8	42
9	25	9	40

duction functions on the same graph, which is shown in Fig. 3.15.

The relationship shown in Fig. 3.15 is a competitive one between the two outputs. There are other types of relationship that exist between outputs, which are described below.

Competitive relationship

A competitive relationship is where the switch of inputs from one livestock enterprise to another leads to the increase in the livestock output of one enterprise and decrease in output of the other. An example of this type

Table 3.10. Relationship between sheep meat and beef production with only seven units of feed available.

Units of feed (X) used to sheep meat (Y_1)	Output of sheep meat (Y_1)	Units of feed (X) used to produce beef (Y_2)	Output of beef (Y_2)
0	0	7	43
1	7	6	42
2	13	5	40
3	18	4	36
4	22	3	30
5	25	2	22
6	27	1	12
7	28	0	0

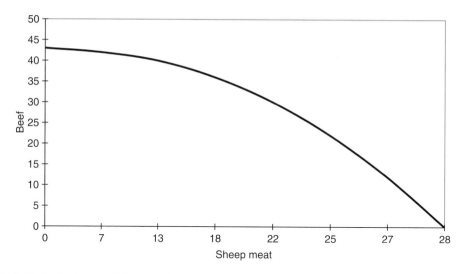

Fig. 3.15. Production possibility curve for sheep meat and beef production with only seven units of feed.

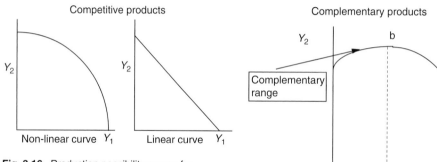

Fig. 3.16. Production possibility curves for competitive relationships.

Fig. 3.17. Production possibility curve where products have a complementary relationships and range.

of relationship would be concentrate feeding to different animal breeds, species and ages. The competitive relationships are usually *non-linear*. There are also *linear relationships* and an example would be the transfer of land between livestock enterprises.

Figure 3.16 presents the production possibility curves for competitive relationships.

Complementary relationship

Where the production of one livestock product can increase the production of another product, this is said to be a complementary relationship. An example is cattle being fed the straw from a cereal crop and producing manure and draught power to produce the crop in the

future. From a crop situation, legumes planted with a cereal crop either as a rotation or as mixed cropping increase the yields. However, complementary relationships eventually end up being competitive. Figure 3.17 presents a complementary production possibility curve. As can be seen the complementary range is only for a part of the production possibility curve.

Supplementary relationship

There are also instances where expansion of one livestock enterprise will leave other enterprise production levels unaffected. This

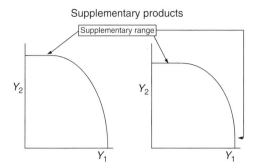

Supplementary products

Joint products

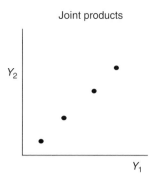

Fig. 3.18. Production possibility curves where products have a supplementary relationship and range.

Fig. 3.19. Production possibility curves with joint products.

could be when resources are not fully utilized throughout the year, and during slack resource use an extra enterprise can be added. Examples would be sheep fattening over the winter on an arable farm; chicken and pig fattening on a mixed farm, the growing of crops during the dry season using irrigation. Figure 3.18 presents two possible production possibility curves with different supplementary ranges. Similar to the complementary relationships, they become competitive.

Joint products

In a livestock production system, it is common that two products are produced, which are distinct and different. Good examples of this type of production are meat and wool, manure and milk, calves and milk, eggs and meat. For duck systems in South-east Asia, there are systems that produce three products, eggs, meat and feathers. Production of one is not possible without the production of the other. No substitution is possible between the products and the inputs are used in fixed proportions. Figure 3.19 presents a joint product relationship.

The objective of the product–product relationship is to determine the combination of enterprises that best meets management objectives, given the resource limitation. The primary use of the production possibility curve is to determine the most profitable combination of enterprises for a limited amount of input.

Revenue Maximizing Combination of Products

Similar to the two variable input relationships there is a concept known as *marginal rate of product substitution* (MRPS), which is the slope of the production possibility curve. This is analogous to MRTS for the variable inputs. The MRPS can be represented as the general equation:

$$\text{MRPS of } Y_1 \text{ for } Y_2 = \frac{\mathrm{d}Y_2}{\mathrm{d}Y_1}$$

A negative MRPS indicates a competitive relationship between products; a positive MRPS indicates a complementary relationship. If the MRPS is zero then the products are supplementary.

The *isorevenue line* is the point where the total revenue from the two products is constant. This is analogous to the isocost line for the two variable inputs. The isorevenue line can be represented as a general equation:

$$\text{Total revenue (TR)} = P_{Y1} * Y_1 + P_{Y2} * Y_2$$

Figure 3.20 presents the isorevenue line in a graph.

The revenue maximizing combination of two products is the point where the production possibility curve and the isorevenue line touch. This is known as a point of tangency and at this point the slope of the two lines is

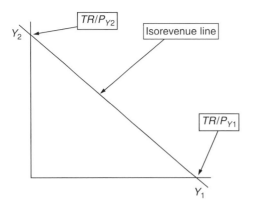

Fig. 3.20. The isorevenue line for two outputs.

equal. The slope of the production possibility curve is given by the MRPS (see Fig. 3.21).

The slope of the isorevenue line can be calculated by dividing the rise by the run. For an isorevenue line the rise is equal to zero minus the point where the line crosses the Y_2 axis. The point where the line crosses Y_2 axis is:

$$Y_2 = \frac{TR}{P_{Y2}}$$

Therefore, the rise can be represented in the following way:

$$Rise = \frac{0 - TR}{P_{Y2}}$$

Similarly, the run is equal to the point where the isorevenue line crosses the Y_1 axis minus zero. The point where the line crosses the Y_1 axis is:

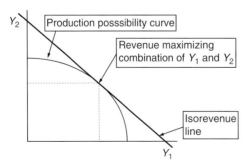

Fig. 3.21. The revenue maximizing point for the combination of two livestock products.

$$Y_1 = \frac{TR}{P_{Y1}}$$

Therefore, the run can be represented in the following way:

$$Run = \frac{TR}{P_{Y1} - 0}$$

The slope of the line is:

$$\frac{Rise}{Run} = \frac{\left(\dfrac{0 - TR}{P_{Y2}}\right)}{\left(\dfrac{TR}{P_{Y1} - 0}\right)}$$

$$= \frac{\left(\dfrac{-TR}{P_{Y2}}\right)}{\left(\dfrac{TR}{P_{Y1} - 0}\right)}$$

$$= \left(\frac{-TR}{P_{Y2}}\right) * \left(\frac{P_{Y1}}{TR}\right)$$

$$= \left(\frac{-TR}{P}\right) * \left(\frac{P}{TR}\right)$$

$$= \frac{-P_{Y1}}{P_{Y2}}$$

Therefore, at the revenue maximization point for two products:

$$MRPS \text{ of } Y_1 \text{ for } Y_2 = \frac{-P_{Y1}}{P_{Y2}}$$

$$\frac{dY_2}{dY_1} = \frac{-P_{Y1}}{P_{Y2}}$$

where dY_2 is negative.

$$dY_2 * P_{Y2} = dY_1 * P_{Y1}$$

This implies that at the revenue maximizing point the switch of resources from Y_2 to Y_1 will mean that the fall in revenue generated from output Y_2 will be equal to the increase in the revenue from Y_1.

Returning to the above example with sheep meat and beef, if the price per unit of sheep meat (Y_1) = US$2 and beef ($Y_2$) = US$1, it is possible to calculate the MRPS of beef (Y_2) for sheep meat (Y_1) and the revenue, and determine the revenue maximizing point (see Table 3.11).

Table 3.11. The marginal rate of product substitution for sheep meat and beef with a set number of feed units.

Units of feed (X) used to produce sheep meat (Y_1)	Output of sheep meat (Y_1)	Units of feed (X) used to produce beef (Y_2)	Output of beef (Y_2)	dY_1	dY_2	MRPS (Y_1), (Y_2)	Revenue
0	0	7	43				143
				7	−1	−0.14	
1	7	6	42				56
				6	−2	−0.33	
2	13	5	40				66
				5	−4	−0.80	
3	18	4	36				72
				4	−6	−1.50	
4	22	3	30				74
				3	−8	−2.67	
5	25	2	22				72
				2	−10	−5.00	
6	27	1	12				66
				1	−12	−12.00	
7	28	0	0				56

Note: The revenue maximizing point is where the MRPS of Y_1 for Y_2 equals the price ratio of Y_1 to Y_2.

General Revenue Maximizing Point

The change in the output of Y_1 and Y_2 is caused by the switch of a small amount of input X (dX). If we divide both sides of the above relationship by dX we get the following equation:

$$\frac{(dY_1 * P_{Y1})}{dX} = \frac{(dY_2 * P_{Y2})}{dX}$$

which can be rearranged to:

$$MPP_{XY1} * P_{Y1} = MPP_{XY2} * P_{Y2}$$
$$MVP_{XY1} = MVP_{XY2}$$

Finally, if we divide by the price per unit of input X:

$$\frac{MVP_{XY1}}{P_X} = \frac{MVP_{XY2}}{P_X}$$

This allows us to make the statement of the equimarginal principle:

The general equimarginal principle states that the ratio of the value of the marginal product of an input to the unit price of input (MVP_x/P_x) be equal for all inputs in all outputs (enterprises).

Time and the Production Process

The general introduction to the subject of production economics has excluded time, and livestock production processes were taken as instantaneous, with inputs disappearing and outputs appearing as if by magic. This is obviously unrealistic for any production process, but was necessary to develop an economic framework for analysing decision making. In Chapter 6, there will be an introduction of tools that also do not take into account time such as gross margin analysis. This limits certain aspects of how both the tools and the production economics theory that underlies them can be used, and it is important to recognize these limitations.

Reintroducing time gives a more realistic three-dimensional feel of the production process. The value of time will be further discussed when the subject of investment and cost–benefit appraisal is presented in Chapter 6. It should not be forgotten that even with time introduced, where profit maximization is the main objective, there is a search for the point at which every dollar spent on an input will return a dollar.

When considered as a function of time, inputs and outputs may be classified as:

- Point inputs would be fertilizer, seed, vaccination, worming drugs and examples of point outputs would be grain, meat, replacement heifers.
- Sequential inputs would be rainfall, feed, vitamins and examples of outputs would be milk.
- Continuous inputs would be temperature.

For each of the three types of time-dependent inputs, timeliness of application can be important. In the animal health field at a farm level, timing the application of deworming drug in a sheep enterprise can be critical to ensure that the parasites are removed and do not return before lambs are fattened. In national animal disease control campaigns, the speed of detection and response becomes critical in stopping a disease spreading.

Costs and revenues can occur at single points or sequentially. At farm level, the farmer must maintain funding for family expenses, production costs and mortgage payments. For disease control programmes, having access to funding so that vaccination campaigns can be targeted at certain high-risk times of the year can be critical for the success of the campaign. Cash flows within the production period or year therefore become important. Even when yields and prices are known with certainty, revenues and expenses could be poorly timed, resulting in unpaid bills. Capacities of durables, such as machinery, storage bins, milking parlours or laboratory equipment, become important for planning the timeliness of farm-level production, marketing and national animal decision making.

The introduction of time into a production process adds an additional complexity to the assessing decisions. Some aspects of examining this are shown in the preceding examples on a fattening unit and the purchase of durable input. For further examples please refer to Doll and Orazem (1984) and Dillon and Anderson (1990, chapter 6).

Profit maximization for a variable production process

Two issues need to be addressed when examining a variable production process:

1. Is the objective of the farmer to maximize the profit over the single production process? or
2. Is the objective of the farmer to maximize profit over a set period of time?

The latter option implies that the production process can be repeated a number of times over the set period. For many commercial farmers, the set period will be a year, because of the need for financial and tax accounting of the farm business. Having a set period of time to maximize profits may have little or no relevance in many smallholder situations. However, pressures such as yearly school fees may make this a growing issue for farmers with children. For the remainder of the discussion, it will be assumed that the critical time period for a farmer is a year.

If the production process takes exactly a year, then equating marginal revenue with marginal cost will maximize profit for the production process and for the year. However, most production processes do not last for a year. This raises the question of whether the length of the production process is fixed. If it is fixed, for example most cropping activities will be fixed, the profit maximization for the production process is the same as the profit maximization for the year.

If the length of the production process is not fixed, then the profit maximization of the production process is not the same as the profit maximization for time. The appropriate objective in this situation is the maximum profit per unit of time.

Livestock feeding operations, such as broiler production, pig fattening and feedlot fattening for cattle, are typical examples of an agricultural process that can be varied in time. The important decisions the farmer has to face in this situation are:

1. What type of ration and feeding system should be used? Will the choice of diet affect the rate of gain and time when the animal is marketed?

2. When should the animals be marketed to obtain the best possible price? (Are there seasonal prices for the output?)
3. Given the ration and market price, how long should the production process be to maximize profits per unit of time?

In the following example of drylot cattle feeding system, the last question will be examined in detail. The feedlot buys in animals that are 600 lb (1 lb = 0.45359237 kg) in weight. To simplify the analysis only the costs of animal purchased and feed are considered, and all other costs are assumed constant. Any animal can be bought or sold at US$0.20/lb. The possibility that the quality and hence the value of an animal will vary with time is also ignored. Once an animal has been fattened and sold, it will be immediately replaced with another animal.

The total time costs (TTC) of keeping an animal in this feedlot has been estimated as follows:

$$TTC = 120 + 2N + 0.0067N^3$$

where N = time in 10-day feeding units.

The total time revenue (TTR) from the sale of the animal at any time is estimated to be the following:

$$TTR = 120 + 0.6N^2 - 0.02N^3$$

where N = time in 10-day feeding units.

Table 3.12 presents the revenue and costs for the enterprise with different time units.

With the introduction of time, there are different profit maximization points. If the farmer is trying to maximize profit for a single animal then the point is 131-day fattening per animal. This would allow the farmer to raise 2.8 animals per year, assuming that there was no need for time between animal lots. This profit maximizing point assumes that feed is the variable input and that the animal is a fixed input.

However, if we consider that time is limited, then the farmer should be interested in the point where the average profit per unit of feed is at a maximum. For this relation, this would be 112 days, which would allow 3.3 animals to be fattened per year. The profit in a year with this solution for a single animal unit would be US$50.66 versus US$46.87 for the 2.8 fattened animals per year when looking at the profit maximizing point for feed.

The solution of 131 days assumes feed to be the variable input, the animal the fixed input and time to be available in infinite quantities. The solution of 112 days is determined assuming feed and animals to be variable and the amount of time to be limited. In this solution, the farmer is applying feed and animals to a fixed amount of time. If the farmer does not intend to repeat the feeding operation, i.e. if they feed just one lot a year, then he should maximize returns to the animal and feed rather than to time.

Table 3.12. Revenue and costs of a feedlot operation with estimates of profitability and economic productivity with varying lengths of fattening time.

Units of time (10 days)	Total costs	Total revenue	Profit	Marginal profit	Average profit
0	120.00	120.00	0.00		
2	124.05	122.24	−1.81	−0.91	−0.91
4	128.43	128.32	−0.11	0.85	−0.03
6	133.45	137.28	3.83	1.97	0.64
8	139.43	148.16	8.73	2.45	1.09
10	146.70	160.00	13.30	2.29	1.33
12	155.58	171.84	16.26	1.48	1.36
14	166.38	182.72	16.34	0.04	1.17
16	179.44	191.68	12.24	−2.05	0.76

Production Economics: Durable Inputs

A durable input is something that can be used over a period of years on a farm. Examples of durable inputs are tractors, buildings, oxen for draught power, etc.

If a durable input lasts for 10 years then it does not mean that it can be purchased in ten bits, it will have to be purchased as one piece. To charge the cost of a durable input during the year of its purchase would distort the cost structure of the farm for the first year and for the next 9 years. To remedy this, an annual depreciation charge should be levied against the farm expenses each year of a durable input's productive lifetime. When the durable input is worn out, it should be completely 'paid for' by depreciation, thus ensuring that capital will be available to purchase another. When farmers are unable to make depreciation payments because of low farm earnings, they are said to be 'living off their investment'. They use the depreciation fund to pay annual living and farming expenses and are unable to replace durable equipment when it wears out.

Depreciation of durable resources used only on one enterprise can be charged directly to that enterprise; depreciation should be charged each time the production process is repeated. On a farm, durable assets such as tractors, trucks and combines are commonly used in several enterprises; i.e. they are involved in several production processes. In such cases allocation of depreciation among the enterprises is difficult, and depreciation can only be charged against the farm business as a whole.

Depreciation deals with the money required to repurchase the durable input at the end of its life. However, it is also necessary to take account of the value of money that is invested in the actual machine. This can be done by charging interest at the local bank lending rate on the purchase price of the durable input.

Therefore, depreciation is the money required to replace the durable input when it can no longer be used and interest is the cost of the capital that is invested in that durable input.

Purchasing durable inputs

When purchasing a durable input, it is important to have some method of assessing what size of durable input to invest in (75 hp versus 50 hp tractor, draught bullock versus draught cow) and what price to pay for the input. Three methods are available for assessing durable inputs:

1. Using a production function for a durable input, it is possible to determine the number of durable inputs to purchase.
2. Using purchase and salvage values for the durable input and examining cost curves for different output levels, it is possible to determine the price to pay for that input.
3. Using a durable input budget, it is possible to determine the average fixed cost per unit of physical output and total cost per unit of physical output.

The first two techniques require a knowledge of production function for the durable input and, as it is unlikely that this will be available in most livestock situations, these techniques will be ignored. The third technique requires knowledge of creating an enterprise budget, but the general technique is relatively easy.

The costs first need to be considered as either fixed or variable. The fixed costs for a durable input include:

- depreciation;
- interest;
- taxes;
- insurance;
- housing.

The variable costs will be different for the different durable inputs being assessed. The following example develops the issues of durable assets and how they can be assessed. A feeder wagon has been purchased for US$6000 and Table 3.13 presents the depreciation, interest, taxes, insurance and housing costs on an annual basis.

If the feeder wagon is expected to handle 500 t of silage per year the average fixed cost per tonne can be calculated as follows:

$$\text{Average fixed cost per tonne} = 960/500$$
$$= \text{US\$1.92/t}$$

Table 3.13. Annual costs of depreciation, interest, taxes, insurance and housing for a feeder wagon.

	Percentage of the purchase value	Fixed costs per year
Depreciation	9	540
Interest	5	300
Taxes	1	60
Insurance	0.5	30
Housing	0.5	30
Total fixed costs per year		960

The variable costs per tonne of silage have been calculated to be US$1.56 so the total cost per tonne of silage would be as follows:

Total cost per tonne of silage =

Average fixed cost per tonne +

Variable cost per tonne

= 1.92 + 1.56

= US$3.48/t

To help a farmer make a decision on the purchase of the feeder wagon, they should be looking for contractors who would offer a price of less than US$3.48/t of silage handled.

However, it may also be necessary to consider the convenience of having the feeder wagon on the farm.

Comparison of draught oxen and draught cows

Table 3.14 contains information on the use of oxen and cows for draught power production in two villages of India. Information is also given on the cost of hiring a team of draught animals for a day in each village.

The cows in Golahally are kept primarily for draught power production and milk production is secondary. The price of milk is Rs 5.8/l and cattle feed is Rs 5.0/kg. Table 3.15 presents the enterprise budgets for the different sources of draught power in the two different villages.

The table shows that only the owned oxen in Golahally have a lower cost per day than hired oxen. However, if the output of milk is included then the owned cows also have lower daily costs than the hired oxen in Golahally. Including milk production in the calculation is justified as the cows were kept

Table 3.14. Information on the draught animal markets and use of animals in two different villages in India.

Item	Golahally			Byatha	
	Local cows	Local oxen	Hired oxen	Local oxen	Hired oxen
No. of animals per team	2	2	2	2	2
Purchase value (Rs/animal)	2250	3000	–	5500	–
Hire price per day (Rs)	–	–	60	–	80
Output					
Draught power days	65	105	1	85	1
Milk output/cow/year	150	–	–	–	–
Variable costs					
Feed/day of work (kg/animal)	0	0.75	0	1	0
Fixed costs/animal/year					
Feed (Rs)	1000	1000		1250	
Labour (Rs)	250	250		250	
Vet cost (Rs)	22	25		60	
Building (Rs)	100	100		100	
Depreciation as a percentage of purchase price	20	20		20	
Interest as a percentage of purchase price	15	15		15	

Note: Rs = Rupees.

Table 3.15. Enterprise budget per team of animals.

Item	Golahally			Byatha	
	Local cows	Local oxen	Hired oxen	Local oxen	Hired oxen
Output					
Physical output (days worked/year)	65	105	1	85	1
Financial output (Rs/year)	1740				
Variable costs					
Feed	0	787.5	0	850	0
Hire charge	–	–	60	–	80
Total variable costs	0	787.5	60	850	80
Fixed costs					
Feed	2000	2000	0	2500	0
Labour	500	500	0	500	0
Vet cost	44	50	0	120	0
Building	200	200	0	200	0
Depreciation as a percentage of purchase price	900	1200	0	2200	0
Interest as a percentage of purchase price	675	900	0	1650	0
Total fixed costs	4319.00	4850.00	0.00	7170.00	0.00
Total costs	4319.00	5637.50	60.00	8020.00	80.00
TFC/physical output	66.45	46.19	0.00	84.35	0.00
TC/physical output	66.45	53.69	60.00	94.35	80.00
TC minus other output/physical output	39.68	53.69	60.00	94.35	80.00

primarily for draught power and the difference between the daily rates for using their own cows and hiring animals translates to a large increase in milk production.

$$\text{Difference in daily rates} = 60.00 - 39.68$$
$$= \text{Rs } 20.32$$

Multiplying by the number of draught power days the cows are used per year, an annual saving can be calculated:

$$\text{Yearly saving} = 65 * 20.32$$
$$= \text{Rs } 1320.8$$

Finally, the extra milk yield per cow needed to switch from the cows being used primarily as draught animals to primarily for milk production is as follows:

$$= 1320.8/5.8$$
$$= 227.71/\text{team}/\text{year}$$
$$= 113.91/\text{cow}/\text{year}$$

This is a 75% increase in the annual milk yield per cow and is an unlikely target for these animals to achieve. The daily cost of owned bullocks in Byatha is much higher than the hire charge. This indicates that:

1. Data are incorrect; bullock prices may be too high; number of days worked is too low; etc.
2. The hire price is not a true reflection of the demand for draught power.
3. The importance of timely cultivation during critical times may mean that it is worth paying more than the hire price for draught power.

Summary

The basic elements of production economics have been covered in this chapter with the aim to introduce the theory behind the tools that will be described in detail in Chapter 7. The concepts of points of profit maximization and least cost combinations are important to recognize either when assessing a decision-making environment in the role of someone studying why people within a livestock sector react in certain ways; or as an adviser to a livestock farmer or livestock policy on what would be economically more favourable as an action.

The most important message from what has been covered is that when advising people in the livestock sector it is not sufficient to look only at the technical relationships between inputs and outputs. The conclusion if only the technical relationship was used would be to use more inputs if they are producing more output. As resources for the livestock sector are limited, it is necessary to introduce values to the inputs and outputs. With values, the decision-making process can be refined with an aim to reach a point where the value of each incremental addition of input should return exactly the same value of output. Beyond this point adding more inputs will actually lose value or reduce profit to the livestock activity.

There are some limitations in this general approach that are covered in some detail when the topic of institutional economics is discussed in Chapter 12, cultural and social issues in Chapter 13 and the need to make assessments of impacts on human health in Chapter 14. However, a good understanding of production economics allows for a much greater interpretation and use of economic decision-making tools and therefore stronger levels of advice to actors within the livestock sector. Chapter 4 by Professor Clem Tisdell applies a theoretical framework to animal health economics.

4 Economics of Controlling Livestock Diseases: Basic Theory

Clem Tisdell

Introduction

Economic analysis of the optimal control of livestock diseases is complex. This is because of the diversity of diseases, differences in their epidemiology and in their nature of occurrence as well as considerable variation in preventative measures, treatments and responses. Economic analysis takes account of the monetary benefits and costs of controlling diseases. To do this, it has to combine biological and veterinary knowledge with financial considerations. Consequently, inputs from both economists and non-economists are required for this economic analysis.

Cost–benefit techniques are widely used in economics for determining optimal economic choices at the farm level and on wider scales, such as at regional or national levels. Using this approach, optimality is achieved where net benefits, i.e. economic benefits less costs, are maximized. McInerney (1991), McInerney *et al.* (1992), Tisdell (1995) and others have advocated its use for obtaining the economically optimal control of livestock diseases. Some simple economic models are outlined here to illustrate its use. They draw on, and extend, some of the models in Tisdell (1995).

Economic Benefit from Controlling a Disease as Economic Loss Is Avoided

The economic benefit from controlling a livestock disease can be measured by taking into account the reduction in economic loss from the disease corresponding to different levels of expenditure on its control (McInerney, 1991). In Fig. 4.1, for example, OA is the economic loss from the disease if there is no expenditure on its control, and ADF represents the economic loss as a function of control effort measured by variable expenditure on control of the disease. Therefore, the difference between line AG and curve ADF, shown by the shaded area, represents the economic benefit from controlling the disease for possible levels of expenditure on its control. Given available knowledge, it is assumed that for any level of expenditure on disease control that expenditure is undertaken in a way that maximizes economic benefits. To ensure this, however, is not always an easy task.

Optimality in a Very Simple Economic Model and Threshold Possibilities

A very simple economic model can be developed from the above. Mathematically, the

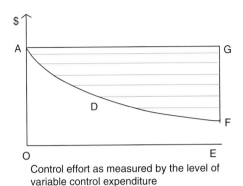

Control effort as measured by the level of variable control expenditure

Fig. 4.1. An illustration of the economic benefit from the control of a livestock disease by the level of economic loss avoided.

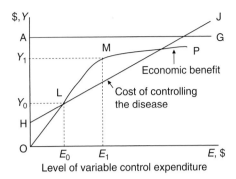

Level of variable control expenditure

Fig. 4.2. A cost–benefit model for livestock disease control in which start-up costs give rise to a threshold effect.

type of economic benefit relationship illustrated in Fig. 4.1 can be expressed as:

$$B = a - g(E),$$

where B is economic benefit, a is the level of economic loss in the absence of control of the disease and E represents the level of variable cost of (expenditure on) control of the disease. The total cost, C, of control of the disease, can be envisaged as consisting of possible start-up, fixed or overhead costs, k, and variable outlays, E. Thus:

$$C = k + E,$$

where $k \geq 0$. Therefore, the net benefit from disease control is:

$$NB = B - C = a - g(E) - (k + E)$$
$$= f(E) - (k + E)$$

If the benefit function increases at a decreasing rate, i.e. if $f' > 0$ and $f'' < 0$, net benefits from disease control will be maximized when the value of E, expenditure on control, is such that the extra economic benefits from control equal the extra costs of control, i.e. for the value of E for which:

$$f'(E) = 1$$

This is so, provided that for this value:

$$f(E) - (k + E) > 0$$

i.e. total benefits exceed total cost. Otherwise, no expenditure on controlling the disease is optimal. Other things equal, the higher k is, the more likely it is that no control is optimal.

However, even if $k = 0$, it is possible that no control of a disease is optimal because the marginal benefit of control of the disease, $f'(E)$, is always less than its marginal costs of control.

The presence of start-up or overhead cost for controlling a disease, $k > 0$, creates a control threshold. If it is economic to control the disease, control must be on a minimum scale before benefits cover costs. This can be illustrated by Fig. 4.2. In this figure, start-up costs are shown as OH and line OHJ (a 45° line) represents the total cost of controlling the disease. The curve marked OLMP shows the total benefit of controlling the disease, and OA is the loss caused by the disease in the absence of its control.

From Fig. 4.2, total expenditure of less than Y_0 on control of the disease, involving a variable expenditure of E_0, can be seen to be uneconomic. At least this level of outlay on control is required before benefits cover costs. However, net benefits are maximized for a total outlay of Y_1, or an operating outlay of E_1, and the optimum corresponds to point M in Fig. 4.2. Other things equal, the larger the start-up costs, the larger is the control outlay required before benefits cover costs.

A Second Economic Source of a Disease Control Threshold

The economic benefit curve from expenditure on the control of a livestock disease may not be strictly concave everywhere, unlike in the model considered above. It may, for example, take a logistic form like that shown in Fig. 4.3 by curve OKLMP. In this example, start-up or overhead costs for control of the disease are assumed to be absent and therefore the 45° line OLJ represents total outlay on control of the disease.

The net benefits of control are maximized when $E_1 = Y_1$ is spent on controlling the disease. Furthermore, a minimum of $E_0 = Y_0$ must be spent on controlling the disease before the costs of its control are covered by the benefits gained. This threshold, created by initially increasing returns from undertaking control on a greater scale, arises in the absence of start-up or overhead costs.

Discussion

Empirical evidence is of course needed to establish which types of benefit and cost functions are relevant to the control of particular livestock diseases. There may even be some cases where it is economic to eliminate all losses that could arise from a disease by eradicating it. In such cases, the benefit functions would actually meet line AG in Fig. 4.2 rather than merely approach it. The modelling can also be extended to take account of the simultaneous control of several diseases as suggested in Tisdell (1995) and more

specific allowance can be made for time. Nevertheless, the above simple models provide policy insights.

They highlight the potential importance of thresholds for the control of livestock diseases. When such thresholds arise, they can be lowered by reducing fixed, start-up or overhead costs of control or by increasing the productivity of control outlays in securing benefits, depending on their source.

It is also important to realize that the benefit and cost curves for disease control do not remain stationary in time. For example, if the economic value of particular types of livestock increases, then greater benefits are obtained by controlling diseases that afflict these livestock. The models outlined can also be used to show that diseases causing great economic loss may be less economic to control than those that cause less economic loss. Often the presence of a large loss from a livestock disease is used as a political argument in favour of its control and for spending more on its control than a disease that causes smaller economic loss. However, this may not maximize net economic benefits from the control of livestock.

A major problem in deciding on levels of optimal expenditure in controlling livestock diseases is uncertainty about the economic cost and benefits involved. Trial and error may be used to search for the economic optimum, but this will be risky if large thresholds occur before benefits exceed costs. The search procedure can, however, be undertaken by small steps in the case illustrated by Fig. 4.1 if $k = 0$ or is small, i.e. if start-up costs are zero or very small (see Tisdell, 1996, chapter 3).

More information may also be collected about the nature of the benefit and cost curves, for example from trials or experiments. However, even the collection and processing of information has an economic dimension. Baumol and Quandt (1964) suggested that it is only economic to collect and process information up to the level where the extra cost of this equals its expected extra economic value (see also Tisdell, 1996, chapter 1; Ramsay et al., 1999).

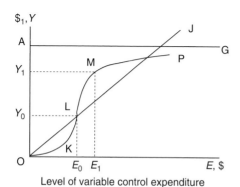

Fig. 4.3. Another cost–benefit model in which economies of scale rather than start-up costs of control give rise to a threshold effect.

Thus, even if it were possible to collect enough information to obtain perfect knowledge of the benefits and costs of controlling a livestock disease, it may not be economic to do that. Or, in the case of public administration, less funds may be provided to obtain information about the benefits and costs of control of livestock diseases than are optimal. Consequently, much decision making about the economically optimal level of control of livestock diseases must be made under conditions of uncertainty. Therefore, it is also important to analyse the optimal control of livestock diseases under conditions of uncertainty, for example, by drawing on decision-making models, some of which were stimulated by the development of the theory of games (von Neumann and Morgenstern, 1953; Tisdell, 1968, chapter 2).

5 Data Collection

Introduction

When performing an economic analysis of animal health and production, it is easy to forget the need to carry out data collection. Sophisticated analyses can be meaningless if the data used are of poor quality either through badly planned data collection exercises or the need to use estimates due to a lack of data. Planning and implementation of data collection itself are economic exercises where there needs to be a balance between the costs of collecting the data versus the extra benefits of refining information provided through analysis. The principles described in Chapter 3 of marginal costs and benefits should be applied to a data collection exercise. This chapter briefly describes the important elements of data collection, from descriptions of what data are to the need for careful management of a data collection exercise. This is followed by a contribution from Rommy Viscarra with an overview of the data collection tools available for the economic analysis of animal health and production. First a brief introduction on the familiarization of an area is presented.

Familiarization of an area

Before beginning an economic data collection exercise, it is recommended to carry out a thorough familiarization of the area where the work will take place. Three activities are highlighted in this initial phase:

1. Check all available secondary data through:
   (a) A *web search* for the area and the livestock sector.
   (b) *Organizations*: find out which organizations have been working in the area, e.g. government, cooperatives, aid organizations, etc., and check if they have records or reports.
   (c) *Individuals*: find out if the farmers keep records of their activities and enterprises.
   (d) The important data to find are:
       (i) prices of agricultural commodities and agricultural inputs;
       (ii) quantity data from local markets, purchasers and suppliers of agricultural produce;
       (iii) population data (both human and animal);
       (iv) farm size data;
       (v) weather data to determine important seasons.

2. Visit the area with a guide and make careful observations *using your eyes and ears*; do not miss an opportunity to observe what is taking place in the fields. Turn these initial observations into questions to your guide and to the farmers you initially visit. A note of caution at this stage, check if your guide is

familiar with the area and if the farmers you talk to are representative of the area.

3. Record all observations in a diary.

Once familiarization of the area has taken place, develop a list of questions that need to be answered on the topic of interest. These should be given to your guide and it is useful to question a small selection of farmers on future visits. Notes should be made at the time of visit to allow for clarification of the answers. This first stage will help to place the purposes of the data collection into perspective. It should help to determine what is feasible and what is infeasible to collect in a more formal approach. It will also direct the most appropriate methods that will be used.

What Are Data?

Data are a series of observations, measurements or facts that can be either qualitative or quantitative, the former generally being thought of as 'subjective, verbal and descriptive' and the latter as 'objective, numerical and amenable to mathematical analysis' (Moris and Copestake, 1993).

A distinction is made between data and information. Data are collected and turned into information by analysis. For quantitative data collection an analysis structure is usually an important aspect in directing data collection. Therefore, information plays a key role in directing data collection.

Who Needs To Collect Data?

Data are collected in many forms. For example, a farmer is constantly collecting data on their livestock, farm and household systems. These data are analysed to manage existing and plan future livestock enterprises and household activities. These data may be stored on record sheets, computer databases or in most cases around the world these data are simply stored in the farmer's head.

Data are also collected by governments in order to assess the importance of the livestock sector in terms of its contribution to the general economy and employment.

Governments require such data to plan development initiatives, programmes and projects and monitor the impact of policy.

The agrobusiness companies, either providing inputs or marketing and processing outputs, also need data to manage their activities and plan for future services and investments in the livestock sector. These data may also be used to lobby governments on the need for policies, programmes and projects that support the livestock sector in general. The storage of data by large organizations generally has a formal structure and usually requires computerization.

Is Livestock Data Collection Different from Other Types of Data Collection?

Poate and Daplyn (1993) state that 'livestock data collection does not present different problems from other farming activities' but they go on to say that the long production cycle of large animals requires a different strategy for data collection. They specifically recommend that production parameters such as mortality and fertility rates are estimated by 'recording historical life cycles for a number of animals'. In addition to these differences two other aspects complicate livestock data collection:

- nomadic or semi-nomadic livestock-owning communities present special problems for sample selection and enumeration; and
- continuous production activities such as milk or eggs require frequent detailed recording.

These problems will be discussed in more detail in the tools available for data collection.

Different Levels of Data Collection

Data collection for the economic analysis of livestock systems can be conveniently split into three levels: the animal, the herd/flock and the farm/household (Fig. 1, Preface, this volume). The types of data to be collected at each level will be different, and data collection methods used at the different levels will need to reflect these differences. In addition to the levels of data collection for the livestock systems, there is also a need to consider the input and output markets that livestock producers use, and the influence of government policies and programmes on the livestock sector in general (see Fig. 5.1).

Fertility data and recording of inputs such as drugs would not require such regular recording. Animal data can be used to determine physical productivity parameters, input–output coefficients and epidemiological information.

Animal

At the animal level, data collection can include:

- age;
- milk or egg production;
- weight gain or loss;
- fertility;
- feed intake;
- disease; and
- drug usage.

Feed intake, milk or egg production requires frequent data collection from the same farms.

Herd/flock

At the herd/flock level, data can include:

- numbers of animals in a herd/flock;
- herd/flock age structure;
- herd/flock inputs.

Herd or flock data can be used to assess breeding performance and characteristics, sales and purchases and life cycle events. Livestock numbers may be used as an indicator of wealth, to assess pressure on grazing or feed stocks or as a measure of draught available in the community.

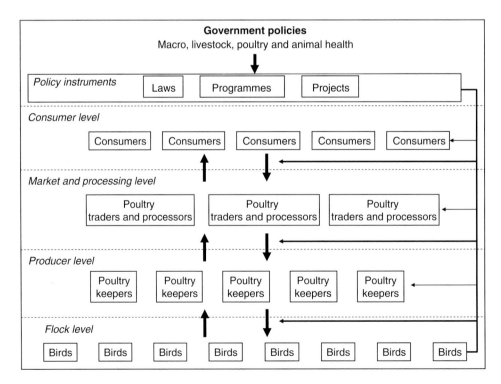

Fig. 5.1. The different levels of data collection for the livestock sector.

Farm/household

At the farm/household level, data can include:

- labour availability;
- competition for resources with the live-stock enterprise of interest;
- the use of livestock products by other farm/household activities;
- attitudes to the livestock such as interest, status, etc.; and
- knowledge of livestock management issues including local knowledge systems.

These data are required for determining farm management strategies and assessing the potential for adopting new technologies.

Markets

It is also important to recognize that market data are required to carry out economic analysis in order to convert production into monetary values. In some cases this is straightforward, as a disease may affect growth or production but have no impact on the quality of product produced and hence the price received per unit. However, diseases such as mastitis do affect the quality of product and in situations where producers are rewarded for good-quality milk and punished for bad quality there is an impact on price. Another example is pig meat with cysts, which has a much lower value than meat that is free of cysts. Therefore, market information needs to recognize prices for quantity and quality.

The economic analyses that are concerned with the impact of diseases in a much wider national or regional sense need to estimate the impact on the changes in production levels on prices. With changes in output of livestock products there is likely to be a change in the price of that product. The shape of the supply and demand curves will determine if an overall change is positive and who are the winners and losers within the society.

Again there are different levels of market data collection:

- Household market data. These are needed in situations where much of the produce from an enterprise is being consumed by the household members.
- Local market data. These could be from villages or local towns. The source of the data will depend on the infrastructure connecting the place where the goods are produced and where they are sold.
- National market data. These data may indicate the differences in market structure for a country and help to explain reasons for the concentrations of certain specializations in different areas of a country.
- International market data. These data are required for analysis on protection or taxation of agricultural production.

Policies

Much valuable discussion and specification exists of what needs to be achieved in livestock development, but there is much less on how this should be achieved (Omamo, 2003). One of the reasons is the lack of knowledge of how policies influence changes in the livestock sector and how these subsequent changes affect the livelihood strategies of the poor and have an impact on poverty reduction. However, such changes in livestock sectors are taking place (planned and unplanned) and there exists evidence to improve the understanding of the impact on poverty of these changes and the policies that encourage or constrain these changes. In order to explore how policy affects access to public and private goods by livestock producers and people involved and affected by the livestock sector, it is necessary to identify the political, institutional and technological constraints that affect livestock development.

The institutional domain refers to *'how people organize themselves and relate to each other'*. Formal and informal organizations and institutions with influence on livestock-keeping systems and livestock keepers are considered. In addition, there are social, cultural and economic factors that can influence people's relations. In particular, the research examined how people:

- Promote, adopt and adapt technology and inputs.
- Make market transactions.
- And if there are differences in the nature of these relationships between poor and non-poor groups within the society.

The policy domain is part of the production environment created by governments, non-governmental organizations (NGOs) and private companies. Policies on their own are just statements. To have an effect or impact, these policies need policy instruments such as laws, programmes and projects. The key question here is what are the key policies for the livestock sector? The focus is on specific livestock policies, but there is also a need to consider policies that affect livestock systems and institutional relationships such as credit policy, land tenure, education, etc. There is a need to investigate how livestock systems and the relationships between actors are affected by policies. These impacts can be positive, neutral or negative, and should be differentiating by socio-economic group. The important end point with policy data collection and analysis is to determine the impacts on the poorest and look for means of poverty reduction.

The above identified levels are an enabling environment where policies are made and are implemented through laws, programmes and projects. Examples of these are:

1. A policy to increase livestock production may be implemented through a project that introduces high-yielding breeds of animals that directly affect the herd or flock level.
2. A policy to increase the efficiency of feed resource use could be implemented by improving herd or flock fertility management in order to generate more young stock per breeding female. This would influence the relationship between the herd or flock and the livestock keepers.
3. A policy to empower women may be implemented by extension messages that target women with training and information. This would influence the intra-household dynamics of the livestock keepers.

4. A policy to increase government revenues could be implemented through laws that put value-added tax on livestock and livestock products. This would affect the relationships between livestock keepers, livestock traders, livestock processors and also consumers.
5. A policy to improve the nutrition of urban consumers could be implemented through the introduction of subsidies on livestock products. This would influence the relationship between livestock product traders and processors and consumers.

Data collection requires searches of reports, policies, laws, programmes and projects.

A note: there are different ways of measuring inputs and outputs

Standard units for livestock inputs and outputs would be litres, kilograms and tonnes. Plus it is common practice to convert the monetary estimates into American dollars. However, not all countries or regions within countries use these measures to estimate the quantities of inputs and outputs.

Milk in many countries is not sold in metric units. In the USA, measures used are quarts and gallons. In Nepal, milk is sold in units known as 'Mana' that are equivalent to 0.598 of a litre. In the high Andes of Bolivia, sheep are small and sold by the head not by weight, which would require data collection on an average weight.

In many developing countries, farmers slaughter animals on their farms and sell the meat. The offal is eaten by the family, so an estimate of the number of animals slaughtered with the weight and nutritive value of the offal is required to estimate the family consumption of protein from such sources.

Manure and draught power are common livestock products used within a farming system. In countries such as India, markets exist for draught power and farmers will be able to say how many days' work are required to plough an area of land and how much 1 day of an oxen team is worth. This can then be converted into monetary value or a measure of horsepower used. Similarly, the bodyweights of animals and the types of housing and grazing systems can be used to estimate the availability of manure for a family's cropping system. If this information is combined with information on the chemical composition of manure, estimates of chemical availability of the manure can be made.

Which monetary unit to use for international estimates has also been made more complicated with the fluctuations of the American dollar. Any analysis that is present in dollars needs to recognize that a rise in the value of output may partially reflect the devaluation of the dollar. Similarly, in the past a reduction in the value of the output may have been related to a very strong dollar.

The Management of Livestock Data Collection

The key to obtaining good livestock sector data is a well-managed collection exercise. This is an area that is frequently ignored once survey and questionnaire design have been completed. If the data collection exercise is not properly managed data will be missing and data quality will be poor. The key components to achieving good data collection management are:

1. Clearly defined organizational structure;
2. Recruitment of appropriate enumerators and supervisors;
3. Good training and retraining procedures;
4. Provision of appropriate facilities and equipment for staff;
5. Appropriate level of public relations to encourage respondent's and local organization's cooperation;
6. Effective supervision of data collection procedure and early checking of data;
7. Appropriate data input and preliminary analysis procedures;
8. Timely report writing.

Informal survey

Informal surveys are normally small and the teams implementing them are usually highly skilled and motivated. Therefore, it is unlikely that organization will be a problem. However, beware of lags in the report writing from such surveys, as one of the strengths of such work is the timeliness of the information they provide.

Formal surveys

A number of decisions have to be made with formal surveys. Enumerators have to be recruited and their quality will play a vital role in the quality of the data collected. Decisions have to be made about: Where to recruit the enumerators from? What form of organization to construct? Use personnel from an existing body? Recruit personnel specifically for the survey and establish a permanent body?

All decisions will be dependent on the:

1. Resources available for the survey;
2. Data to be collected;
3. Organization in the area;
For example, the presence of a veterinary college would allow veterinary students to be employed to collect data. The advantage of this approach would be that they would know the subject area. However, the disadvantage is that their own interests may influence the data collected.
4. Length of time the data collection will run.

There is little point in establishing a permanent body for the completion of a cross-sectional survey.

Whether establishing a permanent body or utilizing personnel from other organizations, it is important to establish a clear, explicit, complete and unambiguous structure of responsibilities, reporting and communication. Organizational charts are useful to ensure that each person is responsible to one and only one supervisor. It is also necessary not to have too many subordinates. An absolute maximum should be seven and a minimum five. The ratio, however, will depend on the ease of access of the subordinates. For example, if enumerators are based in close proximity to each other it would be feasible for a supervisor to supervise seven. However, in sparsely populated regions where enumerators are widely spread, journey times to visit enumerators will increase and subsequently the number of supervisors to enumerators should be reduced. Provision of clear duty statements or terms of reference is recommended for reducing conflict.

Recruitment of field workers

Recruitment of field workers requires the consideration of the following issues:

- Educational level:
  Reading, writing and arithmetic, but also method of thinking.
- Formal skills:
  Use of equipment, map knowledge, interviewing skills, rural knowledge/ background, and language skills; rural knowledge particularly of livestock and livestock issues may be critical for farmers to take an enumerator seriously.
- Personal skills:
  Self-reliance and motivation, maturity, courteous, flexible, honest.

It should be noted that good education levels are not the only criteria for selection of field staff. Where staff are selected who are overqualified for the data collection work, it can lead to frustrations and difficulties in completing the work satisfactorily.

Informing stakeholders of the data collection exercise

Before a survey begins, the respondents need to understand the reason for the survey being done. It will be useful to outline the benefit to the respondents, but beware of raising expectations too high. Farmers should not be told that they will receive a miracle medicine or gift. Reassurances that the data collection will be confidential and will not lead to tax assessments may also be necessary. These messages may be presented to local leaders and farmer organizations, or through media such as posters, radio and television. After initial introduction of the survey, it is important that the enumerators are properly introduced to the local people. It may be necessary to ask the local leader to come with the enumerators during the first visit to an area.

Training and supervision

Training should include material on the:

- reasons for the survey to be carried out and its relevance to national and local development;
- rationale of sampling employed;
- purpose of particular measurement techniques or topics.

Course material should be compiled as an enumerator manual, which can subsequently be used as a reference guide in the field.

Supervision of data collection procedure and early checking of data

Supervision of fieldwork needs to be carried out in the field and in the office. Field visits should be random to check on the activity of enumerators and the visits should include supervision of the actual data being collected, not just a brief chat and a handover of completed forms. Forms should be scanned by the supervisor before being hand on. This will allow a check of the data being collected. It is usually relatively easy for a trained eye to see data that are being fabricated or data that are not being taken correctly. Questions that are generating the wrong data need to be carefully assessed. Although it may be possible to retrain the enumerator, it may be necessary to consider dropping the question from the survey. The following considerations have to be made before coming to a decision:

- How important is the question?
- How large a part of the sample has already been wrongly enumerated?
- How costly in resources and time it would be to go back and gather data again?
- Whether it is physically possible to repeat the measurement or interview?

Other possible errors relate to the sampling frame used. Bad questions need to be changed or dropped. The list for making a decision is similar to the one above.

Data checking, entry and storage

Establishment of good data input facilities and procedures will facilitate data analysis. This is vital for the production of timely reports. It is important to make best use of computer facilities for repetitive checking of data and assessment of its quality. There should also be a good level of feedback to field staff. This is important for both good- and bad-quality data. Do not use the feedback to tell bad news; use it as a means of telling the staff they are doing a good job. Maintaining good morale in the field staff is a large part of the battle of maintaining data quality.

Summary

Data and data collection are not the 'sexiest' of subjects, particularly in the field of economics and agricultural economics, where more and more emphasis is given to complex analytical methods. However, it is worth reflecting that all analytical methods require data either for their development and/or their verification. The quality of an appraisal is as much to do with the quality of data as it is with the analytical structure. The quality of data is related to the planning and management of the data collection. Once available, data need to be analysed using an open and flexible approach, where interesting and less obvious trends in the data set should be analysed. In such an approach, it is important to place the data analysis and the appraisal of the livestock system within the socio-economic and cultural environment of the livestock keepers. The end point of such analyses is to provide information that can be used by livestock keepers, technical staff working with livestock keepers and political decision makers. The latter groups are in positions of allocating resources to the livestock sector and their decisions can only be improved if they are provided with information generated by good data collection systems, data and appraisal methods.

Chapter 6 includes a contribution from Rommy Viscarra, who has a broad experience of primary livestock sector data collection in Bolivia and of secondary data collection in Latin America. It will present a broad overview of the main types of livestock data collection methods available.

6 Livestock Data Collection Methods

Rommy Viscarra and Jonathan Rushton

Primary livestock data collection methods can be classified into the following categories:

1. Informal data collection methods:
   - participatory rural appraisal (PRA);
   - rapid rural appraisal (RRA).
2. Formal data collection:
   - cross-sectional;
   - longitudinal.
3. Combination of informal and formal data collection methods.

The following discussion will detail some problems of sampling for the different livestock data collection methods. However, it does not include statistical sampling methods. Those requiring more information on sampling and statistical design are referred to Poate and Daplyn (1993, chapters 2 and 3), Casley and Lury (1981, chapter 4) and Putt et al. (1988). For those more interested in general sampling biases that can be introduced by informal methods please refer to Kumar (1993, pp. 16–18), and for biases created by rapid execution of these methods to Heffernan et al. (2003, 2005).

In addition to primary data collection methods it is important to mention that much data and information already exist and are more accessible than ever before through the use of web searches. Before investing time, money and energy in planning primary data collection exercises, the authors recommend doing searches for available data and information.

Informal

Informal data collection methods use unstructured or semi-structured methods of collecting data, and do not concern themselves with obtaining a representative sample of the study population. A number of general reference works are available on informal methods (McCracken et al., 1988; Theis and Grady, 1991; Kumar, 1993; Narayan, 1996) and there are some reference works for livestock (Waters-Bayer and Bayer, 1994; RRA Notes, 1994; Conroy, 2005).

Rapid rural appraisal (RRA)

According to McCracken et al. (1988), RRA are methodologies 'which make use of a multidisciplinary team, working with farmers and community leaders to develop in a quick, yet systematic fashion, a series of hypotheses for such purposes as:

1. Assessing the agricultural and other development needs of community;
2. Identifying priorities for further research into those development needs;
3. Assessing the feasibility (on both social and technical criteria) of planned interventions and innovations;
4. Identifying priorities for development actions;

5. Implementing development actions; or

6. Monitoring development actions'.

In some instances, as the above description demonstrates, there is very little to distinguish RRA from PRA. However, they can be distinguished by the role of the data providers in the data analysis. RRA gathers data and the analysis is performed by the researcher.

RRA is useful where the researcher has a lack of time and resources available to carry out more formal methods of data collection. If well done, RRA can generate data of as good a quality as more formal methods. An example of an RRA method used for livestock data collection is livestock interviews or progeny histories. This method has been used by livestock professionals for many years, but has only recently been documented.

Livestock interviews or progeny histories

Progeny histories can be used to collect data on mortality and morbidity rates, reproductive and sale rates. They provide a means of structured memory recall.

The following list of questions can be used for this:

1. For each adult in the herd/flock ask:
   Where did it come from?
   How many times has it been pregnant?
   How many abortions has it had?
2. Then for each birth ask:
   Was it a single or a twin?
   What happened to the offspring?
   Why?

These questions should generate information on abortions, offspring disposal and mortalities. There is a potential bias with this method. The better animals will stay the longest on the farm and therefore there is greater chance of them being interviewed. Also, if the herd/flock is large the question arises which animals do you interview. Again the farmer is likely to select the best, as he/she will probably want to impress an outsider. It may be worth asking to see the best, the worst and the average animal. Finally, in a flock of sheep or a herd of goats, individual performance details may not be available. Therefore, the use of this method needs some caution, and in some instances modification.

Participatory rural appraisal

PRA is a process 'which actively involves the rural people in identifying their problems, seeking solutions and evaluating results. PRA combines local capacities for development planning with those of external development agents' (Waters-Bayer and Bayer, 1994). Narayan (1996) also describes participatory research as 'an approach to data collection that is two-directional (both from the researcher to the subject, and from the subject to researcher). The process itself is dynamic, demand-based and change-oriented'. Therefore, PRA requires the farm household members to be involved in both data giving and data analysis.

Information generated from PRA exercises should then be available to the local community in order to plan their own development. This empowerment of the target groups is the basis for long-term success of data collection activities. The more appropriate the data collection activities for assisting households with their development, the more likely the data collection will continue to be used. These activities do not need to be confined to informal data collection methods. For example, formal methods such as dairy recording systems are successful because the information generated allows farmers to plan their enterprise future with greater certainty.

Livestock in general

Waters-Bayer and Bayer (1994) produced an excellent review of the rapid and PRA methods available for livestock data collection and development. Many of the main tools are well described in their manual and have changed little since this publication.

Conroy (2005) has added to the Waters-Bayer and Bayer book with another excellent review of two general methods: participatory situation analysis and participatory experimentation. The former is a subject area that has been developed from RRA and PRA, which are subjects that have been at the forefront of livestock development since the late 1990s. Participatory livestock experimentation in his book is well covered with examples from different regions. The only limitation of Conroy's book is that it does not include the organizational or institutional context of farmer participation and experimentation; nor does it go into detail on general livestock development issues.

Heffernan *et al.* (2003, 2005) have worked extensively on poverty and livestock development, collecting data from three different continents. Their models of how to bring these data together and produce information are based around conceptual ideas of interlinking layers of the livestock sector. While useful, these models have yet to be tried in a development context and only recently has the group moved into extension and information provision. The latter has been on the basis of providing information through touchscreen computer information points.

Animal health

Mariner (2001) has been very successful in developing participatory methodologies in searching for rinderpest in the Horn of Africa and Pakistan. These methods have involved a mixture of key informant interviews and prioritization methods of diseases and treatments, combined with scientific disease investigation. In the FAO manual Mariner produced details on his field experiences in the latter stages of the worldwide rinderpest eradication programmes. Catley (1999, 2005) details the key participatory methods

for collecting data on animal health and their overlap with conventional methods.

Rushton and Viscarra (2003) present how participatory methodologies can be used within a more general epidemiology and data collection framework that combines participatory and scientific data collection to help prioritize disease at local, regional and national level in order to direct animal disease control policies. These methods have been applied in a Bolivian context.

Many informal PRA methods exist for livestock systems. Two examples are provided that illustrate how these techniques can be used to help community development. For a complete list readers are referred to Waters-Bayer and Bayer (1994, chapter 2).

Preference for livestock

Mukherjee (1994) describes the use of the matrix method to determine the preference for different types of livestock. Cattle, goats, poultry and donkeys were ranked according to six attributes: number kept; utility; hardiness; security; ease of acquisition; and ease of marketing. Ideally a farmer, or group of farmers, would be given a set number of counters and asked to place appropriate quantities on the attributes of each species. The resulting matrices could then be used to assess how important each species was. The final table may look something like below and the percentages have been calculated to give some impression of the importance of each attribute (Table 6.1).

Table 6.1. Results of a matrix ranking exercise.

	Species							
	Cattle		Goats		Donkeys		Poultry	
Attributes	Number	%	Number	%	Number	%	Number	%
Numbers kept	3	10	10	20	5	13	9	17
Utility	9	29	18	36	7	18	14	27
Hardiness	5	16	6	12	13	34	10	19
Security	10	32	7	14	7	18	6	12
Ease of acquisition	2	6	4	8	3	8	6	12
Ease of marketing	2	6	5	10	3	8	7	13
Total	31	100	50	100	38	100	52	100

Production priorities

The production priorities method links two important aspects of PRA, a ranking exercise with a simple causal model to stimulate discussion and prioritize further data collection and analysis.

A group of farmers are asked to participate. This group should have representatives from the different socio-economic groups. The groups are asked to list the outputs from a livestock enterprise. The outputs are written or drawn on the ground. Each farmer is given a set number of counters and asked to allocate the counters according to the importance of each output. The results are recorded. A similar approach is then applied to livestock enterprise inputs. The results are then examined to find the important inputs and outputs. Farmers are then asked to discuss how the important output(s) is/are related to the important input(s). If the understanding of the relationship is poor then longitudinal data collection and further analysis can be suggested so that development opportunities can be assessed.

PRA summary

Successful use of PRA often requires a change in attitude of people involved in the exercise. Outsiders are likely to find this easier to achieve as they are willing to listen and learn about new systems. However, it is a method that may be difficult to apply by a researcher who has been, or is, living, working and possibly farming in the area of study for two reasons. First, the researcher will have a good idea of the farming systems, constraints and requirements for the area. Second, for such a researcher to carry out a PRA, it will be difficult to remain impartial as their perceived value judgements may differ from people interviewed, or where priorities raised or ignored could affect the researcher's own livelihood. Waters-Bayer and Bayer (1994) also note that 'participatory planning with local people is the commencement of a long process and should not be started unless there is a commitment from the initiators to continue'.

Summary

Both RRA and PRA data collection methods are valuable in allowing livestock keepers to set agendas and establish target groups. They are also often presented as techniques that require fewer resources and time than formal data collection methods. If informal data collection techniques are well applied, it has also been argued that they can produce more appropriate data than formal approaches (Franzel and Crawford, 1987). However, the representative nature of the findings from such studies relies on the knowledge and abilities of the team carrying the RRA and PRA surveys. The one-off nature of RRA could create a data bias.

Formal

Formal data collection uses structured methods of data collection, often with statistical samples of farm households, a prepared questionnaire and trained enumerators. The method is seen as a more quantified approach than the informal methods of data collection. Formal approaches to data collection are well described in a number of general data collection textbooks (Casley and Lury, 1981; Poate and Daplyn, 1993). These books have sections on the different types of formal survey work such as censuses, sample surveys and case studies. The books also include important details of designing questionnaires, managing a data collection team and managing and analysing the data.

Survey design will depend on the purpose of the enquiry. Production studies within a settled community would probably involve longitudinal data collection, with a stratified multistage sample design and static resident enumerators. For data collection activities that require an inventory of livestock from a large area, a cross-sectional survey or aerial survey may be used. Aerial surveys are of importance for pastoral systems where it may be difficult for enumerators to locate farmers. These types of surveys are also vital for wildlife number estimations (see Poate and Daplyn, 1993).

Sampling

Many descriptions of formal sampling procedures are available in textbooks (Casley and Lury, 1981, pp. 42–64; Putt *et al.*, 1988, pp. 30–37; Poate and Daplyn, 1993, chapters 2 and 3). These descriptions provide information on the difficulties of applying sampling methodologies for household surveys. However, only Putt *et al.* (1988) address the problems of sampling of livestock populations. They raise the problem that in most situations a sample frame for animals will not exist. Their solution is to adopt a multistage sampling methodology, which is essentially cluster sampling. Household or village lists are used as the sample frame for the initial sampling. Once chosen, all animals in a village or household will be surveyed. This has the advantage of reducing travelling time. The disadvantage is that the sample size for such a cluster sample has to be larger than a random sample if an estimate of a parameter is to be produced with the same reliability. These issues of sampling relate to individual animal information, but the problems with sampling methods for other levels of livestock data collection will be similar to other types of survey.

Interviews and questionnaire design

No formal survey can be properly conducted without a well-designed questionnaire and interview protocol. This section will present some issues relating to interview protocol, questionnaire design and the use of cross-sectional and longitudinal data collection procedures for livestock data collection.

Good questionnaire formats and interview protocols are vital for the success of a formal data collection exercise (Putt *et al.*, 1988). The questionnaire 'forms should be orderly, with related items grouped together (calf number, date of birth, place of birth), convenient to use (the form should fit on a clip board), and technical words not likely to be understood by field staff avoided' (Putt *et al.*, 1988). The forms should also have a section to record the date, place, farm and enumerator. Questions can be improved and

ambiguities reduced if the names of inputs, outputs, diseases and common treatment methods are accurately translated into the local languages. Some data such as capital assets, i.e. livestock, will be sensitive information and farmers may not be willing to give accurate figures if they are suspicious of the use of the data. This type of data therefore requires careful questioning, an element of trust of the data collection process and in some cases a means of double-checking if the figures generated are correct.

General points on questionnaire design and interview protocol would be:

1. Provide an explanation of the survey purpose.
2. Do not ask leading questions. This will produce answers that the data providers think you want to hear.
3. Do not make the questionnaire too long.
4. Questions that produce subjective data should be avoided.
5. Long complicated questions tend to create misunderstandings and wrong answers.

Finally the questionnaire and interview protocol should be tested and modifications made before proceeding.

Cross-sectional

A cross-sectional formal survey involves a one-off visit to livestock-keeping farms to collect data. Such activities may involve a sample of farmers or alternatively all farmers may be included, i.e. a census. For a census, data would usually be collected on the number, species and possibly sex and age of the livestock held by each household. This type of inventory data collection is prone to problems. First, such data collection has very little participation of the local communities and its use is usually for wide-scale planning needs of areas. Second, concealment of land, crops and animals is a constant problem. Land and crops have the advantage of being immobile, but animals can be walked away. If the main purpose of the survey is to count animals, a combined approach, making use of household interviews and ground or aerial transects, should be considered (Poate and Daplyn, 1993).

Cross-sectional studies that involve collecting data from a representative sample of livestock keepers can provide important details of herd structure. These can be used to make estimates of the herd production parameters such as offtake and fertility. These methods require an understanding of livestock system dynamics, but, as discussed by Matthewman and Perry (1985), there are limitations with the approach. A minimum set of data for such analysis would be total livestock numbers, age and sex structure, fertility and mortality. Such data require considerable resources and ideally involve return visits at yearly or biyearly time periods. Methods to reduce the amount of time for surveys are to use local terminology for ageing animals and to shift the focus of survey work to individual animals. Individual animal performance can then be used in livestock models to estimate herd performance (Poate and Daplyn, 1993).

Cross-sectional formal surveys are probably the least participative method of data collection. Data are taken from the local groups and usually analysed by the researcher. The information generated is usually the basis of further research or development action. However, it is unlikely that the analysis involves discussion with the providers of the original data.

Longitudinal data collection

Formal longitudinal data collection is probably the most satisfactory method to obtain data that can be used to generate livestock production parameters, inputs and outputs. However, there are limitations and problems with this approach: it is expensive in terms of enumerator staff and it requires careful thought to ensure that the data providers remain committed and enthusiastic about the survey.

Continuous production such as milk, eggs and weight gain and continuous inputs such as feed require longitudinal data collection methods to obtain accurate information. From a sampling point of view, the recording frequency should be chosen to suit the accuracy and precision required from the survey. The choice is between daily visits, frequent less-than-daily visits and a single point esti-mate. A single point estimate by memory recall will tend to produce a long-run average estimate of output and may not reflect the specific period accurately. However, frequent visits are expensive in terms of resources and time. Very frequent visits may also run into problems of farmers having to commit too much time to providing data. While it may appear most accurate to have daily visits, to avoid farmer fatigue, it is usually best to limit to fortnightly or monthly visits. If data are required between visits, farmer involvement should be sought. In some cases, this can be achieved by involving school children in collecting daily milk or egg production or recording the feed and forage given to livestock.

Longitudinal data collection works best where there is an analysis system in existence, supporting the data collection. This allows information to be returned promptly to the farmers. The analysis system may be centred on a model. Alternatively, many systems are based on generating reports that can be used by farmers to plan routine fertility checks, identify high-performance animals and keep accurate records on critical inputs. Livestock systems where this two-way process has been most successful are dairy cattle systems. These systems require information on the herd and individual animal performance which can be used to produce accurate livestock parameter information and help to prioritize information for livestock development.

To summarize, longitudinal data collection requires a two-way flow of data and information if it is to be successful. If such data collection is implemented where no relevant information is taken back to the livestock keepers, it is unlikely that the farmers will continue to participate, and if they do they will probably provide poor-quality data.

Summary

Formal data collection methods require greater resources and time to be completed than informal methods, but are capable of producing a more quantified approach. The choice of analysis method is dependent on the skills and interests of the investigator.

Combination of Formal and Informal Methods

Informal data collection techniques can be used to determine the constraints of a system. These, in turn, can be used to develop a questionnaire for a formal study. Preliminary analysis can then be carried out by the researcher and presented to the data providers for discussion and clarification of the findings.

The description of the production priorities method described above provides a good example where informal and formal methods can be combined. This method has been used in Java, Indonesia, to identify a need to investigate the relationship between grass intake and manure production. This investigation required the use of formal longitudinal data collection methods and results were then presented to the livestock farmers concerned.

Summary

Livestock data collection methods can be distinguished by how data are collected, either informally or formally, and by how the data are analysed. For informal data collection, RRA and PRA methods are distinguished. RRA is seen as a process of data gathering and analysis by the researcher, whereas PRA data are both provided and analysed with the target group. For formal data collection a distinction is made between cross-sectional and longitudinal data collection methods. It is recommended that a combination of methods is used in any study.

7 Economic Analysis Tools

Introduction

As stated in Chapter 3, the conceptual basis of farm management, enterprise and business analysis techniques is production economics. For those unfamiliar with this conceptual background to these techniques, it is recommended that they refer back to Chapter 3. Enterprise management, be it for a large commercial company or a small subsistence farmer, requires judgements about the level of input use that is appropriate. To answer this question, information is needed on the technical relationship between the inputs and the output and the prices of the inputs and the price of the output.

The underlying process of a livestock operation is biological. The level of output is directly related to the amount of input. The type of relationship can take on various forms and has been explained in Chapter 3, in the description of the input and output relationship (see Figs 3.1–3.3, Chapter 3, this volume). This is of interest because it can help to determine the efficient area of production and the optimum level of input use. However, the biological optimum level of input use is not necessarily the same as the economic optimum. To calculate the latter requires input and output prices. An enterprise budget is a representation of the relationship between inputs and outputs as a single point on a production function (see Fig. 7.1).

The interest for someone involved in the livestock sector is first to be able to describe the current enterprise through the simple representation of its inputs and outputs in the form of an enterprise budget. This can then be used to determine important inputs and examine efficiency questions of the key outputs and inputs. Finally, if data have been collected from different people involved in the livestock sector, it will be possible to see variation in enterprise budgets between these people. This information can be used to determine if some people are able to achieve better levels of profitability than others and if changes in production of the less good people are profitable or not.

This is a very basic explanation of the relationship between production economics and farm management tools. Readers who require a more in-depth study of this are recommended to refer to Boehlje and Eidman (1984, pp. 86–127).

The remainder of this chapter will focus on an explanation of the main farm management analysis techniques, which for convenience have been split according to the classification adopted by Dorward (1984) into conventional and complex farm management analysis techniques.

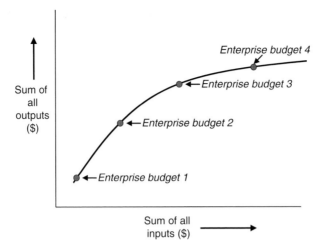

Fig. 7.1. Relationship between an enterprise budget and the production function.

Conventional Farm Management, Enterprise and Business Analysis Techniques

Conventional farm management, enterprise and business analysis techniques such as input and output analysis, gross margin analysis, enterprise budgets and whole-farm budgets are well explained in a number of farm management textbooks (Barnard and Nix, 1979; Brown, 1979; Boehlje and Eidman, 1984; Dent *et al.*, 1986; Upton, 1987; Rae, 1994). These techniques are widely used in developed countries to identify production improvements and assess the value of change. Conventional farm management analysis techniques, however, have not been widely adopted in developing countries. The reasons for the poor adoption can only be placed in context with a brief description of conventional farm management analysis techniques.

Gross margin analysis

Gross margin analysis is a technique used to evaluate and compare the profitability of different enterprises. It is based on actual records and each gross margin is essentially a single point of an enterprise production function (Kletke, 1989). Gross margin analysis assumes

that there is a set of fixed assets on the farm and it only considers inputs that vary according to the scale of the enterprise. The analysis period is usually a year, or less if the enterprise is completed in a shorter time period. To allow enterprise comparisons, it is normal to divide a gross margin by the major limiting resource used by the enterprise.

Gross margins can be used to perform price sensitivity analysis, and a collection of gross margins can be used to select the best combination of enterprises. Dent *et al.* (1986) recommend that the selection of enterprises for a farm system should be on the basis of choosing the enterprise with the highest gross margin first, and scaling this enterprise up to the maximum level possible within the constraints of the fixed assets. The second enterprise would be chosen in a similar manner (Dent *et al.*, 1986).

Gross margins can either be generated from on-farm records or taken from standard reference books such as the *Nix Pocketbook* (Nix, 2001). Both sources depend on gross margin analysis techniques being appropriate for the farming system. In smallholder farming systems, gross margin analysis has limited applicability. For instance, gross margins value an enterprise by its final financial output, and this is usually represented as an output per unit of land area. In many smallholder farming systems, financial returns are not the only criteria for enterprise selection. Other constraints, such as the need to generate food grains, can play an important part in decision making. Poor applicability of gross margin analysis at farm level reduces the incentive to collect gross margin data. The lack of data reduces the number of gross margin models available for enterprise comparisons.

Gross margin analysis is a useful technique for livestock and farming systems analysis where quantitative enterprise data are available and farmers are primarily motivated by profit maximization. Where profit maximization is not the main goal, the gross margin analysis structure needs to be adapted. This would probably require graphical output of resource use and production, and less reliance on the final financial figure summary.

Additional issues that need to be taken into account when using gross margins are:

1. Comparisons of livestock enterprises with gross margins are only justified where the production systems are similar.
2. Differences in gross margins, given similar conditions, are due to the level of yield obtained and/or price differences of inputs and output. To make justifiable comparisons in terms of efficiency, the input and output prices used and the climatic conditions of the year the calculation was carried out should be clearly indicated.
3. Gross margin figures should never be looked at in isolation and should always show the workings for the costs. The very nature of how one farmer produces a litre of milk may mean that costs would be variable in one system and fixed in another, e.g. the hiring of labour versus permanent labour to milk animals.

The gross margin is defined as the enterprise output less the variable costs attributable to it:

Gross margin = Output – Variable costs

While this is a familiar technique for most farm management specialists, there are a number of important issues when applying the gross margin model to a livestock enterprise. Livestock outputs should include all animals and produce sold and purchased. For subsistence systems, this requires the monitoring of animals slaughtered for home consumption and milk and eggs used in the house. It will also require the recording of animal gifts to, and from, the enterprise. Finally, the usual time period for gross margin analysis is 1 year, which is shorter than the life cycle of larger animals. Therefore, there is a need to recognize a change in herd value, which is not a cash item but a change in capital value. The following gives a clear statement of what outputs to look for from a livestock system.

Livestock outputs

1. Animals and produce 'out' – these items will be positive. They include:
   - sales of products; milk, meat, hides, wool, hair, draught power;
   - sales of animals;
   - home consumption of products;
   - gifts of animals or products, for payment of labour or presents.
2. Animals and produce 'in' – these items will be negative. They include:
   - livestock purchases;
   - gifts of livestock received or animals transferred into the enterprise or herd from another enterprise or herd on the farm.
3. The change in the value of the herd (can either be positive or negative). This is calculated by the following method:
   - *closing valuation of the herd* (the number of animals at the end of the period multiplied by their value) *minus the opening valuation of the herd* (the number of animals at the beginning of the period multiplied by their value).

Variable costs

Variable costs are those costs that vary in the short run, and vary directly with the amount of output produced, declining to zero if output is zero. In practical terms, variable costs can easily be allocated to individual enterprises. Variable costs include items such as feed, veterinary inputs, seed, fertilizer, insecticide, marketing costs and casual labour (employed specially for certain jobs such as harvesting, in contrast to permanent or regular labour, which is a fixed cost).

Although in theory, fuel and oil consumed by vehicles, gas, water and electricity charges are variable, they are generally not included in variable costs in farm accounting, unless they can be assigned to a specific enterprise and increase in proportion to its output.

Other resources will vary according to the enterprise chosen by the farmer and the scale of those enterprises, e.g. the number of cattle maintained. These resources are described as *variable costs* and are included in the gross margin analysis. The variable costs should satisfy two criteria:

1. Be specific to a single enterprise;
2. Vary approximately in proportion to the size of the enterprise.

For variable costs, it is normal that livestock enterprises split these into forage costs and other costs. Therefore, there will be two gross margin figures, gross margin before forage costs and a gross margin with forage costs. This again requires consideration of data collection required for livestock-related activities and forage-growing activities.

Figure 7.2 presents the gross margin structures for crop, non-grazing and grazing livestock based on a British farm management perspective.

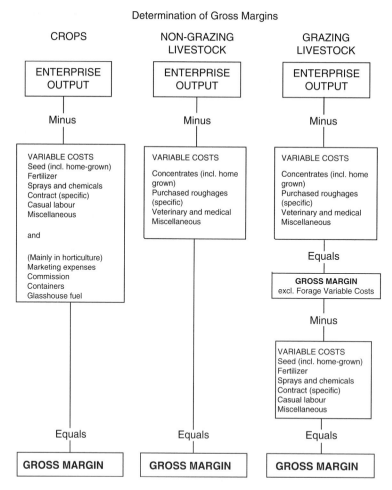

Fig. 7.2. Determination of gross margins for crops, non-grazing livestock and grazing livestock. (From MAFF, 1980, p. 7.)

The power of gross margin analysis: the economic impact of FMD in the livestock systems of the UK

The last two major epidemics of foot-and-mouth disease (FMD) in the UK have had extensive analyses of the impact of this disease across the economy in general (Power and Harris, 1973; Thompson *et al.*, 2002). These studies have much value in terms of valuing the impact of the FMD control measures adopted in both epidemics and in particular the more complex impacts outside the livestock sector. One point of interest is the apparent assumption that across all systems and species the control of FMD is a good thing for producers. During analysis of FMD vaccination strategies for the Royal Society inquiry into the 2001 epidemic, FMD impact was assessed at farm level for different systems and species in order to assess the farm-level incentives to control this disease (Rushton *et al.*, 2002). The analysis model was based on gross margin data for different production systems (Nix, 2001) and the entering of expected changes in the production parameters due to the presence of FMD (see Table 7.1).

Table 7.1. Farm-level impact of FMD in the different production systems of the UK. (Modified from Rushton *et al.*, 2002.)

Species	System	Impact	Comment
Cattle	Intensive dairy systems	Dramatic drop in milk yields for between 7 and 15 days Mastitis with as high as 90% of the herd affected (penalties on milk quality) Increased replacement costs A 10% reduction in milk yield creates a break-even enterprise budget figure	The choice without government intervention would probably be to close the farm or replace the stock. Between destocking, disinfecting the farm and restocking it is likely that the business will be unable to earn income for between 2 and 3 months. An intensive dairy system in the UK could not survive a FMD outbreak. It would be put out of business. Therefore, there are strong incentives to eradicate the disease in areas with large dairy populations
Pigs	Intensive rearing systems	Increased pig mortality Increased abortion Lower milk yields Increased sow replacement	Small changes in the number of piglets per sow can produce a loss in the production system. The system is very sensitive to small changes in fertility rates and it is doubtful that these systems could survive the impact of FMD. Strong incentives to eradicate the disease in areas with large pig breeding populations
Pigs	Fattening unit	Poorer feed conversion Possibly higher mortality	These systems are sensitive to feed conversion rates. Small changes can put the enterprises into a loss
Cattle	Beef suckling systems	Reduced fertility Increased calf mortality Increased replacement rate of breeding stock	Lowering calving rates from 90% to 45% does not produce a negative gross margin. Variable and fixed costs are small in comparison to output. Subsidies are provided according to stocking density rather than production. Less incentive to spend time with the cattle to increase production
Cattle	Beef finishing systems	Possibly slower finishing Some mortality	Protected by subsidy payments
Sheep		Lameness Possibly a reduction in fertility, but there is no information in the literature on this subject	Well protected with subsidy. Reduction in lambing rates has little impact on the gross margins of these systems and in the case of hill flocks the lamb per ewe can be dropped to zero and the gross margin remains positive.

This analysis, using a relatively simple gross margin analysis, shows that the impact in the main livestock systems of the UK indicates that the most severe impact at farm level is in dairy and pig systems. It is likely that FMD would put these types of farm enterprises out of business in a very short time. However, in beef and sheep systems, which have lower variable costs and lower capital investments and are supported by subsidies, the impact at farm level of FMD is much lower. These latter systems could possibly 'ride out' an outbreak of FMD on a farm and manage to survive. This indicates that farm-level incentives for control and eradication are very different in different systems and therefore very different within different areas of the UK. Whether an outbreak can be isolated, however, depends on the movement of animals between the different points of the country.

Enterprise budgets

An enterprise budget is an estimate of the input costs and output returns for producing a unit of an enterprise and the difference between them produces the enterprise profit. Unlike the gross margin analysis the fixed costs are included. In general, it can be calculated on a basis of a certain number of key inputs or outputs in a similar way to the gross margin analysis, which introduces the concept of productivity.[1] In this way it can be considered an extension of the gross margin analysis work that has been discussed and we can define the enterprise profit as follows:

$$\text{Enterprise profit} = \text{Output} - \text{Variable costs} - \text{Fixed costs}$$

The household or farm profit would therefore be the sum of the enterprise profits:

$$\text{Household profit} = \text{Sum of the enterprise profits}$$

A more in-depth explanation of fixed costs is provided below.

Fixed costs

Fixed costs vary only in the long run, and are still incurred even if output is zero. Fixed costs are usually shared by several enterprises. They are sometimes called overheads.

Fixed costs usually include:

- regular paid labour or permanent staff – including both paid labour and an estimate of the value of any unpaid (usually family) labour;
- where family labour inputs are divided into gender and age, this should be recognized in the analysis and labour inputs separated into men, women and children;
- depreciation on equipment, machinery, vehicles, some buildings, etc. (see below for a further explanation of this concept and how to calculate depreciation);
- maintenance and repairs;
- fuel and oil costs, where these cannot be assigned to a particular enterprise;
- rent (both paid rent and estimated or 'notional' rent on land owned by the actor in the chain);
- gas, water, electricity costs where these cannot be assigned to a particular enterprise;
- paid management costs;
- paid interest (see below for a complete explanation).

While discussing payments to labour, it is worth mentioning payments in kind. Where casual or permanent staff is paid partly with produce, the *value* of such payments should be included as a fixed cost.

However, definitions of variable and fixed costs can vary slightly from country to country. Readers working in the Indian subcontinent will probably find that, although at the level of economic theory the definitions of variable and fixed costs apply, at a practical level, the division of farm costs between fixed and variable costs is slightly different. You should check on what the local conventions are, and follow these. In the end, the objective of this type of accountancy exercise is to come up with estimates of output and gross margins that can be

---

[1] Note that productivity is a measure of how efficient an enterprise is and is very distinct from production, which is a measure of how much an enterprise produces.

compared with those made for other farms or by other people. For this reason, what is important is that everyone working in the same geographical area uses the same system.

To complete this section on fixed costs, an explanation is required on depreciation and interest.

Depreciation

Depreciation is not a cash value cost, but an estimate of the amount by which the value of a capital item falls in a given period. Therefore, it represents a cost of ownership of that item. The inclusion of such a cost in an enterprise budget is to recognize that in the future when this object needs to be replaced there is sufficient money available to do so. Where depreciation is not taken into account and the contribution of capital items is important, there can often be a false sense of making large profits in the early years of a business. If this money is not reinvested during this period, problems could well arise when capital items need to be replaced. One of the common problems of many businesses is that replacement costs for capital items are not taken into account.

Depreciation may occur for three reasons:

1. Obsolescence;
2. Gradual deterioration with age;
3. Wear and tear with use.

The first two factors limit the economic life of a machine or capital item and the third limits the life of the item in terms of hours or days of use. In a context where capital items are of relatively low technology, the most important reason for depreciation to occur is the wear and tear with use. Therefore, where the livestock activity is seasonal and practised for short periods of time each year, the number of years of life is likely to be much longer than for an activity that is increasing in intensity.

There are three common ways of calculating depreciation:

• straight line method – estimated by dividing the difference of the purchased and salvage price of the item by the number of useful years of its use;

• diminishing balances method – estimated by taking a percentage of the remaining value of the item as the depreciation year on year. For example:

Depreciation = (Estimated value the previous year [2]) multiplied by the percentage

• sum-of-the-years'-digits method – estimated by multiplying the difference between the cost and salvage value of the item by the number of years before the item will be replaced divided by the sum of the years of useful life. For example, in year 5 of an item with 8 years' useful life for an item that costs 2000 pesos with a salvage value of 200 pesos:

Depreciation (year 5) = (original cost minus the salvage value) multiplied by ((total years of useful life minus year the depreciation is calculated) divided by (sum of the digits of the years of life))

$$(2000-200)*((8-5)/(1+2+3+4+5\\ +6+7+8))$$
$$=(1800)*(3/36)$$
$$=150 \text{ pesos}$$

Table 7.2 presents the estimation of depreciation using the different methods with an example of a capital item that cost 2000 pesos, with a useful life of 8 years and a salvage value of 200 pesos.

The diminishing balances and sum-of-the-years'-digits methods are relatively complicated in comparison to the straight line method. They are also more applicable where there is a need to calculate depreciation for an item with a large degree of obsolescence, e.g. a lorry, a computer or a processing machine; where technologies change rapidly, the value of such an asset will decline rapidly in the first year of life due to the purchased item being quickly replaced by newer versions with different technologies. For capital items such as basic tools, machetes, spades, etc. or buildings, the straight line method is preferred and more appropriate for investments that are basic technologies often used at farm level. However, investments in capital equipment that has rapidly changing technologies

---

[2] This will be the original value in year 1.

Table 7.2. Estimation of depreciation using different methods. (Modified from Barnard and Nix, 1979).

Year of life	Annual depreciation method			Estimated value of the item (Written-down value)		
	Straight line	Diminishing balances	Sum-of-the-years'-digits	Straight line	Diminishing balances	Sum-of-the-years'-digits
0–1	225	500	400	1775	1500	1600
1–2	225	375	350	1550	1125	1250
2–3	225	281	300	1325	844	950
3–4	225	211	250	1100	633	700
4–5	225	158	200	875	475	500
5–6	225	119	150	650	356	350
6–7	225	89	100	425	267	250
7–8	225	67	50	200	200	200

Note: Written-down value = original cost less the sum of the depreciation values. It is an indication of the present value of the capital investment.

should have depreciation methods applied that take into account the need to recognize the sharp decrease in the value of that asset in early years of life.

Interest

In an enterprise budget it is a common convention to estimate interest as the interest charged on half the initial cost of any capital item. For example, if a family invested 300 Bolivianos[3] in equipment to collect rubber and the interest rate in the region was 10%, then in the enterprise budget the cost of interest for this capital investment would be (300/2)*10% = 15 Bolivianos per year. Note that this simple method assumes simple rather than compound interest.

Example: enterprise budget as a tool to examine returns to key inputs and outputs

One of the major difficulties in livestock studies is the valuation of labour and capital inputs to livestock production, processing and marketing activities. While it is possible to collect data on local labour rates, these can

vary according to the time of year and also the gender of the person supplying the labour. In addition, given that labour is such an important input it is important to estimate how efficiently labour is used. Therefore, to overcome these problems and investigate the interesting issues with regard to labour it is possible to remove this input from the enterprise budget, and once the final profitability has been found to divide the final output by the number of labour days used to generate an estimate of income per day of labour. This provides a figure that can be compared with local labour rates and gives an indication of whether the livestock activity is attractive. It can also provide a means to examine the rewards of labour input from men and women.

Similarly, where capital is an important input, but the investment in capital items has come from family resources, interest can also be set to zero and an estimate made on the returns of the investment as a percentage. Again this can be used to compare investment returns in other local activities and also to compare these returns with local available credit sources. The latter will provide information on whether a livestock activity would be able to repay credit to begin the activity.

Whole-farm and business plans and resource allocation tables

Whole-farm and business plans look at all the resources used and produced by the farm or

---

[3] Boliviano is the official Bolivian currency; in November 2005 the exchange rate was US$1 = 8 Bolivianos.

livestock sector businesses, and also the availability of resources throughout the year. The overall structure of whole-farm or livestock sector business plans and resource allocation tables provides a good method for assessing farm and business profitability and examining change. However, to develop individual farm or business plans, either on paper or by spreadsheet, is cumbersome and time-consuming. Performing sensitivity analysis can also be difficult, if it involves a change in enterprise combinations. Finally, adapting a farm or business budget to a new production or marketing system is difficult, and it is usually easier to develop a totally new budget. The lack of flexibility of these methods generally discourages experimentation.

An enterprise gross margin measures the contribution of that enterprise to farm or business profit. The sum of the enterprise gross margins minus the fixed costs of the farm or business equals the farm or business profit (or loss).

Profit = Sum of enterprise gross margins
– Fixed costs of farm or business

However, gross margins do *not* directly measure profit of the enterprise as they ignore fixed costs. They are useful for enterprise comparisons and assessing enterprise efficiency or productivity. Such comparisons may lead to minor plan modifications, where the fixed costs remain the same. Figure 7.3 shows how gross margins relate to farm profit.

However, to assess the change from one enterprise to another requires budgeting methods to compare the marginal benefits and costs from a change. The next section will introduce a partial budgeting, a method designed for such comparisons.

Assessing change in livestock systems and the components of the livestock

The economic assessment tools presented are generally speaking used to assess overall profitability of systems or enterprises. To assess change, there are other methods, which will be presented below.

Partial budgeting

Partial budgeting is a technique used to assess small changes in farming systems, a livestock sector enterprise or an existing organization. Costs and benefits of a change are estimated and compared to give an indication of whether the change is worthwhile. If costs and benefits occur in different time periods, it is necessary to introduce discounting. This marginal analysis is not designed to show the profit or loss of the farm as a whole but the net increase or decrease in net farm income resulting from proposed changes. Partial budgeting is based on expected values and can be used as an evaluation tool, e.g. estimating the economic impact of disease. The economic concept of partial budget is important for cost–benefit analysis of disease control projects, which will be discussed later.

Partial budgets are interested in four basic items:

Costs	Benefits
(a) New costs	(c) Costs saved
(b) Revenue foregone	(d) New revenue

To assess a change, there is need to estimate the difference between (a) + (b) and (c) + (d). If the benefits exceed the costs then it would be advantageous for the farmer or person in the livestock sector to pursue the change; conversely if there were no difference or the costs were greater then the existing system would be better. Compare this to moving along the production function in the one input, one output relationship or the production surface for more than one input. The search is for the point where the last dollar spent returns a dollar. The methods compare marginal costs versus marginal benefits (see Fig. 7.4).

Partial budgets are most often used for considering the use of a new input, enterprise or farm practice. Therefore, it is a useful technique to test the viability of introducing a new medication or a different animal management practice. It can also be used to evaluate the feasibility of adding a supplementary enterprise, for example poultry or pig rearing

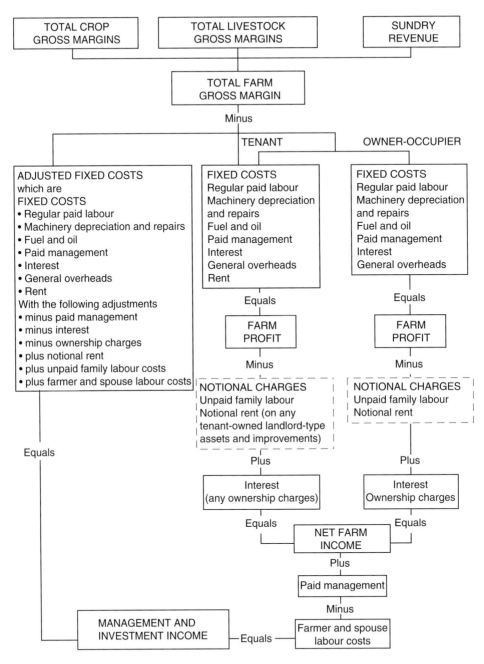

Fig. 7.3. Relationship between farm profit, net farm income and management and investment income. (From MAFF, 1980, p. 9.)

to utilize surplus family labour. Care should be taken to ensure that surplus labour is truly surplus. For example, women may not be working on the farm, but they will be involved in important activities such as preparing food, washing and taking care of the children. The demand for labour may also be seasonal so that surplus labour will only be

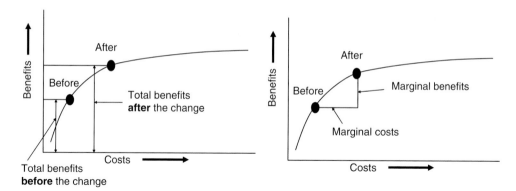

Fig. 7.4. Marginal costs and benefits.

available at certain times. Animals need care throughout the year and if the labour is not available at one time then it will often not be economically viable for the family to take on extra responsibilities. Careful consideration of changes that utilize (perceived) surplus resources cannot be overemphasized. Many suggested changes are poorly adopted because farmers are simply unable to manage them.

The technical feasibility is an essential precondition of partial budgeting. It is completely useless to test the economic feasibility of a change if it cannot be implemented or the technical assumptions made are invalid. A change can only be technically feasible if:

1. The soil, climate and other physical and biological factors are conducive to the proper growth of the livestock.
2. The change made to the system will not put undue strain on the existing organization.

Partial budgeting is an extremely useful technique for examining change, and its conceptual basis is also used when introducing time into analysis to assess change (see section on investment appraisal). However, it is not capable of examining seasonal resource flows, and it is also unsuitable for enterprises that have irregular or lumpy inputs and outputs.

Partial budget example: improvement of dairy enterprise

In the following example, a farm planting 150 decares of wheat and 50 decares of barley has ten dairy cows, and produces ten fattened animals each year. All the straw and 60% of barley grain produced by the farm is fed to the dairy and fattening stock. The farm also purchases 15,400 kg of dairy concentrate feed each year. The dairy cows have a calving interval of 400 days and a lactation yield of 2500 l. The annual milk production from the unit has been calculated to be 22,800 l/year ($(365/400) \times 2500 \times 10$). The average number of calves produced per year is estimated to be 9.125 ($(365/400) \times 1 \times 10$). The labour requirement per year is calculated to be 3777 h or 472 days.

It has been recommended that the farmer should replace 4 daa of wheat for lucerne and feed all the barley grain to the dairy and fattening stock. The lucerne produced will be fed to the fattening stock.

The change reduces the amount of dairy concentrate purchased to 15,000 kg. All the straw produced by the farm will still be fed to the dairy and fattening stock. The change is also estimated to reduce the calving interval to 375 days and to increase the lactation yield to 3000 l. The annual milk production for the unit will therefore increase to 29,175 l/year ($(365/375) \times 3000 \times 10$) and the number of calves produced per year will increase to 9.733 ($365/375 \times 1 \times 10$). The labour requirement per year for this plan is estimated to be 4092 h or 511.5 days.

The following parameters are provided:

- wheat yield 200 kg/decare;
- barley yield 250 kg/decare;

- fattened animal sale weight 300 kg live weight;
- Prices June 1995:
  (a) wheat 6475 TL/kg;
  (b) barley 4900 TL/kg;
  (c) concentrate 7000 TL/kg;
  (d) milk 17,000 TL/l;
  (e) beef 85,850 TL/kg live weight;
  (f) labour 60,000 TL/h;
  (g) calf 3,000,000 TL/animal.
- Costs per decare of crop:
  (a) lucerne 563,000 TL/decare;
  (b) wheat 790,000 TL/decare.

Table 7.3 presents a partial budget for the recommended change.

The change would improve the farm income by 65,112,000 TL/year (116,160,000 – 51,048,000), which would clearly indicate that the change is economically favourable. One note of caution is the large increase in labour that this change requires.

Investment appraisal

Gross margins, enterprise budgets and partial budgets are restricted because they can only be carried out for set periods of time, either a year or production cycle. For assessing a change in management or an investment that affects outputs over a number of years, a different approach is required. Investment appraisal utilizes the basic framework of partial budgets, i.e. identifying costs and benefits of change, but adds the concept of the time value of money. This allows the analyst to examine the impact of a change in disease over a number of years with a flow of costs and benefits.

For partial budgets the following steps were outlined:

1. Identify all the benefits.
2. Identify all the costs.

However, if these benefits and costs occur over a number of years at different points we also have to consider exactly when they will occur. For investment appraisal, this list alters slightly to include:

1. Identify all benefits and *when they occur*.
2. Identify all costs and *when they occur*.

Costs and the benefits of a change are then compared, but investment appraisal recognizes that the value of money changes over time. For example, receiving US$100,000 now is better than receiving US$100,000 in a year's time because US$100,000 could be invested. If the money were placed in a bank account with an interest rate of 10%, then it would be worth US$110,000 next year, US$121,000 in 2 years' time, US$133,100 in 4 years' time, and so on.

Conversely, if a person is to be given a sum of money in the future rather than a sum now, it is necessary to calculate what the sum is worth in present value terms. In the example above, US$121,000 received in 2 years' time would be worth no more than US$100,000 to be received now, so that the present value of US$121,000 in 2 years' time

Table 7.3. Partial budget for a change to improve dairy production.

Costs (000 TL)		Benefits (000 TL)	
New costs		*Costs saved*	
Lucerne (4 × 563,000)	2,252	Wheat costs (4 × 790,000)	3,160
Labour ((4,092 – 3,777) × 60,000)	18,900	Concentrate ((15,400 – 15,000) × 7,000)	2,800
Revenue foregone		*New benefits*	
Barley grain sold ((50 × 250) × 0.4 × 4,900)	24,500	Milk ((29,175 – 22,800) × 17,000)	108,375
Wheat grain sold (4 × 200 × 6,745)	5,396	Calves ((9.733 – 9.125) × 3,000,000)	1,825
Total costs	51,048	Total benefits	116,160

is US$100,000. Converting future values into present values is known as discounting. Discounting requires a rate known as a discount rate. The discount rate does not necessarily equate to the rate of interest offered at banks. The underlying concept of discounting is stated as follows:

> A basic principle is that a US dollar now is worth more than a US dollar to be received some time in the future because that (present) US dollar received can be invested at interest to accumulate more than its original value.

To compare costs and benefits that occur in different years it is necessary to convert their value into a *present value*. This is done by using a technique known as *discounting*. Discounting requires a rate known as a *discount rate*. The formula for discounting is as follows:

$$PV = \frac{X_t}{(1+r)^t}$$

where PV is the present value,

X_t is the amount of money in year t,

r is the rate of discount (expressed as a proportion, e.g. 10% = 0.1), and

t is the number of years from the present date.

When all benefits and costs are converted to present values it is possible to compare them. This is commonly done using three decision-making criteria: net present value, internal rate of return, and the benefit/cost ratio.

The *net present value* (NPV) is the difference between the sum of the present value of the benefits and the sum of the present value of the costs. The formula to calculate the NPV is as follows:

$$NPV = \Sigma \frac{B_T}{(1+r)^t} - \Sigma \frac{C_T}{(1+r)^t}$$

$$NPV = PV_B - PV_C$$

If the *NPV* is negative, then investment is not worthwhile, while a positive *NPV* indicates only that the investment might be considered.

An alternative approach to assessing an investment is the calculation of the investment's *internal rate of return* (IRR). The IRR is the discount rate that will make the NPV equal to zero. In simpler terms, the IRR is the interest rate that will make the investment just break even. In mathematical terms it is the discount rate for which:

$$NPV = \Sigma \frac{B_T}{(1+r)^t} - \Sigma \frac{C_T}{(1+r)^t} = 0$$

If the IRR exceeds the minimum acceptable discount rate or the opportunity cost of money, the project is worth further consideration.

A third criterion, the *benefit/cost ratio* (BCR), is calculated by dividing the sum of the present value of benefits by the sum of the present value of costs.

$$BCR = \frac{\Sigma \dfrac{B_T}{(1+r)^t}}{\Sigma \dfrac{C_T}{(1+r)^t}}$$

An investment is worth considering if the BCR is greater than 1.

Each of these three investment appraisal criteria has strengths and weaknesses (Gittinger, 1982), and for this reason it is common practice to present the results of an investment appraisal with all three measures of project worth.

Investment appraisal provides the basis for much economic impact assessment of livestock diseases and their control. However, it is important to recognize the difficulties with assessing costs and benefits from livestock systems. Livestock are difficult investments to appraise, because of their ability to reproduce and the fact that they take a number of years to reach maturity. These characteristics mean that it is often necessary to model the livestock system being studied to obtain a satisfactory impact assessment.

Carrying out a cost/benefit analysis of disease control projects requires a process similar to partial budgeting. It is not the value of the whole livestock system that is of interest. Instead the analyst examines how proposed changes in health management and treatment will affect the output of the livestock system under study. To do this, it is necessary to calculate the losses being incurred because of the disease, generally either through mortality or morbidity, and to calculate how much it would cost to control or eradicate the disease.

MORTALITY. The cost of losing an animal to disease can in most cases be taken as the market value of that animal, as this should reflect the expected future income from the animal. It is important to recognize that, if the animal can be sold after its death, there may be a salvage value. It is also important to recognize that acutely sick animals may be slaughtered. An animal slaughtered because of illness will probably have a lower value than if it was slaughtered at the time the farmer planned. However, slaughtering sick animals will reduce the mortality rates and increase offtake, which may appear to increase output. In this case, it is important to obtain information from farmers about their attitude to sick animals and to see if they classify the slaughtering of a sick animal as a death or as normal offtake. Their classification can hide the true cost of a death due to disease.

MORBIDITY. A disease is likely to have an effect on those animals that survive. This will usually affect the animals' performance in terms of:

- fertility;
- delays in reaching maturity (for reproduction or sale);
- decreased production of milk, eggs, wool, etc.;
- decreased draught power available;
- decreased weight of fattened or culled animals.

Once the effects have been quantified it is necessary to consider the different control options.

Perhaps the most efficient way of converting observations on morbidity and mortality into livestock outputs and inputs

is through the use of herd models, which will be discussed in more detail later in the book.

The following example presents how mortality and morbidity can be used within an economic analysis framework in order to compare the costs and benefits of FMD vaccination campaigns in Bolivia. These campaigns had differing rates of success, but it was particularly difficult to achieve high levels of vaccination coverage in the extensive beef systems. In order to understand the difficulties encountered with the campaigns, an economic analysis of the impact of FMD was carried out to determine the incentives to participate (Hoyos et al., 2000). A deterministic herd projection model was developed which allows the user to change mortality, fertility and offtake rates and also modify prices. The model has two projections, one for a herd without vaccination and another for a herd with vaccination. The impact of the disease was entered as an outbreak in the first year. Further analysis was then carried out to determine the frequency at which an outbreak would have to occur to make a farm-level vaccination programme attractive. The results are shown in Fig. 7.5.

Figure 7.6 shows the undiscounted costs associated with FMD control and the losses caused by the disease. The costs in the herd without FMD and practising twice a year vaccination are related to the herd size, but are relatively constant. In the herd that had a FMD outbreak in year 1 of the simulation, the losses are similar to the costs of vaccination until years 4–6. The difference is greatest in year 5, which is approximately 4 years after the outbreak.

The reasons that losses are predicted to occur so long after the outbreak relate to the time that an animal is ready for sale in these extensive systems. Male animals are sold at between 4 and 6 years of age and female animals are normally all retained in the herd. An FMD outbreak in such a system has little effect on the male adult animals, but increases calf mortality and reduces fertility in cows and heifers. Therefore, in the year of the outbreak, the calf crop is reduced and this is only felt as a loss when this calf crop matures

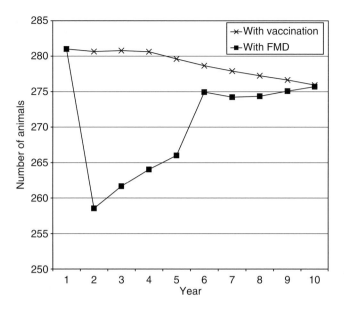

Fig. 7.5. Projections for herds with vaccination against FMD (i.e. no disease) and a herd without vaccination and an outbreak of FMD in the first year of the simulation.

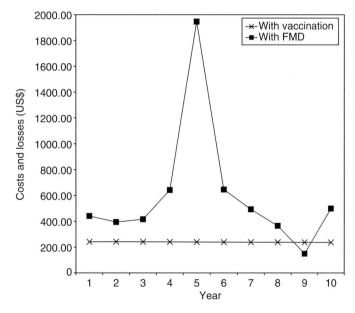

Fig. 7.6. Undiscounted costs and disease losses for a herd with vaccination and a herd without vaccination and an outbreak of FMD in the first year of the simulation (US$).

for sale between 4 and 6 years after the outbreak. The nature of these losses is worrying in that it is unlikely that farmers will recognize the importance of FMD to their sales of animals as the major impact occurs so long after the outbreak. It would be natural for farmers to confuse a low number of animals for sale with other problems such as flooding

Table 7.4. Net present value of costs for each strategy with and without outbreaks.

Vaccination strategy	Outbreak in year 1	No outbreak
Herd that is vaccinated two times a year	1474.17	1474.17
Herd that is not vaccinated	3921.51	0
Herd that is vaccinated once a year	2162.26	1094.38

or drought in the previous years. The NPVs for different vaccination strategies are presented in Table 7.4.

At farm level, the control of FMD in extensive beef systems does not give a positive economic return and the losses caused by an outbreak appear to be greatest some time after the outbreak. A positive return to control is only generated if the disease occurs once every 1 or 2 years, which is probably biologically impossible. Given that these systems also are managed in a way that only allows farmers to see their animals once a year, there is a great need for a vaccine that protects an animal for 12 months, reducing costs of vaccination and improving FMD control.

With the information presented above there is a need to shift the assessment from farm/household implication to broader sector-level impacts of FMD and the control measures proposed. To place this analysis of disease impact and its control at sector or national level, a number of questions have to be answered:

- How many livestock owners have extensive beef systems?
- How many extensive beef farmers vaccinate twice, once or not at all?
- What are the additional costs and benefits from having a sector or national FMD control programme?

The answering of these questions requires a classification of livestock systems and an analysis of the market, social and environmental implications. In some situations, farm/household models that predict livestock owners' behaviour in response to a change in disease status (and hence produc-

tivity of the livestock system) are used. A brief section on these types of models is presented below in relation to the farm level. They are also discussed in relation to analysis at the sectoral and national levels. The complete discounted costs and benefits of this analysis are presented below under different assumptions of disease outbreaks and eradication (see the section on risk and uncertainty).

In summary, investment appraisal takes account of the time involved for a system to reach a steady state and of the time value of money. As most livestock systems have cycles that are longer than a year this technique is extremely valuable in the economic impact assessment of livestock diseases and their control. The framework of investment appraisal is the basis of cost–benefit analysis, which is a method of analysis at the sectoral, national and regional levels. The process of carrying out investment appraisals has been made far easier with the availability of computers and spreadsheets. Those interested in applications of this method with spreadsheets are referred to the farm management book by Rae (1994).

A weakness of investment appraisal for investigating the impact of animal diseases is the lack of a component that can consider the probability of an event occurring. As disease outbreaks are random events, this failing has to be addressed using other methodologies, which are discussed below. It also needs to be stressed that investment appraisal provides an estimate of the economic profitability of a change; it does not, however, go into detail of whether that change is implementable. The following description of financial feasibility provides detail on this.

Financial feasibility

Once the economic profitability of various investments has been analysed and an alternative is chosen, its financial feasibility should be evaluated. The purpose of financial feasibility analysis is to determine whether or not the investment project will generate sufficient cash income to make the principal and interest payments on the borrowed funds used to purchase the asset. However, if the asset is purchased with money that does not need to be borrowed, i.e. equity, then financial feasibility is not necessary.

The steps for financial feasibility are as follows:

1. Determine the *annual net cash flows* for the investment. These should be available from the economic feasibility.
2. Determine the *annual principal and interest payments* based on the loan repayment schedule.
3. *Compare the annual cash flow with the annual principal and interest repayments* to determine if a cash surplus or deficit will occur.

If the investment produces cash surplus, it will be able to meet the loan repayments and it can be classed as financially as well as economically feasible. A cash deficit means the investment is not financially feasible. This does not mean that the investment should not take place; it simply means that the servicing of the loan will meet with problems.

Cash deficits can be reduced or eliminated in a number of ways:

1. Extending the loan terms, i.e. more years to repay the principal, will result in lower annual debt servicing requirements.
2. Increasing the amount of down payment will reduce the size of the principal and interest repayments.
3. Increasing the utilization of the asset; in the example above, more diagnostic tests could be carried out.
4. Subsidizing the investment repayments from other activities:
  • decision tree analysis;
  • modelling.

Those interested in examples of financial feasibility are referred to Boehlje and Eidman (1984, pp. 332–334).

How to deal with risk and uncertainty in the economic analysis of animal health and production

At the end of the example on investment appraisal for a farm-level vaccination strategy, it was mentioned that decisions can be assisted by taking into account uncertainty. Risk and uncertainty were also mentioned in the discussion on production economics. Uncertainty in the livestock sector has three main causes:

  • *environmental variations* causing production and yield uncertainty;
  • *price variation* causing market uncertainty;
  • lack of information.

For livestock enterprises, risks of disease and reproductive disorders are obvious. Livestock farms in harsh climates will also experience the risk of dry seasons or long cold seasons, both of which affect the level of animal production achieved through the year. The lengthy period between making a production decision and obtaining an output in the majority of livestock enterprises means that the prices at the point of sale cannot be known. This is particularly true for beef enterprises where it may take 3–4 years for an animal to reach a sale weight, but it can also be argued that a dairy enterprise which invests in buildings and equipment has the same problem even though the product is sold every day. The price variation can be reduced by promoting more stable markets, for example through dairy cooperatives or quantity agreements with local butchers. Livestock farmers who live in isolated areas and are geographically distant from markets may have large costs to obtain market information. There are also livestock producers who because of low levels of education are unable to obtain information due to illiteracy. Both the latter two groups will experience a lack of information.

Additions to the list of uncertainties in many countries are *state actions and wars*. Many markets in developing countries are controlled by state bodies, and farmers are therefore in the hands of politicians for the sale of their produce. Farmers are also subject to policies from outside the area – for example, livestock farmers in West Africa have been affected by the European Union exporting meat at cheap prices to their zone. Finally a number of countries in the developing world such as Vietnam, Ethiopia, Mozambique, Angola and Sudan have experienced civil war. Where there are wars, farmers are constantly open to the possibility of their animals being stolen, which makes production decisions very difficult. War zones also have problems in terms of access to veterinary services and products and it is no surprise that rinderpest was last encountered in the troubled zones of Sudan, Ethiopia and Kenya.

With all the uncertainty detailed above, livestock farmers and people within the livestock sector cannot plan with certainty – their decisions on livestock production and investments in the sector are subject to risk.

Ellis (1988) presents the following list of impacts of uncertainty on farmer decision making which is applicable for the livestock farmer:

- Uncertainty results in suboptimal economic decisions at the level of the production unit (livestock enterprise) and therefore means that there is no profit maximization. Note that one of the assumptions in the development of a framework for production economics was perfect certainty.
- Uncertainty results in unwillingness or slowness to adopt innovations such as new disease control methods.
- Uncertainty can help to explain farming practices such as keeping a mixture of livestock species. Such practices are successful ways of mitigating the effects of uncertainty.
- The impact of uncertainty is more severe for poor than for better-off farm households, which implies that it reinforces social differentiation.
- Uncertainty can be reduced by increasing market integration through improved information, communication and access to market outlets. However, greater market integration can exacerbate uncertainty as the safety of subsistence is replaced by the insecurity of unstable markets and adverse price trends.

Therefore, the livestock sector has various means to adapt to uncertainty, and the discipline of economics has developed frameworks and tools to support livestock farmers and people involved in the livestock sector in this process.

There is often a distinction made between risk and uncertainty with *risk* being defined as where the decision maker knows the alternative outcomes and can attach a probability to each of them, and *uncertainty* being where the decision maker has less information on the outcomes of a decision and also cannot attach probabilities to their outcomes. At one time the distinction made between the two terms was about their objective or subjective nature. The probabilities attached to a risk situation were thought to be objective in nature, but the probabilities attached to an uncertain situation were subjective due to a lack of information. This distinction has now been discarded, because it is impossible in any situation to determine objectively the probabilities of an outcome. Uncertainty helps to describe the economic situation facing a farmer and the farmer can take a degree of risk in each of the events within that uncertain environment.

Measuring risk

Risk is a measure of the effect of uncertainty on the decision maker. In these terms, it is an attempt to measure the difference between the outcome of a decision made with uncertainty in mind and a decision that produces the optimum outcome. The general opinion on people's attitudes in decision making is that all people are risk-averse. This means they are willing to forego some income or face extra costs in order to avoid risk; they are cautious in their decision making. Two methods will be explained below of measuring risk in order to assist decision-making variation or instability of income and the possibility of disaster or ruin, through the use of an example.

A farmer has the option of two breeds of sheep, a hardy breed and a productive breed. The hardy breed is a good mother capable of withstanding very cold weather, but has a lower lambing rate. The productive breed is not such a good mother and is less able to withstand cold weather, but has a higher lambing rate. A sheep farmer in a marginal area wants to examine which breed to adopt with the information shown in Table 7.5 on the lambing rates of the two breeds in different weather conditions. This table is called a 'pay-off matrix'.

It is assumed that the quality and price of the lambs produced from both breeds are the same. Therefore, the farmer will only be interested in the pay-offs in terms of number of lambs rather than cash. The number of lambs produced per 100 ewes is less variable for the hardy breed than the productive breed. If a decision had to be made just from this information then a cautious farmer may decide to use just the hardy breed. In this way, they guarantee that they will get at least 80 lambs each year even in the worst weather conditions. This is known as the *MAXIMIN* choice as it maximizes the minimum or worst possible outcome.

Such a policy would be very cautious and would assume that the weather is always going to be bad. If the sheep farmer adopts just the hardy breed, they will forgo 60 lambs in warm years, 20 lambs in normal years and only gain 40 lambs in the cold years. There is, therefore, a trade-off between adopting a risk avoidance policy and net gains. The choice for a sheep farmer would, however, be clear-cut if one breed outperformed for all weather types. For example, if the productive breed outperformed the hardy breed in all weather conditions it would 'dominate' the hardy breed.

Table 7.5. Pay-off matrix: number of lambs produced per 100 ewes in different weather conditions.

	Weather conditions during lambing season		
	Warm	Normal	Cold
Productive breed	140	120	60
Hardy breed	80	100	100

This decision can be refined by information on the weather conditions of the area where the sheep farm is found. The meteorological office has predicted the probabilities of warm, normal or cold years as being a warm year 0.2, a normal year 0.5 and a cold year 0.3. These probabilities can be used to calculate the expected lamb numbers for each breed using the following formula:

$$E(Y) = \sum Y_i P_i = Y_1 P_1 + Y_2 P_2 + \ldots + Y_n P_n$$

where Y_1, $Y_2, \ldots Y_n$ are the lamb numbers under the different weather conditions and P_1, $P_2, \ldots P_n$ are the respective probabilities.

The expected number of lambs produced by the productive breed is $(140 \times 0.2) + (120 \times 0.5) + (60 \times 0.3) = 106$ lambs and for the hardy breed is $(80 \times 0.2) + (100 \times 0.5) + (100 \times 0.3) = 96$ lambs. A sheep farmer who is *risk-indifferent* rather than *risk-averse* would choose the productive breed rather than the hardy breed as it gives the highest expected number of lambs.

However, as well as the expected number of lambs it is also important to look at the variation in the output. The variation can be quantified in two ways: either as the variance, which is the square of the 'standard deviation' calculated using the following equation:

$$V(Y) = \sum (Y_i - E(Y))^2 P_i$$

where $V(Y)$ is the variance,
   $E(Y)$ is the expected production level,
   Y_i is the production level in each season, and
   P_i is the probability of that season occurring,
   or as the mean of absolute deviation calculated using the following equation:

$$MAD(Y) = \sum |Y_i - E(Y)| P_i$$

where $MAD(Y)$ is the mean absolute deviation,
   $E(Y)$ is the expected production level,
   Y_i is the yield in each season, and
   P_i is the probability of that season occurring.

The variance and mean absolute deviation of lamb crops for the productive breed are:

$V(Y) = (140 - 106)^2 \times 0.2 + (120 - 106)^2 \times 0.5 + (60 - 106)^2 \times 0.3 = 964$ and $MAD(Y) = (140 - 106) \times 0.2 + (120 - 106) \times 0.5 + (60 - 106) \times 0.3 = 27.6$. For the hardy breed the variance is 64 and the mean absolute deviation is 6.4.

This information just confirms the initial observations that the productive breed although capable of producing more lambs has a much more variable output. Such a situation may make a farmer think carefully before adopting such a breed. However, as mentioned above, it would be a cautious farmer who chooses the hardy breed as in the long run he will lose out.

If, instead of choosing one or the other breed, there is a mixture of the breeds then output and variation of output can be modified. This is diversification of risk by having more than one breed of sheep on the farm at a time. To keep the example simple it is assumed that there is no cross-breeding, but simply having different numbers of the two breeds. Table 7.6 presents the different possibilities of lamb crop, variance and standard deviation for various combinations of the hardy and productive breeds.

It can be seen from the table that the lamb crop from a combination of the 20 productive breed sheep with 80 hardy sheep is less variable than one breed on its own. Examining the data further it is possible to continue a line of study either in terms of the worst possible outcomes or in terms of the variation of outcomes. Examining the table the choice of 20 productive breed sheep and 80 hardy sheep would maximize the worst possible outcome. This combination is the maximum level of production even in the cold and the warm season and is the MAXIMIN strategy of the mixed breed strategy. These points are easier to examine when the lamb crop is presented graphically (see Fig. 7.7). The first chart plots the different outcomes for warm, normal and cold years. The second chart plots only the line that specifies the minimum output for a combination of years. It is clear from this second chart that the maximum output in the worst scenario is 20 productive sheep and 80 hardy sheep.

Adopting the MAXIMIN policy would again be cautious as there are extra returns to be gained by adding a higher number of the productive breed to the flock. Most farmers would probably choose a point somewhere between this solution and a higher level of lamb crop production. What level that is can be examined by looking at the trade-off with risk expressed by plotting minimum return against total expected return. Note that the steepness of the curve is a reflection of the riskiness of the enterprise.

Assuming that the sheep farmer has to have a lamb crop of 70 per year to cover their farm and living expenses, a minimum output can be introduced that restricts the choice of combinations, but still leaves a wide choice. Alternatively, assuming that the sheep farmer's minimum is dependent on his utility function, the optimum level of output can be determined with indifference curves. The steepness of these indifference curves is related to the farmer's attitude to risk.

The range of species kept on a farm may help to reduce risk due to disease as different species will be affected by different diseases. However, for climatic problems, such as drought, it will probably mean that the risk is the same for all species and hence the variation of production is not minimized. In these situations it may be necessary to examine the

Table 7.6. Expected lamb crops, variance and mean absolute deviation for different combinations of sheep.

Number of productive breed sheep in a flock of 100	Number of lambs produced during			Expected yield	Var.	MAD
	Warm	Normal	Cold			
0	80	100	100	96	64	6.4
20	92	104	92	98	36	6.0
40	104	108	84	100	112	9.6
60	116	112	76	102	292	15.6
80	128	116	68	104	576	21.6
100	140	120	60	106	964	27.6

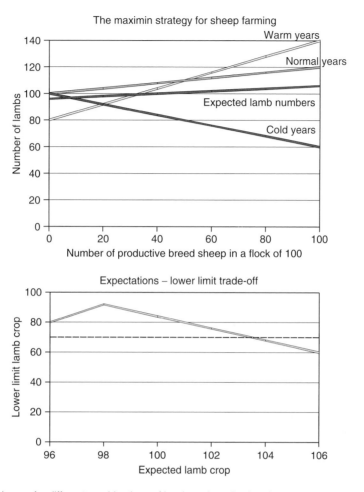

Fig. 7.7. Lamb crop for different combinations of hardy and productive sheep.

possibility of insurance or increased numbers of animals. Insurance may be in the form of some formal policy where money is paid to a company on the possibility that some costly event will occur in the future. In societies where there is no access to institutions that offer such insurance services, families will probably develop more complicated social ties. When times are good the family may give gifts and provide support for other families; when times are bad they will expect similar support from the families they have helped or paid patronage to in the past. Therefore, there are various means of coping with risk, first by reducing variation and second by putting in place mechanisms that alleviate bad situations when they occur either

through formal insurance or through informal social insurance policies.

Another concept that was introduced was a minimum level of output or threshold income required to meet basic requirements. In some situations this may mean a level that provides sufficient food and shelter for the family. In other societies it may be an income necessary to maintain a large house, three cars and private education. People's needs and utilities will generally reflect the expected level of income for the society in which people live. It would appear that if income can be guaranteed above a certain threshold people would accept variation in output or income. However, a large degree of variation may be unacceptable as it makes future planning difficult.

Mace and Houston (1989) present an analysis of the unpredictable environments of pastoralists in Africa and through modelling methods determine what combinations of camels and small ruminants provide a viable household income. The models they use are *stochastic* – a process that is random. The authors describe the long-term viability by minimizing the chances that the basic household needs will not be met. This is similar to minimum income or output discussed above. In their work they found that goats have the greatest variation in output, which means that they are unlikely to provide a good long-term viability. Model runs that begin only with goats and have no possibility of exchange for camels found that less than 1% of families would have a viable flock to maintain a family after a 15-year period. However, goats were important during good years to rapidly build up animal numbers. Once goat numbers have exceeded a level required to meet a basic household threshold, it is then important to convert the extra goats, which are risky, to the more stable camel units. This strategy provides long-term viability. If camel numbers drop below the threshold for minimum basic household needs there is a need to change the camels for goats to try to rebuild the family stock of animals. This is a risky strategy, but the alternative is a constantly reducing camel herd size. These conclusions from the modelling analysis are supported by empirical evidence, which reports that families adopt such strategies when animal numbers fall.

Practical tools for assessing risk

The theoretical aspects of risk and uncertainty described above are supported by a range of economic tools that can be applied when faced with an uncertain situation where risk needs to be quantified. The following will focus on sensitivity analysis, break-even analysis and decision tree analysis and pay-off tables.

Sensitivity analysis

Sensitivity analysis is used where uncertainty exists about prices of both inputs and outputs and where there is variation in the level of outputs due to environmental factors. A range of figures is provided for the parameters that are uncertain and the worst and best scenarios for the project or activity are used to perform separate gross margin analyses, partial budgets or cost–benefit analyses. Such analyses are greatly facilitated by using spreadsheets and being able to quickly change the factors that are known to be most variable.

The output of the sensitivity analysis can then be used to determine how sensitive a project or the activity is to changes in the costs and benefits that cannot be given definite values. In this manner, sensitivity analysis is estimating the risk of the activity and it can help indicate which prices or production levels have the greatest impact on project or activity profitability. If these are known, a farmer or a person involved in the livestock sector can use this information to monitor the most important variables. This is clearly an important method to prioritize data collection.

For livestock product systems that are heavily reliant on concentrate feed inputs such as pig, poultry and dairy units the price of concentrate feed is likely to influence the profitability of the enterprise. Sensitivity analysis can be used to determine the range of prices that an enterprise can support. The analysis will also help a producer to make investments in data collection on sourcing and pricing feed from different locations. In some situations costs of such activities may be borne by a group, perhaps through a cooperative.

Break-even analysis

Break-even analysis is a form of sensitivity analysis where the search is for a value of a parameter, be it a price or a level of output, which will produce a zero profit or NPV. For example, the IRR is actually the break-even rate of return for an investment or cost–benefit appraisal. The technique can be modified to produce an answer which would produce an output value which is an acceptable threshold for an enterprise or a family.

Decision analysis, decision trees and pay-off tables

Livestock production and health decisions often involve a series of events, some of which can be controlled and others happen by chance. For example, the occurrence of FMD on a farm involves chance events like the entry of the virus to a property and also control events such as vaccination of the herd. The decision to vaccinate is often taken through an informal analysis of the risk of the virus entering the farm and the impact of the disease if it occurs on the farm. Similarly, decisions on tick control involve a process of examining the risks of clinical tick-borne disease occurring, the impact of a tick-borne disease once it does occur and the costs of controlling ticks. Such decisions are often taken with informal or 'gut feeling' analysis, but they can be improved by the use of decision analysis.

Decision analysis is a method for formally analysing complicated decisions which involve a sequential series of actions and chance events. It involves the identification of three aspects within the decision: the events which a decision maker can control such as vaccination, treatment of animals or culling of animals; the probability of the occurrence of chance events, which are events such as the entry of a virus in a farm, the biting of a naive animal by a tick infected with babesiosis or the delivery of feed contaminated with meat-and-bone meal from BSE-infected cattle; the value of various outcomes, normally, but not necessarily, expressed in monetary terms. This could be the cost of vaccinating, cost of a disease outbreak without treatment or cost of a disease outbreak with treatment.

Once a decision has identified these three items, a quantitative analysis is performed using either pay-off tables and/or decision trees.

Pay-off tables

The use of a pay-off table is best demonstrated by a simple example. A farmer has 100 ewes and is worried because enzootic abortion has occurred in some of the neighbouring farms. They want to know whether to vaccinate the ewes (at US$1 per head), treat with antibiotics if the disease occurs, or do nothing. The vaccine is known to be 100% effective. The estimated costs of an outbreak of enzootic abortion in the flock, if left untreated, is US$1100 while treatment of the outbreak is estimated to result in losses of US$400 (cost of treatments plus disease losses). Records kept at the regional veterinary office reveal that about 20% of sheep flocks in a district are affected by enzootic abortion once it occurs in the area. The above information could be summarized in a pay-off table (see Table 7.7).

Under each programme are three columns: the net benefit of the programme–outcome combination (US$), the probability of the programme–outcome combination (p) and the expected value of the programme–outcome combination (US$ $* p$). The sum of the expected values of the programme–outcome combinations for a particular programme is the expected value of the programme.

In the above example, the programme with the highest expected value, i.e. the lowest expected cost, is the one involving treatment (–US$80). However, it must be emphasized that this expected cost of US$80 is an average value which will not apply to any single flock in any particular year. Under the treatment option, a single flock will either have no losses or lose US$400. Thus, for a risk-averse farmer, the vaccination programme might be more

Table 7.7. Hypothetical pay-off table for three programmes for the control of enzootic abortion in a flock of 100 ewes.

| Outcome | Programme | | | | | | | | |
| | Vaccinate | | | Treat | | | Do nothing | | |
	US$	p	US$ $* p$	US$	p	US$ $* p$	US$	p	US$ $* p$
Disease	–100	0.0	0	–400	0.2	–80	–1100	0.2	–220
No disease	–100	1.0	–100	0	0.8	0	0	0.8	0
Expected value		–100			–80			–220	

attractive as it is associated with the least maximum loss (–US$100). For an opportunity cost of US$20, the farmer could purchase the freedom from having to worry about the possibility of a US$400 loss. This would be the MINIMAX strategy for this decision. The 'do nothing' programme can be ruled out entirely, as it is associated with the worst expected value and the highest maximum loss. Note that the programme that offers the maximum disease control, i.e. vaccination, is not the programme that offers the maximum expected value.

Decision trees

All pay-off tables can also be presented as decision trees. The advantage of decision trees, however, is that they can explicitly depict the chronology of events and can be used to evaluate a sequence of decisions. The following example serves to illustrate how a decision tree can be used to help make a decision. A farmer wants to know what type of tick control strategy to adopt and whether to treat and retain animals with clinical tick-borne disease symptoms or to treat and cull. The following information has been provided about the situation:

1. There are three tick control options: no control; strategic control, which costs US$10 per animal per year; and all-year control, which costs US$30 per animal per year.
2. The probability of animals showing clinical tick-borne disease for the no control strategy is 40%, for strategic control 20% and for all-year control 10%.
3. The cost of treating an animal with clinical tick-borne disease is US$25.
4. The loss in income if the animal is culled is the difference between the salvage value and the replacement animal cost. A culled animal is valued at US$150 and a replacement animal at US$215.
5. The loss in production from an animal treated and retained in the herd is estimated to be US$35 during the year. This loss is due to a lower growth rate.

Decision trees are constructed from left to right (see Fig. 7.8), beginning with the earliest decision that has to be made.

- *Decision points* (nodes) are drawn as squares, and lines (branches) coming out of such decision nodes represent the complete set of mutually exclusive options being considered.
- Circles represent *chance nodes*. Branches coming out of chance nodes represent the complete set of mutually exclusive chance events that might occur at that point.
- All *branches* must be labelled, and branches for chance events have probability values.
- The *net benefit* of each path through the tree is identified at the terminal branch.

In this example there are two decision node points:

- the tick control strategy;
- cull or retain sick and treated animals.

There is also a chance event node which relates to the probability of an animal getting clinical tick-borne disease.

A decision tree for the above example would look like the one in Fig. 7.8.

The tree is 'solved' by 'averaging out' and 'folding back'. Starting at the terminal decision, expected values are calculated for each decision (averaging out) and the most profitable decision is identified. The expected value of a node is written into the node, and the option which has been discarded is 'folded back' by drawing a double bar through its branch. Ultimately, the paths not blocked by double bars will specify the sequence of decisions that will yield the greatest expected profit.

In the example above, the decision to cull or retain in all cases would be to retain the animal after treatment. The option to cull is therefore discarded. The tick control strategy is slightly more complicated in that the outcomes of each branch need to be multiplied by the probabilities of the chance node. All workings are show in Fig. 7.8 and in this example a strategic control strategy for ticks with a policy to treat and retain any sick animals would give the lowest long-term costs for tick-borne disease control.

In situations where probabilities are not accurately known, as is often the case, the decision tree analysis could be combined with sensitivity analysis to examine how robust the final output is.

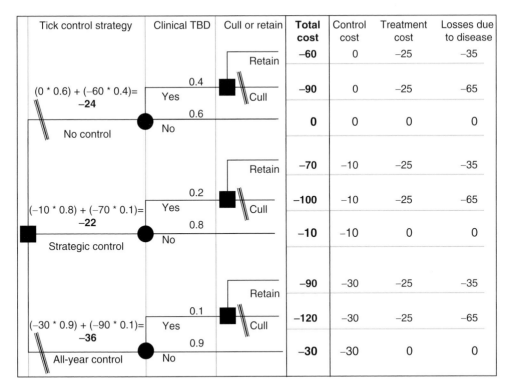

Fig. 7.8. Decision tree for tick control strategy

A thorough decision analysis would involve the following steps:

1. Define the problem and the different actions available.
2. Construct a decision tree for complicated decisions or a pay-off table for more straightforward decisions.
3. Specify the probabilities for each chance event.
4. Calculate the output or costs for each possible outcome of the decision.
5. Calculate the expected values by multiplying the calculated costs or output values with the probabilities at the chance events.
6. Select an option or options for the control points of the decision.
7. Test the robustness of the options by using sensitivity analysis on parameters that are known to vary.

Hardaker *et al.* (1997) present a realistic example of decision tree analysis for decision making on FMD control in a country previ-ously free. Using this methodology they con-clude that culling animals in infected herds and those herds in contact with these herds is superior and less risky than only culling infected herds. They also find that, if an out-break is prolonged, vaccination would reduce risks. Such analyses help decision makers during times of crisis, but it should be noted that because probabilities are introduced they do not provide definitive answers, only guidance on what would be the best solution under different levels of risk.

Mixing risk assessments with time

A country has had reported outbreaks of FMD since the 1930s. Since the late 1990s, a number of campaigns have been implemented to control and eradicate the disease. However, all have failed to come close to the coverage of vaccination required to eradicate FMD. Given the poor support for the campaigns by the livestock owners in areas known to be endemic, an economic analysis is requested for the extensive beef systems in these zones. The initial results show that the main economic impact of a FMD outbreak in the extensive beef systems occurs between 4 and 5 years after the disease has been present.

Epidemiological data indicate that the risk of having a FMD outbreak on a farm is low, and estimates from official data would suggest the risk of an outbreak is every 20 years. Given that these data are unlikely to include all outbreaks, it would be safe to assume that a farm has a risk of having a FMD outbreak every 10 years. It is recognized that some have greater risk where there is greater cattle movement and 10 years would be an average across the cattle rearing region.

With this information a simple risk analysis is presented below. The analysis uses discounted costs and losses for the different outcomes and assumes that once the disease is eradicated the farms can stop vaccination (see Tables 7.8–7.10).

The risk analysis demonstrates that the incentive for the extensive beef farmer to participate in control programmes is small and possibly non-existent. Until a programme is implemented that will achieve short-term results, it would appear that the farmer would be better off taking the risk that FMD will arrive at the farm and treating all animals that become sick. Policy implications are that the Government should not advertise FMD control campaigns until it has the financing and power to implement a strong campaign.

Table 7.8. Discounted costs if FMD is eradicated in 3 years and there is the possibility of an outbreak every 10 years.

	No vaccination control		One vaccination per year		Two vaccinations per year	
	Cost	Probability	Cost	Probability	Cost	Probability
Outbreak	3921.51	0.10	1512.25	0.10	600.50	0
No outbreak	–	0.90	444.37	0.90	600.50	1
Outcome	392.15		551.16		600.50	

Table 7.9. Discounted costs if FMD is eradicated in 5 years and there is the possibility of an outbreak every 10 years.

	No vaccination control		One vaccination per year		Two vaccinations per year	
	Cost	Probability	Cost	Probability	Cost	Probability
Outbreak	3921.51	0.10	1744.49	0.10	913.91	0
No outbreak	–	0.90	676.60	0.90	913.91	1
Outcome	392.15		783.39		913.31	

Table 7.10. Discounted costs if FMD is eradicated in 5 years and there is the possibility of an outbreak every 10 years.

	No vaccination control		One vaccination per year		Two vaccinations per year	
	Cost	Probability	Cost	Probability	Cost	Probability
Outbreak	3921.51	0.10	2162.26	0.10	1474.17	0
No outbreak	–	0.90	1094.38	0.90	1474.17	1
Outcome	392.15		1201.17		1474.17	

Summary

There are a number of analytical tools for handling risk and uncertainty in the study of the economics of animal health and production. Risk is where the decision maker knows the alternative outcomes and can attach a probability to each of them. Uncertainty is where the decision maker has less information on the outcomes of a decision and also cannot attach probabilities to their outcomes.

Conventional farm management analysis techniques summary

The relatively simple structure of conventional farm management analysis techniques makes them an ideal medium to interact and participate with farmers in decision making. They are basically rudimentary simulation models that cannot provide optimal solutions, but they can give information that a family may require to make decisions about their farming system. The output from these conventional tools assumes that the farm decision makers are profit maximizers and, as Dorward (1984) states, these conventional farm management tools, though well suited to 'commercial farmers', are of little use to 'subsistence farmers', who rely more on qualitative data for making decisions.

If the need for a single financial output were relaxed, qualitative data could be provided using the basic structure of conventional farm management methods. For example, resource use and production can be shown graphically to identify resource conflicts. Dorward et al. (1996) discuss the combined use of conventional farm management tools and rapid rural appraisal (RRA) and participatory rural appraisal (PRA) approaches. They suggest new, more relevant smallholder farming systems analysis structures, such as participatory budgeting, resource-flow diagramming and developing appropriate combinations of tools to form simple models. These techniques are still to be tested in the field, but methods that generate a mixture of conventional and qualitative output are seen as being appropriate for assisting smallholder farm planning and management.

Complex farm management analysis techniques

Complex farm management analysis techniques are split into two basic categories: optimization techniques and complex simulation techniques. Optimization techniques identify a solution to a farming system that is optimal to a set objective. Complex simulation methods use a combination of decision structures to determine how a plan will proceed.

Optimization approaches

Construction of an optimization model requires the specification of a resource and activity matrix, which includes all possible activities and the constraints on resource use and production. The matrix is solved according to an objective function, which should reflect the priorities of the manager of the farming system. Early models relied on the assumption that farm families were profit maximizers, or some other simple objective, and that the activity input and outputs were certain and had non-integer output.

The simple objective functions proved unsatisfactory as a representation of farm family priorities. Zuckerman (1973) found that his optimization model generated an unrealistic farming system for the area he had collected data from. Delforce (1994) also found limitations of an objective function based around profit maximization. Lopes (1990) using a linear programming model, with a profit maximizing objective function, to assess smallholder dairy systems in Brazil developed conclusions that appear impractical for such systems.

Other issues are required in the objective function, such as the need to guarantee certain levels of home-grown food grains, social status in the community and dislike of the drudgery of labour. There is also a need for a list of priorities, rather than a single goal (Romero and Rehman, 1984). This has given rise to an interest in the use of multiple objectives, or multiple criteria decision analysis, where an objective function can include more than one goal and the list can be satisfied in some chosen order (Romero and Rehman, 1989). McGregor et al. (1994) discuss the use of this approach for guiding decision making in grazing systems. While this may provide a better method of representing the decision-making unit, it requires careful data collection to determine the objective function.

Zuckerman (1973) also found problems with the type of output generated by his optimization model in terms of non-integer output. He recommended the use of integer programming, a technique described by France and Thornley (1984, pp. 58–59).

The use of activities with uncertain inputs and outputs has been overcome by a number of mathematical techniques, such as parametric programming, to examine the way an optimal solution changes as one or more input coefficient varies (France and Thornley, 1984, pp. 55–57). These models allow the generation of a mean and a variance for different plans. To determine the minimum variance for each expected level of income from a plan, it is necessary to minimize a quadratic statement. This can be done by quadratic programming algorithms (Hazell and Norton, 1986, pp. 81–84). However, this programming method can only deal with a limited number of dimensions, and other techniques have been developed to get around this problem such as MOTAD (Hazell and Norton, 1986, pp. 86–90). The use of these techniques increases the complexity of the optimization technique further.

The literature contains many examples of optimization models applied to farming systems analysis. Bhende and Venkataram (1994) develop a quadratic, risk programming model to assess the effect of adopting a dairy enterprise in a smallholder farming system. They conclude that the adoption is beneficial both in terms of risk and income. However, their analysis lacks a livestock system model, which suggests that the analysis is incomplete. Morrison *et al.* (1986) developed a mixed integer programming model to represent the dry land crop–livestock system in Western Australia. The model was validated through a feedback process involving farmers, farm consultants and technical experts. The model objective function was profit maximization, and the model represents in detail biological, technological and financial relationships and enterprise interdependencies. The model produced a well-balanced farming system, unlike the single enterprise solutions provided by

simpler optimization models. Their work demonstrated that the additional biological information greatly improved the quality of optimization model output.

OPTIMIZATION APPROACH SUMMARY. The identification of an 'optimal' solution and also the availability of shadow prices from optimization models make them an attractive structure to analyse a production process. These models essentially replace the need for a decision maker, and in some instances are used to assess how a general decision maker will react to a change in an environment. Optimization models are, therefore, of interest to researchers investigating decision-making processes, and in particular predicting responses to change.

Constructing and interpreting optimization models is intellectually stimulating and requires considerable skill. However, optimization techniques suffer a number of problems in their application to farming systems. These are highlighted as follows:

1. Optimization models require the specification of an objective function and constraints, which in turn require either:
  • data collection and analysis;
  • trial and error to produce an objective function that can adequately mimic the original system.
2. Given that an objective function can be defined, the subsequent use of an optimization model as a predictive tool has an underlying assumption that the objective function will remain unchanged over time. Evidence of farming systems evolution suggests that objective functions are not always static.
3. The structure of an optimization model does not allow easy adaptation to different farming systems.
4. The complexity of optimization, and the basic idea that an optimization model produces an 'optimal' solution, restricts and confines people's willingness to question the model output. This problem is experienced with highly qualified researchers (Lopes, 1990) as well as with farmers.
5. The provision of an optimal solution discourages researchers to go and discuss results with the people their models are trying to mimic.

6. The assumption that an optimal solution can be found implies that all relevant data are available. This raises the question of whether it is optimal to search for these data.

Complex simulation techniques

A complex simulation is taken to be the process of setting up a model of a real situation and then performing experiments with it (Wright, 1971). The simulation methods include structures such as decision tree analysis, and also models that have specific decision points that are solved according to a criteria list or an interactive process with the user.

The use of simulation models has so far been rather limited (Wright, 1971; Dorward, 1984) because of the difficulty of construction and the specificity of each model (Dorward, 1984). The problem of specificity can be overcome to some extent by modification of existing models, and the establishment of a database of available model structures (Wright, 1971). Some of the issues discussed with the application of gross margin analysis are, therefore, similar to these model structures.

A number of simulation models are reported in the literature. Van Elderen (1987) developed a simulation model for scheduling farm operations with particular reference to wheat harvesting. Finlayson et al. (1995) developed a simulation model to represent a sheep system. Berdegue et al. (1989), Richardson et al. (1993) and Cacho et al. (1995) developed computer simulation models of mixed farming systems, and Thomas (1991) developed a spreadsheet simulation model to examine agroforestry systems. The Berdegue et al. (1989) and Richardson et al. (1993) models will be discussed further in the section on livestock orientated farm/household models (p. 99). Beck and Dent (1987) produced a simulation model of extensive pastoral farming systems found in North Island, New Zealand. They included consumption and production of the farm household in the model, and attempted to use it for policy analysis.

Wilson (1979) and Thomson and Bahhady (1995) attempted a live simulation of backyard poultry and crop–sheep farming systems, respectively. Both studies found it useful to be able to monitor the livestock closely, but found it difficult to mimic the real farm systems on a research station (Wilson, 1979; Thomson et al., 1995).

Dorward (1991) developed an interactive, stochastic simulation model of a smallholder farming system in Malawi. Critical decision points were identified in the calendar of the farming system. Model runs require the user to make decisions at the critical times, and therefore influence the final model output. Dorward (1984, 1986b, 1991) argues that such structures are a good method for the communication and analysis of peasant farm management. He also emphasizes the general importance of decision rule structures for encouraging dialogue between farmers, extension staff and research services. However, the model reported is very specific, and lacks a livestock component.

Jarvis (1974) adapted a simulation model to obtain a suitable age of sale for Argentinean cattle systems. The model selects the optimal age at sale by identifying the point at which the increase in animal value equals the rate of interest. Jarvis (1980) applied the same model structure to an African context in response to what he believed to be a mis-specification of livestock sale response by Doran et al. (1979). Ariza-Nino and Shapiro (1984) and Steinfeld (1988) also used the model to determine the age of sale of livestock in African pastoralist and mixed farming systems, respectively.

COMPLEX SIMULATION MODEL SUMMARY. Simulation models are generally felt to be unsatisfactory because they fail to provide the sort of objective results generated from 'more formal and general optimising algorithms' (Dorward, 1984). However, the inability to find a solution can also be viewed as a strength, as it should encourage discussion with farm-level decision makers.

Complex farm management analysis techniques summary

Complex farm management analysis techniques have generally been rejected by commercial farmers, because they overemphasize planning, are only applicable as a starting point to planning and are of little use during the general running of operations (Dorward, 1984). This suggests that these structures are inflexible, which potentially reduces their value for sensitivity analysis.

Farm management analysis techniques summary

The use of farm management analysis techniques for smallholder farming systems analysis is relevant, but there is a general lack of suitable techniques (Dorward, 1986a). Conventional farm management analysis techniques are limited to simple investigations of smallholder crop–livestock farming systems. In-depth investigations require more information on enterprise interactions, decision-maker objectives and dynamics of the livestock systems. Complex farm management analysis techniques have attempted to address these issues, but in the process have become too complex for easy experimentation. Many of these complex techniques have also failed to adequately investigate the human components of the farming systems (Dent *et al.*, 1995), and lack structures to investigate the dynamics of livestock systems. The next two sections, therefore, review household modelling techniques and livestock systems modelling.

Household Modelling Techniques

The difference between complex farm management modelling techniques and household modelling is, in some instances, not great. Many household models use the same techniques as complex farm management. However, one critical component that sets household modelling apart is the recognition of the value of household time in any production or consumption activity. Many farm household models draw on Chayanov's farm household theory, and on 'new home economics' (Ellis, 1988). The latter subject originates from a paper by Becker (1965) on time allocation within the household.

Nakajima (1986) in his thesis 'Subjective Equilibrium Theory of the Farm Household' introduces the 'farm household as an economic unit into economic theory'. He represents the farm household as three interacting subsys-

tems, 'the farm-firm, the labourer's household and the household consumer'. The theoretical structure developed is a useful basis for quantitative modelling work (Delforce, 1993; Holden, 1993).

Low (1986) applies a household modelling approach to describe the rationale of reduced maize output in Swaziland. The predominant factor in the Swaziland farming systems was the existence of an off-farm labour market for able-bodied males. This reduced the labour available in the farm, which encouraged families to adopt labour-saving activities. High-yielding varieties of maize, which produce high yields per unit land area, were selected because family food grain needs could be satisfied from a smaller land area and less labour.

Barnum and Squire (1979) developed a farm household model in which consumption and production activities were separated. This was justified on the basis of mathematical reasoning and the existence of markets. Their approach used econometric methods to represent the production and consumption sub-models and they applied it to a relatively simple rice-based farming system in Malaysia. Singh *et al.* (1986) discuss the use of this model structure, and present a number of case studies to which the model has been applied. However, Delforce (1993 and 1994) questioned its applicability where econometric techniques are not used for the sub-models.

Household modelling summary

Household modelling has become an increasingly important method for assessing the economic rationale of farm-level decision making, and is an expanding subject, as demonstrated by the recent household modelling book edited by Caillavet *et al.* (1994). However, household modelling approaches have been criticized by Hunt (1991) for:

1. Not fully exploring the production aspects of the household;
2. Ignoring the interactions between production activities;

3. Failing to consider intra-household division of labour;

4. Failing to recognize rigidities and tensions of intra-household resource control; and

5. Failing to give a seasonal value to household time.

In addition to the above criticisms, most quantitative household models attempt to replace the decision-making units, in order to investigate general responses to resource price, resource access or technology change. The results are intended to be of use to policy makers, but do not directly assist farm-level decision makers.

Livestock Models and Their Use in Farming System Analysis

Farm management analysis techniques and household modelling methods provide an adequate structure for analysing economic decision making, but often fail due to poor specification of individual enterprise production functions (Dorward, 1984). This is particularly true for livestock systems, where there are many difficulties in providing simple enterprise input/output relationships. This section, therefore, reviews available livestock models, and examines how some of these structures have either been extended or used within farming systems analysis.

Livestock models

A number of livestock models are reported in the literature (Sanders and Cartwright, 1979a,b; Brockington et al., 1983; Baptiste, 1987; Shaw, 1989; McLeod, 1993; James and Carles, 1996). To assess livestock models it is useful to identify common modelling techniques and classify models accordingly. McLeod (1993) reviews the classification of livestock models and provides a method of her own (Fig. 7.9).

Analytical models

Analytical models are used to investigate how closely observed data fit with a hypothesized relationship. This is mainly applied to determining the effect of management on different aspects of livestock production. Gitau et al. (1994) make use of this approach to investigate the factors influencing daily weight gain in calves. Wood (1967) and Groenewald et al. (1996) use an analytical approach to determine milk lactation curves for cattle and sheep, respectively. Schlecht et al. (1993) also use this approach to develop relationships between the feed management and manure output. Muchena (1993) used production function analysis to estimate the value of non-tradable livestock products in the mixed farming systems of Zimbabwe. Accurate analytical models can, therefore, predict parameters for a livestock system, which could then be incorporated into livestock system models. However,

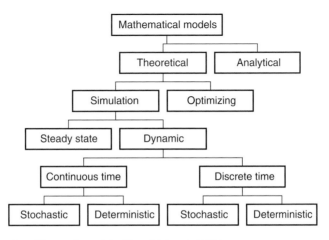

Fig. 7.9. Classification of livestock models. (From McLeod, 1993.)

the approach has relatively limited value to represent the livestock system as a whole.

Optimization models

Many livestock-orientated optimization models exist in the literature, and their structure is similar to the optimization models described above. Kennedy (1986, chapter 7) reviews early optimization models used to evaluate livestock replacement problems. These combine information on feed formulation, growth rates and other productions aspects of a number of livestock species. Nicholson *et al.* (1994) developed a deterministic, multi-period linear programming model to assess the cattle production systems in Sur del Lago, Venezuela. The model produced plans that were more profitable than the traditional farming system. However, these plans were dependent on labour availability. Houben (1995) used a stochastic, dynamic programming model to assess individual cow insemination and replacement decisions in a Dutch dairy system.

Mace and Houston (1989) use a stochastic, dynamic programming model of a livestock production system to evaluate herding strategies. The model relies on input parameters for births and deaths, with sales and slaughter of animals being influenced by household needs. The proportions of camel and small stock in the total herd are optimized according to an objective function that aims to maximize long-term household viability. The model is used to show that goats, while being more prolific, are a riskier enterprise, and that a mixed herd is preferable to specialization (see p. 86 for a fuller description of this model).

The livestock optimization models have similar problems to those listed for the farm management optimization models.

Steady state or static herd models

Static models assess livestock production over a set period, usually a year, and assume that the herd/flock size will not vary over time. Herd/flock size is maintained by altering the level of offtake. The livestock production efficiency calculator (LPEC; James and Carles, 1996) and prying livestock productivity (PRY; Baptiste, 1992) are examples of such models. Static models are particularly useful for assessing livestock productivity (Upton, 1989), but are rather difficult to apply in a smallholder farming system.

LPEC (Livestock Production Efficiency Calculator)

LPEC is a livestock model which is essentially a livestock productivity index calculation. It requires a set of production parameters from a livestock system (large and small ruminants or pigs) and uses these to calculate a herd structure and productivity for that system. The model adapts the herd structure to ensure that the herd size reflects the use of feed resources. The productivity is expressed in terms of the value of herd or flock output per unit of feed intake and therefore is a measure of feed conversion efficiency at herd level.

The main use of LPEC is to compare the productivity of different production systems or the same production system under different conditions, for example a system with different levels of disease prevalence.

According to the developers of this model the system of calculations has two advantages over other models:

1. LPEC expresses productivity as production per unit of feed intake, which means it takes into account the weight of the animals in the system. Conventional systems that express output per unit of animal do not take into account different levels of feed required for different breeds. This aspect is particularly relevant in comparison between indigenous breeds and improved breeds.
2. The LPEC system takes into account all determinants of productivity and their interactions and it can be used to analyse a range of production systems and species (cattle, buffalo, sheep, goats and pigs) taking into account products such as manure and draught power if necessary. This in turn means that LPEC is data demanding; however, missing information can be replaced by assumptions, expert opinion or information from the literature.

In addition to the points mentioned above the author would add that the LPEC model is useful in structuring data collection of livestock information to generate parameters that can be used to assess livestock productivity. This may appear to be a simple task, but in reality, without an analytical structure, data collection for the economic assessment of livestock and the related diseases is very difficult.

LPEC divides the herd or flock into the following categories:

- breeding females – cows after the first day of the first calving;
- replacement females (suckling) – females that are used to replace culled breeding females or breeding females that die;
- replacement females (weaned) – females that are used to replace culled breeding females or breeding females that die;
- surplus females 1 (suckling) – females not needed for replacement and can be sold;
- surplus females 1 (weaned) – females not needed for replacement and can be sold;
- surplus females 2 (suckling) – females not needed for replacement and can be sold;
- surplus females 2 (weaned) – females not needed for replacement and can be sold;
- breeding males;
- replacement males (suckling) – males that are used to replace culled breeding males or breeding males that die;
- replacement males (weaned) – males that are used to replace culled breeding males or breeding males that die;
- surplus males 1 (suckling) – males not needed for replacement and can be sold;
- surplus males 1 (weaned) – males not needed for replacement and can be sold;
- surplus males 2 (suckling) – males not needed for replacement and can be sold;
- surplus males 2 (weaned) – males not needed for replacement and can be sold.

Note there are two categories of surplus animals to allow the possibility of have different management systems for this group. For example, some of the surplus animals may be sold after weaning, while others may remain on the farm until they are fattened or reach maturity.

The model requires the following data:
Mortality and culling rates:

- mortality rate (% per year) for each category;
- culling rate (% per year) for breeding females and males.

Young stock survival and rearing policy:

- percentage survival of young animals to 24 h old (females and males);
- percentage suitable as replacements (females and males);
- percentage of surplus reared as type 1 (females and males);
- percentage remaining as surplus 2 – calculated automatically (males and females);
- percentage of replacement females barren;
- percentage of surplus 1 and 2 females pregnant;
- percentage of surplus 1 and 2 males castrated.

Birth weights, mature weights and ages:

- For replacement males and females and surplus males and females:
  - birth weight;
  - age and weight at weaning;
  - age and weight at maturity.

Metabolizable energy data:

- For all classes of animals:
  - mean feed metabolizability;
  - activity coefficient.
- For milk production net energy required per kilo of milk produced.

Fertility and breeding female management:

- number of breeding females per breeding male;
- parturition rate (similar but not equivalent to the fertility rate);
- mean number of offspring per parturition;
- mean weight lost in early lactation;
- mean weight gain between parturitions;
- mean milk offtake per lactation.

Value of offtake and replacement stock:

- culled and surplus males and females;
- milk;
- mature replacement males and females.

Optional economic parameters:

- salvage value of dead animals for each class of animal;
- other costs per year for each class of animal.

Purchased feed parameters:

- For each class of animal:
  - maximum metabolizable energy (ME) from forage per day;
  - cost of purchased feed.

The model uses these parameters to predict the herd structure according to the energy requirements within the herd and in order to maintain a stable herd structure. Therefore, if parameters such as parturition rate are low and age at maturity is high, the model will automatically buy in replacements to cover the need to replace females within the herd. It will also calculate the need to purchase feed according to the needs of the herd. In addition it produces an estimation of the value of output for a herd that receives 100 MJ of ME per day throughout the year.

The model does not have stochastic parameter input but it is possible to run sensitivity analysis for parameters known to be affected by a disease. For example, parturition rate is a reflection of breeding efficiency and the model will produce a graph showing different productivity levels with varying parturition rate. (Note: the output is a productivity measure and not a level of production.)

For further information on the basic workings of the model readers are directed to the LPEC User Guide (PAN Livestock Services, 1991); for the theoretical aspects of the model to James and Carles (1996).

Dynamic, continuous time models

The dynamic, continuous time models have been used with some success in the study of disease (Anderson and May, 1985). The complex mathematical nature of these models limits their develop and interpretation of their outputs to highly skilled mathematicians. Whilst they can be of value, their complexity can often limit discussion.

Dynamic, discrete time models

A dynamic, discrete time livestock model simulates a herd/flock over a time period often specified by the user. Herd/flock size is usually not constrained and is dependent upon the mortality, offtake and fecundity parameters used. There are two basic types of dynamic live-stock models: deterministic and stochastic. The distinction between these two types of model is the treatment of data input parameters.

Dynamic, deterministic models take no account of input parameter variability, and have no structure to take account of chance outcomes. The output from a dynamic, deterministic model for any set of production parameters will always be the same. The final herd/flock numbers will usually not be integers. CLIPPER (Shaw, 1989) and the livestock models used in TIES (Richardson et al., 1993) are examples of dynamic, deterministic models. Dynamic, deterministic models are of greatest use where the herd size is large and the numbers can be converted to whole numbers without much loss in accuracy.

CLIPPER

CLIPPER (Shaw, 1989) is a spreadsheet-based model which is capable of comparing a herd or a flock with and without a disease. The model contains a dynamic, deterministic herd model and cost–benefit analysis structure. The basic data required are:

- initial number of animals divided into males and females and age categories of 0–1, 1–2, 2–3 and greater than 3 years old;
- mortality and offtake rates for different categories of animals;
- fertility rates.

This information is required for the herd or flock with and without disease. This model is suited to assessing cattle or buffalo disease problems and is recommended as a good starting point for assessing large ruminant disease impact. Modifications are needed for small ruminants, pigs and poultry and users need to be aware that often benefits become large simply because of herd or flock growth and the model is not able to calculate the extra feed requirements.

The model reported by Sanders and Cartwright (1979a) is also a dynamic deterministic model. Animal performance and mortality in this model are determined by the availability of feed. However, livestock models driven by availability of resources, rather than estimated outputs, are data-demanding and dependent on the quality of the available information on the relationship between inputs and outputs. The latter will often be affected by local environments, making such models difficult to apply generally.

Dynamic, stochastic livestock models do take account of production parameter variability. Parameters such as mortality and offtake can be represented as probabilities of events occurring. These model input parameters are not variable, but the model can use them to produce a stochastic output. This can be achieved by comparing the probability of an event occurring with a randomly generated number. A slightly different method is to allow parameters such as offspring live weight, inter-oestrus periods to be specified as a mean and standard deviation. A model can use the mean and standard deviation to select a value from a normal distribution curve.

A stochastic model output for any set of production parameters will not be the same for each run, and the final herd/flock numbers produced will be integers. The output from a number of model runs can be used subsequently to produce a mean output with a standard deviation. Dynamic, stochastic models are useful where a simulation needs to generate integer output on animal numbers. Such models are also of great potential use in the assessment of risk, as their output provides an indication of variation.

McLeod (1993) developed a stochastic, discrete time dynamic model to analyse the epidemiology of infectious disease. Brockington et al. (1986) describe the use of a similar model (Brockington et al., 1983) to analyse short-term feeding and breeding management decisions of smallholder dairy producers in Brazil.

Jalvingh (1993) uses a model that combines aspects of stochastic and deterministic models for an on-farm decision support system. The model uses a 'finite-state Markov chain approach', which includes probability distributions. It requires the specification of the possible states (i.e. production levels) that an animal can be in and the possible transitions between these states. This model generates technical and economic results for a herd by combining numbers of animals per state with the simulated performances per state. Such a model produces a single output, which is effectively a weighted average. However, it cannot generate a standard deviation and therefore could not be used for risk assessment. It also is not possible to use this model structure to produce integer output.

Livestock model summary

Many livestock models are available, but very few incorporate farming systems components. The importance of the farming system for livestock development is well recognized, and has stimulated the development of livestock-orientated farm/household models.

Livestock-orientated farm/household models

Four livestock-orientated household models are identified as being potentially useful for assessing farming systems with livestock: TIES (Richardson et al., 1993), GRANJAS (Berdegue et al., 1989), 3WAY and PCHerd (Udo and Brouwer, 1993) and a spreadsheet model developed by Gulbenkian (1993).

Udo and Brouwer (1993) developed a database and analysis structure, 3WAY, and a livestock model, PCHerd, during a project in Bangladesh. PCHerd is a stochastic livestock model capable of simulating ruminant species to predict livestock production performance. The model can either be run to examine herd dynamics or to look at individual animal performance. Predictions of animal performance are based on a series of rules about feed availability and animal response. The model also includes a traction component, which requires a specification of the draught power requirements of the farm. The selection of animals to perform draught power tasks is on the basis of animal weight and condition, and every animal is assumed to be available to perform a task.

PCHerd has been shown to be useful for livestock research prioritization. However, the rule structure for performance is based on a limited number of feed trial experiments, and the traction module does not appear to allow farmer preference for traction animals. The model also looks at how livestock production is constrained by the farming system, but not how the farming system may in turn be affected by the livestock system. Udo and Brouwer (1993) state that modelling the whole farm requires extra modules to examine resource flows and solutions using optimization or multi-criteria analysis techniques.

TIES (Richardson *et al.*, 1993) is a stochastic household model developed by a team from ILRAD (now ILRI) and Texas A&M. TIES has been used to assess East Coast fever control in Kenyan smallholder farming systems (Nyangito *et al.*, 1994, 1995, 1996a,b). The stochastic elements of the model are yields and prices. The livestock modelling structure is dynamic and deterministic with a constraint on herd size. The model has important merits, in that it is capable of examining the variability of farm output due to either price or yield fluctuations. However, as a tool to examine in greater detail the improvements of the livestock system within the whole-farm system, it is not entirely satisfactory. This problem was shown during a study by van Schaik (1995) in Murang'a District, Kenya, which used a separate livestock model to examine livestock changes more thoroughly.

GRANJAS was developed by a team at the Catholic University of Louvain, and applied to a Chilean peasant farm situation (Berdegue *et al.*, 1989). It simulates household resource use and balance for each month over any specified period. The user can specify the initial quantities of resources, the levels of activities and the simulation period. The model appears not to have a component to model the livestock system. Therefore, GRANJAS is useful for examining resource flows, but cannot examine, in depth, a livestock system.

Gulbenkian (1993) developed a dynamic sheep model on a spreadsheet. It included modules to represent flock growth, on-farm forage-growing activities and a least-cost ration programme to determine feed management. This model generated an enterprise gross margin, which was combined with simple gross margins of other enterprises to develop farm gross margin, profit and net farm income.

Livestock and livestock-orientated model summary

Livestock models that are useful for examining the livestock enterprises have been developed, but it is often difficult to apply them to farm-level analysis problems. Some livestock-orientated household models have been developed. Of those highlighted in this review, PCHerd (Udo and Brouwer, 1993) provides an inadequate structure for the farming system, and also complicates the livestock model with decision structures based on limited experimental work. TIES (Richardson *et al.*, 1993) and GRANJAS (Berdegue *et al.*, 1989) have limited economic analysis and livestock system modelling structures. Finally, Gulbenkian's (1993) model is of great interest, but it is area- and species-specific.

Economic Assessment of the Role of Livestock in Mixed Farming Systems

A number of empirical studies have been carried out to assess the economic importance of livestock in mixed farming systems. These generally use a mixture of the techniques described above.

Steinfeld (1988) studied the mixed farming systems in the Midlands and Masvingo districts of Zimbabwe. He claims to build models of resource use and production in mixed farming systems to improve planning and policy making for livestock systems. However, his work concentrates on quantitative analysis of livestock outputs and inputs. He makes a clear distinction between 'flow products', such as draught power and manure, and 'stock products', such as meat and milk. For the main livestock inputs such as feed, Steinfeld uses harvest indices to estimate feed resources available for the livestock systems. For the mixed farming systems studied by Steinfeld, the 'flow products' were found to be of much greater importance than the 'stock products'.

Barrett (1992) utilizes some of Steinfeld's work to make estimates of the value of keeping cattle in the mixed farming systems in

Zimbabwe. He includes outputs such as draught power and manure, as well as meat. The results clearly show that low cattle offtake rates from the communal farming sector in Zimbabwe are due to the value of on-farm cattle outputs, such as draught power and manure.

Muchena (1993) studied the economic role of cattle in the mixed farming systems of Chiweshe and Gokwe Communal Areas of Zimbabwe. Her study attempts to take the cattle system out of the mixed farming system to value its economic contribution. Before doing this, an analysis structure to value the 'flow products' was devised. Muchena (1993) examined three basic methodologies for this purpose:

1. The cost of replacing the products using the local market;
2. Production function analysis of the activity in which the intermediate products are used;
3. Determining a physical equivalent for the products, such as the mineral content of manure, or the energy output from draught power.

She adopted methodology 2 to estimate the price (marginal value product) of manure and draught power from the crop production functions. Herd growth was estimated using McLeod's (1993) dynamic, stochastic livestock model, and this was combined with estimates of manure and draught power production to produce a discounted cash flow.

Rocha *et al.* (1991), assessing cattle production in smallholder farming systems of southern Mozambique, found that the contributions of draught power to the farming system more than compensated for the lower offtake rates found in these systems compared to commercial systems.

Conceptual Models of Energy Flows, Nutrition Flows for Other Types of Analysis

Livestock systems can also be represented as conceptual models, which have no physical or quantitative structure. These models can be ideas in the mind or diagrams. Such mod-els are usually the starting point for the development of quantitative model structures, but they can also be used for determining data to be collected to assess a system. The development of conceptual models may require data and information. These models can then be used to direct further data collection. Conceptual livestock models can be developed without data, as there are a number of biological events that are known to take place for a herd/flock to survive. By developing a diagrammatic representation of a system or process it is possible to identify the critical parameters to be measured and also to determine the data required to generate those parameters. Figure 7.10 provides an example of a conceptual model of a poultry system, which indicates the rates of interest and the types of data required to generate the rates.

An Example of Combining Farm Management Tools, Modelling Methods and Conceptual Thinking

Rushton (1996) developed a household resource model, from the point of conceptualization to the development of a computerized, quantitative model. The step-by-step development is seen as critical to maintain a clear perspective during model building. While the model developed is ideally suited to analyse the physical flow of resources through a household system, it also has a facility to incorporate resources that do not involve either cash income or expenditure, and in some cases are intangible. Examples of such items would be soil quality, social status and community credits. In many farming systems these variables are critical in decision making.

The input screens were based on gross margins with outputs and variable inputs. A separate input section dealt with major investments. The outputs generated were based on investment appraisal outputs of NPV, IRR and benefit/cost ratios for the entire household economy (see Fig. 7.11).

The household resource model has been developed to examine smallholder crop–livestock farming systems. Given empirical

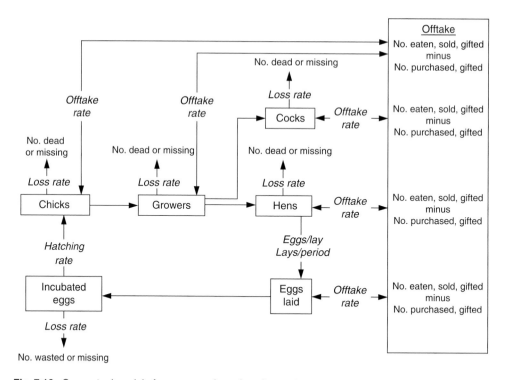

Fig. 7.10. Conceptual model of a scavenge-based poultry system.

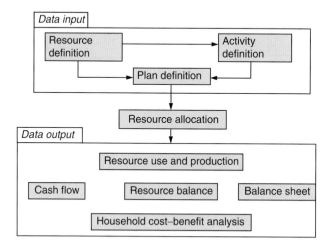

Fig. 7.11. A simplified conceptual household resource model showing input and output structures.

data, the household model was capable of providing information on some aspects of livestock keeping in smallholder farming systems. However, it is well recognized that empirical data on a number of livestock inputs and outputs are either impossible or difficult to generate. To assess the contributions of livestock, and the impact of livestock system changes, requires the livestock system to be represented as a model. Therefore,

Rushton (1996) developed a dynamic, stochastic herd model to simulate a livestock system within a general farming system. The outputs and inputs required for this model were first conceptually developed for the type of livestock systems of interest. From the conceptual model (see Fig. 7.12), a quantitative livestock model was constructed to generate monthly totals for livestock inputs and outputs for cattle, sheep and goat systems. It could also be modified to reflect seasonality of breeding, mortality, offtake, movement and feed quality.

The livestock model output produces information that can be read directly into the household resource model activity definition screen. This information includes:

- milk, manure and draught power production;
- animal offtake;
- herd/flock value;
- ME and protein requirements;
- and labour requirements.

The livestock model output can in turn be used within the household resource model, either to calculate the livestock enterprise profitability, or to examine the use and production resources of the livestock systems within a household resource system.

The model can be used to generate household cost–benefit analysis results for the whole-household system. These can be compared between households with and without livestock (Table 7.11).

The dynamic nature of the model also allows for a month-by-month balance sheet to be developed for different systems. The stochastic nature of the livestock requires the need for different runs of the model and the results are best displayed graphically as there is a spread (see Fig. 7.13).

A predicted cash flow is also available over the period of the analysis and this is shown in (Fig. 7.14).

The models developed were applied to two South Indian smallholder crop–livestock farm household data sets. Both households kept cross-breed cattle, and this activity was simulated using the livestock model. Ten simulations of the each livestock system were performed, and the output was used to estimate the enterprise and household cash flow, balance sheet and profitability. The livestock enterprises gave a positive mean NPV, indicating they were both economically profitable.

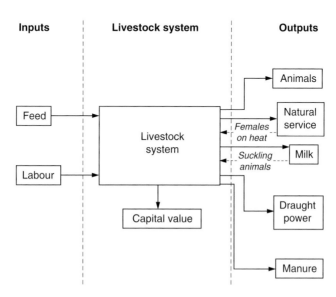

Fig. 7.12. A simple, conceptual, ruminant livestock model was developed to determine a list of livestock inputs and outputs.

Table 7.11. The cost–benefit analysis results for an Indian household system with and without livestock.

	Total	Mean	Minimum	Maximum	SD
Household system including capital costs and benefits					
NPV	−288,231.64	−28,823.16	−35,599.01	−23,629.69	4,191.33
BCR	7.72	0.77	0.72	0.81	0.03
Household system excluding capital costs and benefits					
NPV	−212,844.35	−21,284.44	−26,732.70	−15,358.59	3,721.95
BCR	1.35	0.14	0.03	0.36	0.11
Household system without livestock including capital costs and benefits					
NPV	–	−40,471.59	–	–	–
BCR	–	0.66	–	–	–
Household system without livestock excluding capital costs and benefits					
NPV	–	−12,723.07	–	–	–
BCR	–	0.22	–	–	–

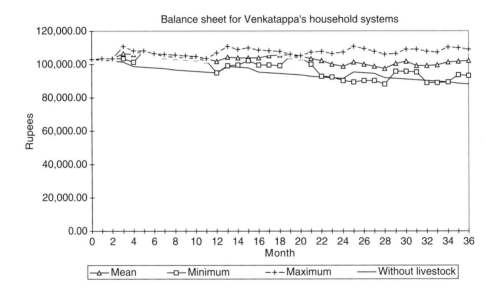

Fig. 7.13. Aggregated balance sheets for an Indian household system with a dairy cow.

However, a number of runs generated a negative NPV, and no livestock activity had a positive cash flow. The results were compared with the actual livestock management. One household, Venkatappa, sold their cattle when their value was highest, and the other household, Nanjappa, fed limited rations to their cattle, and subsequently suffered fertility problems. Both responses were considered rational, given the cash-flow constraints, with the Nanjappa household making a misjudgement on the best strategy to apply to make a profit from the enterprise.

The whole-household model output indicated that the livestock activity had a positive impact on the household profitability. However, the results from the household runs were dominated by an inflated land value, and also indicated that data were lacking on other household income-generating activities.

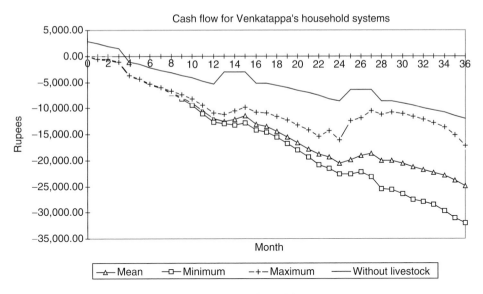

Fig. 7.14. Cash flows for an Indian household system with a dairy cow.

While the livestock systems had an overall profitability it was doubtful if they were viable due to the negative cash flow. As milk was the main cash output from the livestock system, this raises the question of whether the milk price is high enough. The milk sale price used was the rate offered by the local milk cooperatives, and this, in turn, was set by the local government. During the data collection period many farmers expressed dissatisfaction with the milk price, and the model output shows why. The model could be used to determine a milk price that could generate positive cash flows, and would provide a pointer for future milk price policy. Alternatively, sensitivity analysis could be performed on input resource values. This would highlight the resources that need to be provided at lower rates to achieve enterprise viability.

The predicted balance sheets and NPVs were dominated by the value of land. A high land value was used, because it reflects the demand for land in the area. The neighbouring city was expanding rapidly, and many urban dwellers were buying land plots, either for future housing developments or as an investment. The true agricultural worth of the land was much lower than that specified. The whole-household model runs indicate that these inflated land prices will probably change the nature of the farming systems. It will only be worth cropping the land for high-value crops, which will probably require irrigation. Irrigation in this area requires the sinking of borewells, and many farmers were willing to pay large amounts of money to do this, even for small areas of land. Such reliance on underground water supplies, to guarantee attractive agricultural returns, is likely to have detrimental effects on the water table.

Summary

Many approaches have been used and are available for the analysis of livestock farming systems and other components of the livestock sector. These cover elements of enterprise or business profitability either in short time periods or over time, the assessment of change and the analysis of uncertainty and risk. However, one approach alone cannot provide a complete economic analysis of animal health and production; often what is needed is a combination of approaches. These holistic, systems approaches are employed in the livestock-orientated household/farm models presented. To truly capture all elements for the quantitative assessment of livestock systems integrated into household systems, three elements are identified as critical:

- sufficient transparency in the decision-making process to allow its use by technical specialists;
- sufficient flexibility for farming system experimentation through modelling;
- and an adequate livestock model to assess a livestock system.

The list of parameters needed by such models can prioritize the data that need to be collected. The models can also be used for returning information to the livestock keepers and people within the livestock sector supplying the data and hence ensuring their continuing cooperation in data collection exercises. This area is further expanded in the following contribution by Andrew James. This is followed by an explanation by Alistair Stott on how optimization models may be used in policy analysis and decision making in animal health.

8   Modelling and the Generation of Information

Andrew James

Introduction

Models have been increasingly used in animal disease control policy in recent years, at both national and individual herd levels. The purpose of this chapter is to review the strengths and weaknesses of some of the modelling techniques that have been used, to assess the prospects for future development of models and to provide indications of when it is likely that the use of models would be appropriate to assist decision making.

Key Tools and Case Studies

Epidemiological models

Whenever economic analysis of animal health policy is undertaken, an epidemiological model is implied. It is necessary in *ex ante* assessment to make assumptions about the effect of any policy on the pattern of disease in the population. Similarly, in *ex post* evaluation it is necessary to make assumptions about the outcome if an alternative policy had been adopted. These models range from the purely conceptual, to simple extrapolation of results from a sample to the whole population, to complex computer models. All bring benefits and risks to the analysis.

A large number of formal epidemiological models have been developed, and some have been used to guide disease control policy, both at national and individual herd levels. Sometimes these have been linked to formal economic analysis of the predicted outcomes, but even where formal economic analysis has not been used, economic evaluation is implicit: the preferred policy would be the one that produced the best economic outcome.

Recent applications of epidemiological models have highlighted the fact that it is difficult or impossible to estimate some of their parameters, especially those relating to frequency of contact between animals or herds. In any case, such contact rates vary according to local conditions and over time. Usually epidemiologists are forced to use 'guesstimates' of these parameters and the result is that the model will simply forecast their own preconception of the progress of the disease. For example, if the modeller judges that short-distance spread is more frequent than medium-distance spread, the model will predict that such policies as ring-vaccination or pre-emptive culling will be relatively effective. In the opinion of the author, this constitutes a serious lack of objectivity, and the risks are especially severe when decision takers do not understand the logical basis on which the forecasts are being made.

An example of this situation is found in the UK foot-and-mouth disease (FMD) epidemic of

2001. One model in particular, that of Ferguson *et al.* (2001), played a key role in the decision leading to the British Government adopting a contiguous cull policy. A newspaper article from the time reproduces outputs from the model under the caption 'scientific predictions' (*Daily Telegraph*, 11 April 2001). However, this, and other models, contained simplifications and assumptions which heavily influenced the conclusions about appropriate control strategies (Taylor, 2003). Critical assessment of the models within the FMD Science Group was difficult and discussion of their possible limitations did not appear to feature greatly in the decision support process. One interpretation is that decision makers were seduced by the illusion of truth provided by mathematics (Gupta, 2001), with the result that the models were taken as prescriptive tools, providing a ready-made solution to a decision problem.

It is much easier to develop epidemiological models of endemic diseases than of epidemics. The reason for this is that, particularly in the early stages of an epidemic, inherently unpredictable events have a dominant effect on the development of the epidemic. Stochastic modelling techniques do not provide a complete answer to this problem. They tend to produce the answer that 'anything could happen', which is of limited value in economic analysis and decision making. Furthermore, most models have to assume that the population of herds is homogeneous, or composed of homogeneous groups of herds, with uniform contact rates. This is very far from reality.

Endemic diseases, on the other hand, are a much easier subject for epidemiological models. They are usually modelled within herds, where assumptions of homogeneity are more realistic. And more data on critical factors such as contact and transmission rates are usually available. Despite the more predictable behaviour of endemic diseases, stochastic simulation is still important. One of the earliest applications of epidemiological modelling to disease control policy remains an excellent example. Hugh-Jones (1976) developed a model of bovine brucellosis in the UK to ascertain why farmers were not joining the voluntary eradication programme. Brucellosis-free herds received a valuable premium on the milk price, but had to bear the cost of culling reactors. The model showed that on average farmers would benefit from joining the scheme, but that there was a very small risk of an individual farmer suffering major loss. Stories of such cases in the farming press were sufficient to deter many farmers from the programme.

Epidemiological models do have a very important potential application in evaluating *ex post* data to estimate actual transmission rates, and evaluate the reasons for increased and reduced rates over time and space. In this way, it is possible to identify policies and conditions apparently influencing transmission rates, and learn lessons for future control and prevention strategies.

Perhaps the most valuable application of epidemiological models, including purely conceptual models based on diagrams, is to clarify understanding of the mechanisms of disease transmission and maintenance during the development of the model. The process of having to specify possible transmission pathways and interactions is often very instructive. Even where it is not possible to assign values to probabilities and frequencies, it is often clear that one transmission pathway is far more important than others, and this can suggest more effective control strategies. A good example of such a process was a recent study to determine the duration of animal movement standstill regulations to contain the spread of exotic diseases such as FMD (Risk Solutions, 2003). A relatively simple spreadsheet model was produced and, predictably, the model predicted outcomes reflecting mainly the animal movement and disease detection assumptions supplied to it. However, examination of the model structure and the results made it clear that any movement standstill regulation was highly effective in containing spread, almost regardless of the duration. A clear policy recommendation emerged from the logic of the model, and independent of any assumed values of parameters that could not be estimated or predicted (Taylor and James, 2003).

Livestock databases

The availability of low-cost networked computers and stronger regulation of livestock producers have led to the widespread use of livestock databases, both at national and herd levels. These provide a very effective platform for modelling of both disease and production, and therefore the impact of the disease on production. A good example of this is a model used by National Milk Records plc (NMR) to forecast future milk production, both for individual herds and for groups of herds supplying milk buyers. This information is of value to individual farmers managing their quota, and to milk buyers in planning the allocation of collection vehicles and their production schedules. The forecasts are made on the basis of the present herd composition in the NMR database, and recent actual performance parameters, such as fertility, culling policy and lactation performance. The forecast covers not only milk quality but also protein and fat content, which is important to farmers and milk buyers. By applying variations to the policy and performance parameters, it is possible to predict with great reliability the production impact of management policy changes. It is planned to make this facility available as a management tool for farmers in the near future.

The NMR database does not contain complete movement data: animals are only recorded when they are in customers' herds. However, national livestock traceability databases could provide a powerful basis for modelling animal diseases. They contain complete data on the real host population and real animal movement patterns.

If the database also held production information, such as that held by NMR, the economic impact of the disease could also be assessed. While such integrated livestock databases raise issues of confidentiality and security, these can be resolved by effective control of data security and statutory restrictions on the availability and use of information. The Government of Chile, for example, is planning to provide facilities for breed societies, milk recording organizations, milk buyers and private abattoirs within its regulatory database.

A great advantage of database-hosted simulation models is that they tend to be conceptually simple compared to mathematical models. They simulate large numbers of simple events, and technical staff can be fully involved in their development, allowing them to understand and assess the assumptions that are being made.

Risk analysis

When conducting economic evaluation of exotic disease prevention policy, it is necessary to estimate both the risk of disease introduction and the economic impact of an outbreak if it were to occur.

Risk model-building software based on spreadsheets is widely available and relatively easy to use. However, it is very easy to make two types of error in constructing risk models. The first is to assume that successive event probabilities in the risk pathway are independent of each other. This is frequently not the case, and if there is a positive association between the two events (i.e. if the first event occurs, the second is also more likely to occur) then the joint probability of both events occurring obtained by multiplying the two probabilities will be an underestimate. These errors can be compounded through the model, producing serious errors in the risk assessment.

A second, even more serious, criticism of many quantitative risk assessments is that there is no objective way of estimating many of the key event probabilities. In fact, these are not risks but uncertainties. Expert opinions may be sought, but these are often conflicting with the result that the outcome of the risk assessment depends on which expert opinion is believed.

Another difficult issue in quantitative risk assessment is the calculation of the economic cost of a risk. Usually, this is calculated as the product of the expected number of adverse events per time period and the average cost of such an event. The problem is to predict the cost of events such as the introduction of an exotic disease agent. This could range from nothing to billions of dollars, depending on disease preparedness and, to a large extent, chance. To use the historical average cost of such rare events (even if any had occurred) would not be appropriate, as both the livestock industry and disease control services would be likely to have changed over the years.

Humans are by nature risk-averse. The perceived cost of a risk is often greater than the average loss per time period. This is especially true of exotic disease risks, where the potential losses are enormous, both to the economy as a whole and the individual officials who could be blamed for not protecting the livestock industry. In reality, veterinary services wish to pursue zero-risk strategies in relation to exotic diseases, and are likely to seek risk assessment results that would justify the banning of trade where they perceive any risk of exotic disease.

A more constructive approach to disease risk management could be provided by applying the methods of Hazard Analysis Critical Control Points (HACCP) to the problem. This methodology was developed for the food processing industry, where the objective is to establish procedures, control points and monitoring that should eliminate the possibility of food contamination or other hazards. This approach is much better aligned with the real objectives of veterinary services. Where a risk or uncertainty is identified, even if it cannot be quantified, it can usually be prevented by appropriate controls and monitoring. Many countries importing animal products already demand that exporters have HACCP systems in place to control food safety hazards, and there seems no reason why similar measures could not control animal disease risks. The HACCP methodology is applicable not only to preventing the importation of exotic disease agents, but also to their containment in the importing country.

Discussion and Conclusions

Epidemiological models have great potential to guide decision making by individual farmers and governments. However, there are risks that unrealistic models may continue to misguide policy makers. It is critical that the technical decision makers understand the mechanisms, limitations and assumptions of the models and are able to assess for themselves the validity and reliability of the results that they produce. If this means that models should use less-sophisticated simulation techniques, then so be it. The availability of livestock databases offers great potential for more realistic epidemiological and economic models. It is also the case that models developed on such databases tend to be conceptually far simpler than mathematical models.

9 Optimization Methods for Assisting Policy Decisions on Endemic Diseases

Alistair Stott

Why Optimize?

Assisting policy decisions ranges from individual farm health planning right through to international agreements designed to combat global pandemics. At all levels, it will be necessary to allocate scarce resources between competing activities in order to achieve the most appropriate objectives in the best way. In other words, economics is at the heart of this decision support process and optimization of the guiding principle. Unfortunately, optimization models, using for example the loss–expenditure frontier approach, demand considerable data that are rarely available (Bennett, 2003). However, by teaming up with scientists, systems modellers and epidemiological modellers, the data required by economists can often be obtained by computer simulation (e.g. Stott et al., 2003; Gunn et al., 2004; Santarossa et al., 2005). Some applications have also been based on field data (e.g. Yalcin et al., 1999; Chi et al., 2002).

Decision Analysis and Optimization

The analysis of McInerney et al. (1992) assumes complete information and unimpeded optimizing behaviour, assumptions that are not likely to be satisfied in practice (Tisdell, 1995). Tisdell (1995) therefore extends the special case of McInerney et al. (1992) in a number of ways including dealing with multiple diseases and situations where disease control funds are in short supply (see Chapter 4, this volume). An alternative approach is to focus on decision making rather than on disease and so draw on the wide range of generic decision analysis techniques available (Ngategize et al., 1986). The original and best known decision analysis technique is linear programming (Jalvingh et al., 1997). Although little used in animal health economics, linear programming captures the essence of decision support, i.e. it addresses the resource allocation problem.[1]

A more common application in animal health economics is the decision tree (Marsh, 1999; Chapter 7, this volume), which provides a visual representation of the decision choices faced. The decision maker can get directly involved, drawing on his/her experience to estimate likely outcomes and risks (Boehlje and Eidman, 1984) and thus overcoming some of the data problems mentioned previously.

---

[1] Stott et al. (2003) used linear programming to incorporate biosecurity options into whole-farm planning in order to achieve a farm income target at minimum risk.

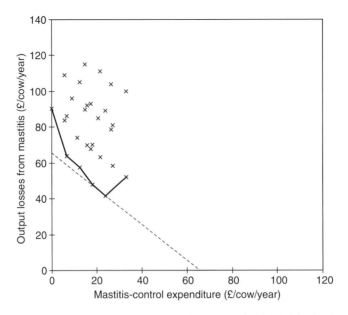

Fig. 9.1. Loss–expenditure frontier for subclinical mastitis in a sample of 750 dairy herds.

These features are of real benefit in practical decision support and are far more likely to result in progress at farm level than more sophisticated 'black box' methods. However, once sufficient branches have been added to capture the full impact of a present decision over the many cycles of animal production likely to be affected, including future decisions and chance outcomes, decision trees become very difficult to handle. This is where dynamic programming (DP; Bellman, 1957) steps in. It finds the optimum route through a decision tree in a computationally efficient way.[2]

Optimization for a Single Disease: the Loss–Expenditure Frontier

Figure 9.1 drawn from Yalcin *et al.* (1999) provides an example of the approach of McInerney *et al.* (1992). Each cross on the graph represents the average performance of farms in the sample using the same approach to controlling subclinical mastitis. Those with

the highest control expenditure tend to have the lowest losses from the disease. The solid line is the loss–expenditure frontier, joining the most efficient treatment strategies at each level of control expenditure. The optimal strategy is on the iso-cost (hatched) line tangential to the frontier. It has the lowest total cost (output loss + control expenditure), in this case £66/cow/year. Average total cost in this sample was £100/cow/year. This gave an avoidable loss (true cost) of £34/cow/year.

Dealing with Multiple Diseases and Restricted Control Funds

Figure 9.2 shows an example of the method of Tisdell (1995) based on data for bovine viral diarrhoea (BVD) in beef suckler herds generated by the model of Gunn *et al.* (2004) and using the function for biosecurity costs set out by Stott *et al.* (2003). The graph deals with a hypothetical allocation of expenditure on biosecurity between beef suckler farms that are either free of BVD or of unknown BVD status but otherwise identical. Expenditure is fixed at £12/cow/year. If this entire sum is given to the BVD-free herds the net benefit

---

[2] For an explanation based on the animal health decision-making scenario see Stott *et al.* (2005a).

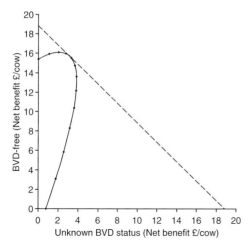

Fig. 9.2. Alternative allocations of £12/cow/year biosecurity expenditure between beef suckler herds of different BVD status.

(output loss avoided less cost of biosecurity) will be just over £15/cow/year. If given to the herds of unknown BVD status the net benefit is just £1/cow/year. The iso-net benefit (hatched) line shows that giving £8/cow/year and £4/cow/year to the BVD-free and BVD-unknown herds, respectively, yields the highest net benefit (£19/cow/year).

The technique could deal with different diseases competing for fixed control resources on the same farm, and can be used to help decision makers at regional level. In this example, by offering twice as much support to farms free of BVD would not only deliver the best regional outcome but would also act as a considerable incentive to 'free-riders' (Holden, 1999) who might otherwise be tempted not to act against the disease.

Multiple Objectives

Most decision analysis techniques seek to maximize financial gain, but this is not always the primary objective of decision makers. For example, at a policy level for endemic disease prevention, motives such as improved animal welfare, human welfare and environmental gain need to be considered. These are not easily expressed in monetary terms and are

therefore liable to be neglected in a decision analysis that emphasizes private cost–benefit. Some decision analysis techniques can handle multiple objectives, and have been successfully applied to the conflicts that can arise between farm profitability, animal welfare, human health and the environment in the control of ectoparasites of sheep (Milne, 2005) and the trade-off between the short-run productivity of natural assets and their long-run value (sustainability) in dairy farming (Santarossa *et al.*, 2004).

At farm level, the trade-off between risk and profit is of particular concern as demonstrated by Stott *et al.* (2003). They concluded that risk and decision maker's attitude towards risk are important considerations when choosing the optimum BVD prevention strategy, and these considerations are likely to apply to other farm-level endemic disease control decisions. Santarossa *et al.* (2005), using a contingent claim analysis method (Stinespring, 2002), incorporated risk reduction and decision makers' attitude towards risk into the BVD control choice decision (see Fig. 9.3).

The contingent claim analysis method calculates the level of (hypothetical) insurance cover necessary to maximize the decision makers' expected utility of wealth (psychological satisfaction of holding wealth) under risk. The more effective the BVD control strategy, the less is the risk and the lower is the excess insurance cover required. For example, in Fig. 9.3, the excess insurance for B80 and V80 was not significantly different from zero, i.e. these options provided adequate protection from the risks of BVD while the others did not. Hypothetical insurance requirements therefore become a proxy for measuring the relative value of alternative endemic disease prevention options in terms of the trade-offs between profit and risk as perceived by the decision maker. The main point to emphasize here is that the results depend on the decision maker's attitude towards risk, which is affected by income and wealth.[3] Another decision maker with different

---

[3] For the values for these parameters used to derive Fig. 9.3 see Santarossa *et al.* (2005).

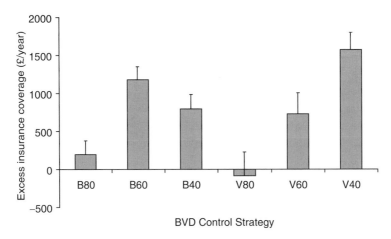

Fig. 9.3. Excess insurance coverage needed to offset risk from BVD under alternative control options. (B80/B60/B40 assumes that biosecurity strategies have a 0.8/0.6/0.4 probability of avoiding virus introduction in any one year. V80/V60/V40 assumes that vaccine ensures that 0.8/0.6/0.4 of all adult cattle are effectively immunized each year. Strategies are hypothetical. Results are mean and SE of 100 Monte Carlo simulations in each case using the model of Gunn *et al.*, 2004.)

values would have a different Fig. 9.3 and make different disease control choices. With such understanding animal owners will be able to act in their own best interest but they may not all act in the same way and their actions may not always be in the best interests of other stakeholders.

Discussion and Conclusions

The aim of sustainable development dictates that the resources required to implement policy are allocated as efficiently as possible. This means that optimization methods for assisting policy decisions on endemic diseases are obligatory, not an optional extra. Such obligation extends from the international policy maker ensuring value for public money through to the private business that must remain competitive to survive. However, for the reasons highlighted above, optimization methods should rarely, if ever, be used to determine policy decisions. The dangers of over-reliance on economic optimization techniques are all too evident in the history of the financial markets of the world (MacKenzie,

2004). This paper therefore highlights more pragmatic approaches to the use of optimization methods in the context of endemic disease decision support.

Data are rarely available to realize the full potential of economic optimization methods in support of endemic disease policy decisions (McInerney, 1996). This problem can be alleviated by closer collaboration between scientists, modellers and economists. However, even with perfect knowledge, problems will almost invariably involve reconciliation of competing objectives rather than optimization of independent objectives. The predominance of multiple objectives in endemic disease decision problems does not reduce the value of optimization methods in decision support. Multiple objectives can be handled as shown in the above examples based on Tisdell (1995), Stott *et al.* (2002), Stott *et al.* (2005b) and Santarossa *et al.* (2005). Cost minimization methods based on sound economics also have vital roles to play. They establish benchmarks against which to measure the opportunity cost of alternatives to the optimum solution. Perhaps more importantly, they demonstrate clearly to decision makers the vital role that economics can play in this field. They highlight the cost of complacency and question traditional assumptions about an issue that has important implications for us all.

It is also important to appreciate that optimization methods can play a wider role in decision support than their name implies. For example, decision analysis techniques focus on decisions rather than on disease. By doing this, they can widen the perspective and draw in decisions not normally associated with disease prevention but potentially vital to it. For example, better support for the replacement decision in dairy cows may allow us to better control endemic diseases such as *Staphylococcus aureus* mastitis, which is unresponsive to antibiotics and/or reduces the use of antibiotics in agriculture with less risk to animal welfare (Stott *et al.*, 2002). The wider perspective therefore captures some of the externalities of conventional approaches to animal disease, thus providing another means to contribute to sustainability.

10 Tools That Go Beyond the Enterprise, Farm or Business Level: Investigating Markets, Market Trends and Assessing Public investments in the Livestock Sector

Introduction

Chapter 7 (this volume) presented and reviewed some of the most important farm and business-level tools available to the people involved in the livestock sector. However, these people need to use markets either to buy their inputs or to sell their outputs. For them, understanding how markets operate, how to assess if a market is changing and who is involved in setting the rules for the markets is as important as understanding enterprise, farm or business-level profitability. Therefore, three parts of this chapter will present tools and information required to carry out rapid market assessments and review the livestock value chains that the people in the livestock sector are part of. The chapter also includes a very brief review of the economic concepts behind markets.

The other important actor in the livestock sector is the State. The role of the State was mentioned briefly in the different levels of data collection (see Chapter 5, this volume) and will be returned to in this chapter in the section on tools for assessing State-level investments (p. 122). However, like the individual farmer or person involved in the livestock sector, the State needs tools to determine if an investment, i.e. a change, in the livestock sector will be worthwhile for society in general. The most commonly used tool for such appraisals is

cost–benefit analysis and this chapter presents an overview of the main aspects of this tool along with a discussion of the additional tools required to estimate the costs and the benefits of a proposed change. This includes how market analysis can be used to estimate how the benefits and costs of a large change in the livestock sector are transmitted through markets to both consumers and livestock producers.

This chapter will also discuss a relatively recently recognized tool in the economics of livestock and health value chain analysis. This can be useful for both the farm, agrobusiness person and the State in assessing components of the livestock sector.

Market Concepts

In a market there is a problem of *scarcity*. In countries where shop shelves are never empty, very few people go without food and the majority have adequate housing, it is difficult to believe that markets can be concerned with scarcity. If someone were asked if they wanted more money their response would undoubtedly be *yes*. What would they do with the extra money? It will be spent on extra goods and services. This response is true of both rich and poor people. Even very wealthy people with a big house and an expensive car would probably like a bigger home, a luxury yacht, etc. The important point to be noted is that human wants are *virtually unlimited*. Yet the means of fulfilling human wants are limited. The world has a limited amount of resources, which means that at any one time only a limited number of goods and services can be produced. Demand and supply and the relationship between the two actually lie at the centre of economics:

1. Demand – related to wants:
   If goods and services were free, people would simply demand whatever they wanted.
2. Supply – related to resources:
   The amount that firms can supply depends on resources and technology available.

With the definition of scarcity above, it is possible to state that human wants exceed what can actually be produced, therefore *potential demands* will exceed *potential supplies*. This is a continual problem and has to be dealt with by society. There is a need to match demand and supply. In the majority of societies the matching of supply with demand is achieved through prices. In general, when prices increase demand will reduce, but supply will increase as actors involved in livestock production, processing and marketing realize that additional profit can be made.

The characteristics of how demand changes with a price change is related to a good on offer, cultural preferences for that good and the alternative goods that have similar characteristics. For example, goats are an important species for religious ceremonies and have few substitutes. The demand for this good is strong and people are willing to pay high prices per head at certain times of the year. In the case of milk, the goods produced from this livestock product compete with similar products made from vegetable oils and soya. Similarly, wool can be replaced by other types of fibre. Substitutes are an important aspect of market structures and recognizing how to address such competition is an important aspect of livestock product marketing.

Looking at supply, a change in prices will change the profitability of a livestock activity, which can be investigated using gross margin analyses and enterprise budgets. An increase in prices will mean that the profitability of the livestock activity will increase not only in absolute terms (i.e. the quantity of money produced by the activity), but also in relative terms (i.e. in comparison with alternative activities). Where the change in profitability is sufficiently large, the impact will be for the current livestock producers and people in this part of the livestock sector to dedicate more time and resources in the livestock production and marketing and also to attract new people to these activities. Their combined action will be to increase supply. This is called the supply response, and how quickly the response takes place is dependent on the characteristics of the baseline production of the livestock production, which as outlined in the production economic chapter (Chapter 3, this volume) is biological, and the speed at which resources can be switched from other activities to the livestock production and marketing activity.

The general relationship between supply and demand with the price and size of the market is represented graphically in Fig. 10.1.

In the situation described where potential demand exceeds supply, how can actual demand and supply be made to balance? There are three ways:

1. Demand has to be curtailed.
2. Supply has to be increased.
3. A combination of (1) and (2).

Market Analysis: from the Point of View of the Producer

Ideally market analysis should build on the data and information generated from the livestock producers using the gross margin analyses and enterprise budgets of their livestock activities. Information on the livestock producers will indicate their resource management and use, the organization of the producers. Information on the processors and traders would also be useful as would the contact of the producers with markets and traders. The farm-level analyses will provide a basis to assess how well the livestock producers and processors can supply livestock

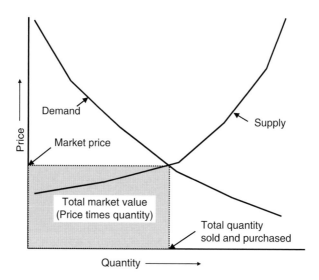

Fig. 10.1. Relationship between the characteristics of supply and demand, market price, quantity of a product bought and sold and total market value.

product demand and how quickly they could change to growing demand.

Much of the market analysis will be dedicated to examining markets for the livestock products. However, when investigating the commercialization of livestock products there is also a need to investigate key input markets. Here the link between market analysis and enterprise budgets is crucial; the latter will help an investigator identify which are the key inputs for the livestock producers and others involved in the livestock sector. In this way it will also determine which input markets need to be further investigated for issues such as seasonality of availability, variations in quality, number of suppliers, etc. Outside the standard list of inputs that can be easily quantified, it should also be remembered that the market for information on prices and technology is important in ensuring that the livestock chain works smoothly and equitably.

The analysis proposed in this section will be centred on community-level issues, with more wide-ranging aspects of the market introduced in the value chain analysis below. The analysis described will also be largely qualitative, for those interested in more quantitative analysis please refer to Ferrell *et al.* (1998) or Weiers (1986).

Objectives

The objectives of market analysis are to:

- Identify the key input markets for livestock production activities.
- Identify the key output markets for livestock and livestock products.
- Characterize the input and output markets, identifying the numbers and types of traders involved.
- Assess the level of understanding of the livestock producers of market demands in terms of:
  - the existing options for livestock and livestock product trading;
  - changes in marketing structures over time;
  - sources of market information used at producer level;
  - perceived constraints of the existing markets.
- Assess the competition in the production of livestock, livestock products or livestock product substitutes.
- Determine the commercialization margins for livestock.
- Improve the producer-level understanding of livestock and livestock product markets by combining local and external knowledge data sets.

With whom?

Market analysis of livestock or livestock products should be carried out at different levels if it is to generate information that will be useful for production-level decision making.

1. All analysis should begin with the producer of the livestock in order to discuss access to input and output markets.
2. To supplement this local knowledge set, secondary data should be sought from key informants and organizations on large-scale trends of the livestock or livestock product market.
3. Information generated by the analysis should be returned to the producers and discussed in terms of how it can be used to increase the success of livestock and livestock product marketing.
4. Where appropriate, information should be disseminated to livestock policy decision makers.

Step 1: Data: where to find them

Data for market analysis can be divided into data that are collected by the investigators and the community, which are called primary data, and data that have been collected and documented by other people and organizations, which are called secondary data. There will be a need to combine both types of data, unless the market analysis is for a very local market. In the latter case primary data will suffice. Please refer back to Chapter 5 (this volume) for further information

Step 2: Analysis of the internal environment of the livestock producers

An important part of the market analysis is the understanding of the objectives, goals and production methods of the livestock producers. The following checklist is suggested:

- Objectives:
  (a) Who are the producers?
    (i) availability of land and natural resources to produce livestock;
    (ii) socio-economic status;
    (iii) skill and education levels;
    (iv) other available resources;
    (v) access to markets for inputs, outputs and knowledge;
    (vi) ability to raise finance.
  (b) What are their objectives and goals in the marketing of livestock and livestock products?
  (c) Do these producers have a good market?
  (d) Is their market growing, staying the same or shrinking?
- Production costs – available from the enterprise budgets:
  (a) quantity, quality, price and total value of the livestock or livestock product;
  (b) quantity, price and total value of inputs (variable, labour and fixed costs);
  (c) the livestock activity's profit, productivity and efficiency;
  (d) the livestock activity's sensitivity to changes in input and output prices.

It is noted that this internal environment is largely under the control of the producer and therefore has some degree of flexibility. The internal environment also sets the parameters in terms of what can be supplied by the producer in terms of quality and quantity of the livestock produced.

Step 3: Analysis of the external environment

The external environment is largely out of the control of the producer, but it is important to understand how the producer engages with this environment and where necessary how this can be strengthened. Information and data for this environment can be sought first from the producer, but ideally should be supplemented with secondary data from livestock sector organizations. The analysis of the external environment can be broken down into:

- *Competition* (this can be other livestock producers and also producers of products that are substitutes for livestock products). The key questions are:
  - Who are they, what are their strengths and weaknesses, capacity, product, distribution, prices, promotion, their reaction in the face of a change, their likely changes in the future?

Failure to understand the competition puts in danger the success of any future investments in livestock activities.

- The *economy,* with data from the producer and supplemented with secondary data sources. The key issues are:
  - The growth of the economy and where this is focused, i.e. is it across all socio-economic groups or concentrated in certain groups? This needs to be related to who are the current and potential consumers for the livestock products and what happens to livestock product demand when these clients get richer.
- *Political, legal and cultural* issues will be discussed in more detail in Chapter 11 (this volume).
- *Technology* changes – data should be collected from the producers on their views of how livestock activities may be improved, and information should be sought from other organizations working in similar areas. The key issue is:
  - Could a technological change affect the quantity and/or the quality of the livestock or livestock product? Could a technological change allow the livestock product to reach new markets? For example, processing, storage, transport or marketing of the livestock product.

Step 4: Client and consumer analysis

Some key questions need to be asked of the livestock producers in order to understand how well they understand the demands of the end clients and consumers. A suggested list of questions is as follows:

- What does the consumer or client do with the livestock or livestock product?
- Where do they buy the livestock or livestock product?
- When do they buy the livestock or livestock product?
- Why does the client or consumer buy the livestock or livestock product from the producer or the area where this producer farms?
- Why do potential clients or consumers not buy the livestock or livestock product from the producer or area where they farm?

Market classification

It may also be helpful to classify the clients in terms of whether they want the livestock or livestock products for:

- consumption – milk, meat, cheese;
- industrial use – broken eggs, hides, specific offal parts;
- wholesaling – some livestock markets attract traders who buy large batches of animals and then distribute them to many farmers;
- generation of national and international public goods – Governments in the payment to farmers for maintaining the countryside.

Clients and markets can also be classified by geographic location:

- international, which can also be divided into Latin America, USA, Europe, Asia;
- national, which can be divided into the main cities or regions;
- regional;
- local.

It is also important to state if the clients of the livestock or livestock products are real, i.e. they are buying the product now, or potential, i.e. they may buy the product in the future, and if the demand for the product is constant, i.e. the same each month or week, or seasonal.

It may be helpful with the community to fill a simple table to express this type of classification (see Table 10.1).

Market integration and commercialization margins

Equitability along the marketing chain is an important aspect of success for livestock production and marketing. The question is how to assess if the distribution of the value of the product is equitable or not? In a market where there is equitable distribution the difference between actors in the chain should reflect the costs of transport, processing and storage of the livestock or livestock product plus a level of profit which reflects the returns of similar activities within the economy. The starting point for this analysis is therefore information

Table 10.1. Simple market classification for some livestock products in Bolivia.

| Product | Market location (local, regional, national, international) | Which country, city or region? | Who are the clients? | |
			Livestock sector	Final
Finished pigs	Local, regional	The Altiplano and the cities of Sucre and Tarija, Bolivia	Local traders	Local and city-based consumers through restaurants
Turkey	Regional	Main Bolivian cities	National company	City-based consumers in Bolivia
Llama fibre	Regional, international	Main Bolivian cities, UK, Italy, China	National and international fibre brokers	City-based consumers in all parts of the world

on the price paid and received for livestock inputs, livestock and livestock products by each actor in the chain from the input provided to the producer and then on through to the consumer. These data can then be used to calculate commercialization margins, which are based on information of the final unit price for the livestock product. The formula for calculating the margin is shown below:

$$\text{Commercialization margin} = \frac{\begin{array}{c}\text{Difference between} \\ \text{sale and purchase} \\ \text{price of the product}\end{array}}{\text{Consumer price}} \times 100$$

The commercialization margins for the milk value chain with cheese as the end product is presented in Table 10.2.

The calculation of the margin is made difficult for products that are processed or transformed when passing through the supply chain, and also for products which do not have a standard unit of measure throughout the supply chain. Therefore, it is not always possible to present this type of analysis for every finished livestock product. For example, a finished steer will be slaughtered and processed into meat, offal and hide. The meat will be consumed, some of the offal processed and the hide cured and then used in manufacturing processes.

An alternative to the commercialization margins is to calculate the proportion of the final price taken by the different actors in the chain. The estimation of the proportion of the final price taken by the different actors in the chain requires information on the end price for the product. There are difficulties in calculating these proportions if the product is processed or transformed when passing through the supply chain and if the unit of measure for a product changes.

Table 10.2. Commercialization margins of the different actors in a milk value chain.

| Actor | Price (Bolivianos/l milk) | | Margin (per litre milk) | |
	Buying	Selling	Boliviano	%
Producer	3.41[a]	4	0.59	
Processor	4	12.03	8.03	43.72
Trader	12.03	18.37	6.34	34.51
Consumer	18.37			
Total			14.37	78.22
Final product value			18.37	100.00

[a]Unit cost of producing a litre of milk.

While the commercialization margins and the proportion of the final price taken by the different actors are of value in some situations and for some livestock products, the fact that they do not take into account costs incurred by each actor in a chain can lead to a distorted impression of who gains and who loses. Where there are significant costs, be they transaction, transport or processing costs, these measures from the marketing chain can give distorted information about the apparent 'profitability' of each actor in the chain. Such analyses should be the starting point of a much deeper cost and profitability analysis based on enterprise budget analysis of the livestock activities of each actor along the chain. In addition there is a need for an understanding of the institutional context in which each actor is found and works. This will be discussed in more detail in the section on value chain analysis in this chapter and in Chapter 12 on institutional economics.

Market trends

Markets are not static, in part because economic growth will change the socio-economic status of the livestock consumers and this often leads to changes in the quantity and quality of the livestock products demanded by these consumers. The trends in the livestock market can be examined at local level with discussions on quantities of the product sold over a historical time period. It is also important to assess if the quality demanded has changed and if such changes have been accompanied with incentives to provide better quality, or whether a livestock product that does not meet a certain quality either is not purchased or has a lower price. What should be remembered when carrying out such local-level analysis is that the information at community level may be incomplete. This may be related to how traders pass on information from consumer to producer, or it may be a lack of skills in analysing data available on the market. In all cases it is recommended that the researchers visit markets outside the communities, preferably with community representatives, to gather extra data and

information on market trends. Ideally, these data should be supplemented with secondary data and information. The local and external data sets then need to be assessed in terms of the community's ability to satisfy present and future demands for quantity and quality of the livestock product. The combination of data and information from the producers, traders and markets is key to generating successful livestock marketing strategy plans.

Summary

The market analysis for producers should provide the basis for developing a marketing strategy on how to improve the success of livestock and livestock product marketing in the future. Table 10.3 shows how a market analysis can be summarized.

Tools for Assessing State-level Investments in the Livestock Sector

The effectiveness of economic impact assessment at State level depends on the specification of the decision problem, and the objectives of the various people in the livestock sector who will be affected. This obviously requires discussions with these groups and some authors such as Carney (1998) and Scoones (1998) have proposed a more holistic means of doing this through a livelihoods framework. However, the most widely used tool for assessing State-level investments is cost–benefit analysis. On its own this is simply a framework for comparing costs and benefits to society that occur over time. Given the complexity of economies that most societies have developed, this requires additional tools to generate information on who gains and who loses and what are the overall costs and benefits to society. Therefore, in addition to an explanation of cost–benefit analysis in general, economic surplus methods, mathematical programming or optimization methods, and simulation and systems analysis are described. These methods will be further discussed with their strengths and weaknesses by Martin Upton in Chapter 11 (this volume).

Table 10.3. Summary of the information from a rapid market assessment for pig and turkey producers in the Cintis, Bolivia.

| Product | Competition | | | | For the locally produced product | | Recommendations and comments |
	Actual product	Substitute product	Important organizations	Exports	Local demand	Current markets	Potential markets	
Pork and pork products	Monteagudo for local breed pigs Santa Cruz for industrial breed pigs Argentina for pig fat (manteca)	Other white meat Vegetable oil	—	No exports due to animal health status. There are imports of manteca	Industrial breed pigs in the main cities. Local breed pigs in Sucre and Potosi	Local in Camargo, small amounts to Sucre	Sucre, Potosi, Tarija,	Animal health status needs to be improved first for cysticercosis, but also classical swine fever An analysis of manteca production
Turkey meat	Chile, Peru and Cochabamba Small-scale producers in Sucre and Tarija	Chicken Other meats	Santa Rosa	There are imports of turkey meat	Demand for turkey in the main cities during Christmas	Does not exist	Tarija and Sucre Christmas markets for whole birds and pieces	Turkey production needs to be directed to finished birds for Christmas A cost analysis of processing the birds in pieces

This is by no means a comprehensive classification of methods available, but is meant more as a practical set of major headings under which to discuss various approaches and issues. All economic impact assessments require methods to identify and determine costs and benefits. In a broad sense, cost–benefit analysis can be seen as the overarching framework into which the outputs from other tools and methods can be incorporated.

Cost–Benefit Analysis

Cost–benefit analysis, or what Bennett (1992) terms 'social cost benefit analysis', is one of the most common methods of State project appraisal (Gittinger, 1982; Winpenny, 1991) and is analogous to investment appraisal described for the farm and business enterprises (see Chaper 7, this volume). It is used for projects or activities that involve public expenditure and values the costs and benefits to society as a whole (Dasgupta and Pearce, 1978). The basis of cost–benefit analysis is social welfare, but its outputs include similar criteria to those of investment appraisal.

Cost–benefit analysis provides a rigorous and comprehensive framework that incorporates the costs and benefits that arise. The costs and benefits produced from State-level interventions may be economic, environmental, biological and from human health changes. No other framework forces the analyst to consider the major impacts of a project, programme or policy change. It is not uncommon that the term cost–benefit analysis is used for analysis of a change using public or private funds. In this book, assessments of private investment over time are described as investment appraisal, as generally speaking they will not consider the wider implications for society of a private investment. However, it is suggested that changes in company reporting to include issues of corporate social responsibility mean that the methods that will be outlined for cost–benefit analysis are equally applicable to the assessment of large corporate investments. In addition, Alston et al. (1995) argue that, when cost–benefit analysis is used to assess research benefits in a partial

equilibrium framework, then it is in effect a special case of the economic surplus method outlined below.

Dijkhuizen et al. (1995) note that, for State investments in long-term disease control programmes either at the regional or national levels, cost–benefit analysis is typically the analytical structure of choice. In general, this involves estimating streams of costs and benefits associated with a particular control programme, which are then discounted using the methods described above in the investment appraisal section. The discount rate to use in cost–benefit analysis is often a source of considerable uncertainty, but for practical purposes the real rate of interest is used. The real rate of interest can be more easily calculated by estimating the difference between the rate of inflation and the current interest rate on saved money.

Cost–benefit analyses are typically carried out to compare and contrast different strategies within the livestock sector, and the outputs of such analyses include a set of investment criteria introduced above, such as the net present value (NPV), internal rate of return (IRR), and benefit/cost ratio (BCR). For example, Kristjanson (1997) projected future costs and benefits for the development and implementation of a vaccine against East Coast fever (ECF) in sub-Saharan Africa. This analysis estimated the maximum benefits possible from such an intervention (Mukhebi et al., 1992). A series of factors or assumptions on the estimated adoption rate, the probability of a vaccine being developed, and a depreciation factor for the vaccine effectiveness were then used to obtain the adjusted benefits and the total costs of the research programme. In a 30-year investment period the NPV was estimated to be US$160 million, the IRR 31%, and the BCR 15:1.

Various published examples of cost–benefit analysis being applied to animal health problems exist (Power and Harris, 1973; Hugh-Jones et al., 1975; Ellis et al., 1977; Rich and Winter-Nelson, 2007). The data requirements of social cost–benefit analysis are very high. The final analyses are often very sensitive to small changes in assumptions of discount rates, adoption rates and changes in livestock production parameters.

Some of the costs and benefits may also be extremely difficult to value appropriately, particularly where there are impacts on human health and the environment.

The term cost–benefit analysis has been used to include studies that look at individual as opposed to societal costs and benefits. For example, Bennett et al. (1997) use a standard methodology to study the economic importance of non-notifiable diseases of farm animals in the UK. This was set up in a spreadsheet for various diseases of cattle, sheep, pigs and poultry. The methodology involved looking, for each disease, at the systems affected, the livestock population at risk, the disease incidence and resultant disease effects, and then calculate the financial loss and the total cost of the disease, together with treatment and control costs. Similarly, McLeod (1995) estimated the costs of the major parasites to the Australian livestock industry using a simple spreadsheet of costs and benefit, which was then used to assess the farm-level profitability resulting from improved parasite management. This spreadsheet model has been extended to assess the importance of tick-borne diseases of cattle in Asia and Africa as well as Australia (McLeod, 1998).

It is assumed that these authors have used cost–benefit analysis to make a financial assessment of a change, whereas social cost–benefit analysis would be an economic assessment. The latter would take a method of analysis for helping society decide what is acceptable and what is not, and take into account the wider implications of change. For example, an intervention that implies a livestock population increase means that there will be pressure on natural resources. Therefore, environmental impacts have to be valued to complete the analysis. Techniques exist for valuing the environment such as the effect on production approach, contingent valuation, travel costs methods, and the human capital approach (Winpenny, 1991). It is noted that the data requirements, especially for the more sophisticated techniques, are considerable.

One of the weaknesses of many assessments of the overall impacts of livestock diseases on a society is a lack of information on the costs to avoid the impacts. The impact of the disease alone is insufficient to take decisions on the allocation of resources and will only give an overall impression of the importance of the disease. In order to take decisions further information is required on:

- the actual situation – a baseline;
- the costs of a change in animal disease status and when they occur;
- the benefits of a change in animal disease status and when they occur.

In many situations the baseline is also dynamic and for State-level interventions it is often important to recognize that the baseline may arrive at similar point to with an intervention. What the State is looking for could essentially be described as short cuts to an improved animal disease status, which in the process requires State investment and generates benefits to society. Examples of possible baselines are shown in Fig. 10.2. To develop a good baseline and also estimate the benefits generated, there is a need to have:

- A good understanding of the technical aspects that make up both the baseline and the intervention line; many of the benefits and costs will be generated within the livestock sector and a thorough understanding of the livestock sector cannot be ignored.
- Information on the incentives for the producers and people involved in the livestock sector to control a disease; a description of value chain analysis will return to this point.

In State or national-level livestock programmes, the objective is to accelerate the development of the sector either through the control or eradication of an animal disease or a change in livestock technology. Given the cost and complexity of carrying out a cost–benefit analysis, there is a need to have additional tools to decide whether it is worth carrying out such analyses. Decisions on whether to carry out a cost–benefit analysis of a State investment in the livestock sector can be refined by determining who benefits from a change. For example, the control of a contagious disease such as foot-and-mouth disease or zoonotic disease such as bovine tuberculosis by a farmer generates benefits to society as a whole and this is described as generating

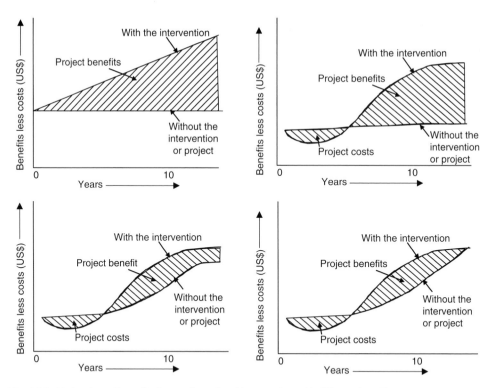

Fig. 10.2. Estimation of benefits from a State-level intervention with different baselines.

public goods. Such actions provide a strong justification for the State to assess whether an overall programme is required. However, there are interventions where the benefits are entirely or largely captured by individual producers. Such interventions generate private goods, and the role of the State is less clear. A possible example would be the control of parasites which have a localized impact. Where the State might play a useful role is in investment on research to control a localized disease and the dissemination of information on best control methods.

A change in animal disease status or the level of livestock technology, production and productivity of the livestock sector will have an impact on livestock product supply and in turn will affect the prices of livestock products. Benefits will accrue across society as most people are livestock consumers and this requires information on the relationship of supply and demand for the product affected. Information is therefore required in the elasticity of supply and demand. For diseases

that affect human health such as zoonoses or food-borne pathogens, changes in livestock sector practices that reduce the existence of these disease agents will lead to an overall improvement of human health status. This will generate benefit in terms of reduced medical costs, a reduction in the number of days lost through illness and with some diseases a reduction in the number of people who die. It has become common to present these benefits as the number of 'disability adjusted life years' (DALYs) saved by an intervention. Interventions in the livestock sector can also create impacts across the economy as a whole and models are required to estimate these impacts such as 'social accounting matrices' (SAMs) or computerized general equilibrium (CGE) models. These will be discussed in more detail below and will be assessed by Martin Upton in Chapter 11 (this volume). A complete cost–benefit analysis should also determine not just *where* and *when* costs and benefits of a proposed intervention to the livestock sector occur; it should also determine *who* bears the costs and benefits. Ideally, a State intervention will leave no one worse off than before and where possible would improve and facilitate the lives of the worse off in society.

It is important to reiterate that cost–benefit analysis provides a framework to assess a change in the livestock sector, either through a direct intervention in terms of a project or programme or through a change in regulations and laws. These are clear expressions of livestock policy. The analysis then requires all the costs and benefits of such a change to be estimated, both when they occur, where they occur and to whom they occur. As can be seen, to reach a final answer of a NPV, IRR and BCR from such complex estimations requires significant data collection and analysis and in many cases the use of a number of assumptions for future change. Therefore, interpreting the output from a cost–benefit analysis requires an understanding of the final output, and the process of analysis used to reach these final numbers. In this, the final numbers produced are an expression of many people's judgements of the value of change. There are no hard-and-fast rules on how to do this, but it is recommended that both people carrying out the cost–benefit analysis and those who have to use its output have a strong understanding of the livestock sector they are assessing and of the economic tools they use to examine farm and agrobusiness change and the wider societal implications. Without such a mixture of technical and economic knowledge there will always be the danger of producing a poor answer, even though the final analyses may involve very complex methodologies. There is no replacement for having good grass-roots knowledge.

The following will give more detailed descriptions of assessing the impact of change on markets and also models to predict the implications of change across society. The outputs of such methods can then be placed into a cost–benefit analysis framework.

Economic surplus methods

In discussing the approaches used to measure the economic consequences of agricultural research, Alston *et al.* (1995) present a relationship (a production function) between:

- current output or productivity, which is dependent on current flows of inputs such as concentrates or fertilizer;
- uncontrolled factors such as the weather; and
- current and past investments in agricultural research and extension.

They divide most of the approaches used into econometric approaches, which seek to quantify such relationships directly, and approaches based on economic surplus methods, which go beyond the production function to look at impacts of change on supply functions.

At aggregated levels in the hierarchy of systems, economic surplus methods have been quite widely used to assess the economic impacts of change. These changes may be brought about by new agricultural technology, such as the application of an animal disease control technology or strategy in a region. For this reason, economic surplus methods have been used in assessing past or future research activities. Rather than trying to assess the algebraic relationship between outputs and inputs, economic surplus methods are based on the premise that change, brought about by new technology or policy shifts, has an effect on the supply of the commodity (or commodities) being produced. This in turn changes the price paid for the commodity by consumers in society. Economic surplus methods attempt to quantify these shifts and to estimate the impact that change has for both the producers of the commodity and the consumers who purchase it.

In a simple example shown in Fig. 10.3 a country produces beef with an inelastic demand for the product and elastic supply for the product. However, the country cannot export beef because it has foot-and-mouth disease. This situation creates a small market and a low price in relation to the international price for beef for producers. The international market for beef is assumed to be unaffected by supply from the country. A plan is developed to control and eradicate foot-and-mouth disease. This has two impacts: there is a shift in the supply curve of beef as no foot-and-mouth disease improves farm-level productivity; and there is access to an international market for beef. The price increases for producers and reduces for national consumers. The benefits are to both groups and can be determined and quantified by examining the relationship between the national and international demand curves and the shifts in the national supply curves (see Fig. 10.3).

The example above is a very simplistic representation of reality and in more complex analyses there is a possibility that changes in the livestock sector may result in more benefits accruing to consumers rather than producers. However, the overall benefit to society could well be positive. The key steps of economic surplus methods are:

- Technological change occurs.
- The change has an impact on the location of the supply curve of the commodity.
- Analysis takes place to estimate this shift in supply and to identify the new market equilibrium.

- The partitioning of the benefits is calculated in some way.

The basic model has been extended in numerous ways. Non-linear supply and demand curves; non-parallel shifts in the supply curve (pivotal shifts, for example); multiple markets for a single commodity; multiple commodities; shifts in the demand curve as a result of quality changes, for instance; all these and more can be incorporated within the economic surplus framework.

Various criticisms have been made of economic surplus methods from both a conceptual and a practical point of view. Some of the conceptual problems are related to the need to make value judgements in such analyses and issues of policy irrelevance. From a practical point of view, the major problem is the substantial effort required in collecting, processing and analysing economic and technical data (Falconi, 1993).

There are various examples of the application of economic surplus methods to assess

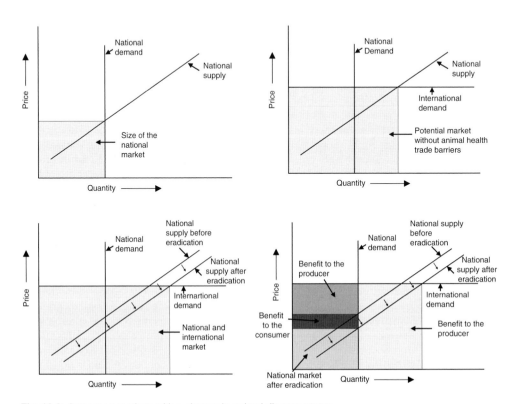

Fig. 10.3. Impact on markets with a change in animal disease status.

economic impacts of animal disease control technology. An example is Kristjanson *et al.* (1999), who look at the potential impact of an as-yet-undeveloped vaccine for trypanosomiasis in Africa using field data from Ghibe, Ethiopia. An economic surplus model was estimated to value increases in productivity and capture the uncertainties involved in ongoing development of a trypanosomiasis vaccine. The lower production costs were estimated to increase meat and milk supplies and at reduced prices to consumers. The value of the potential increase in milk and meat production with trypanosomiasis control was estimated to range between US$420 million and US$1.1 billion per year, with a net present value of trypanosomiasis vaccine research estimated to range between US$170 and US$470 million, an IRR of between 28% and 38% and a BCR varying from 20:1 to 54:1. Ott *et al.* (1995) also used the economic surplus method to measure the national economic benefits of reducing livestock mortality with an example of pigs in the USA.

As mentioned above data requirements for the economic surplus method are considerable. Information is required on:

- Productivity impacts, which may be difficult to quantify.
- Costs and prices and elasticities of supply and demand for the commodities involved.
- Adoption rates of the new technology have to be assessed probably through *ex post* studies either by collecting this through adoption studies or rapid surveys, while for *ex ante* studies expert opinion has to be sought concerning likely adoption lag time and ceiling adoption levels.
- If the study is *ex ante*, then another decision has to be made, again using expert opinion, about the likely success of the intervention (control programme or research activity).

However, such data are required for a complete cost–benefit analysis. What the economic surplus method adds is the ability to examine how livestock sector change affects markets and who will gain or lose in such change. The economic surplus method is reasonably flexible and, for impact assessments that seek to quantify the effects of animal disease control programmes or technology changes at the sectoral, national or international level, there are few realistic alternatives to methods based on notions of economic surplus.

Mathematical programming methods

The optimization methods outlined earlier with regard to the farm level have not been used widely for animal health purposes at the regional or national levels. One example is Habtemariam *et al.* (1984), who investigated the economics of trypanosomiasis control in Ethiopia using linear programming methods. Dynamic programming, which involves the search for an optimal solution involving a sequence of decisions over time, has been used by Hall *et al.* (1998) to model the economics of different animal health control programmes.

In the real world, decision makers do not generally have simple objective functions. Mathematical programming methods have been developed that allow multiple objectives to be dealt with, such as maximizing profit while minimizing income variability, or maximizing profit while minimizing soil loss. Especially when dealing with the regional or national level, the set of objectives that have to be incorporated may become very complicated. The various stakeholders may have competing objectives, which imply that compromises have to be reached. There are very few examples of multi-criteria programming applications to animal health issues at the regional or national level. There would certainly seem to be considerable scope for models such as that of Van Keulen and Veneeklaas (1993) to incorporate animal health issues. That particular model treated animal traction in some detail, and the goals related to physical production, monetary targets and risk in a dry year, employment and emigration, all within an interactive multiple goal programming framework. Indeed, the utility of decision support systems based on multi-objective programming methods would appear to be substantial, in allowing stakeholders the opportunity to investigate 'what-if' scenarios of different options, in an effort to reach compromises interactively between the various objectives of the different groups affected.

The effectiveness of such approaches depends heavily on appropriate specification of the decision problem and appropriate specification of the objectives of the various stakeholders.

Simulation and systems analysis

While modelling and systems analysis have been widely used to address all sorts of problems, including animal health issues, at the animal, herd and farm levels, there are fewer examples of their use at national or regional level. Such models have often been used to help derive input–output relationships that are then used in other analytical frameworks, such as cost–benefit analysis and economic surplus methods. Saatkamp *et al.* (1996) describe a simulation model based on a Markov process designed to evaluate national identification and recording schemes with respect to their epidemiological impact on outbreaks of classical swine fever. Snow *et al.* (1996) used systems analysis to investigate the problem of African animal trypanosomiasis in The Gambia, and identified a few trends as being of major importance: human population growth, declining rainfall, reduced fallowing, etc. The existence of these trends raised serious concerns as to the sustainability of traditional grazing on common land, although it was concluded that improved, intensive management strategies could go some way to alleviating these problems.

Summary of methods at the sector, national and international levels

Table 10.4 presents a summary of the methods covered. It is clear that, at the national and regional levels, the major framework is provided by cost–benefit analysis, often incorporating notions of economic surplus. Mathematical programming and simulation modelling systems analysis can provide useful information for decision making and in quantifying costs and benefits for impact assessments, but generally

require very specific skills. Approaches based on a combination of methods would seem to offer considerable potential for decision makers at the sector and national levels. For example, farm-level information might be generated using optimization or simulation methods, which could then be related to characteristic or 'typical' farms identified from some sort of classification. The response from the farm level could be aggregated to the sector level using cost–benefit and economic surplus methods, to identify impacts of change at various levels in the hierarchy.

For those requiring further information on sectoral- and national-level investment tools please refer to Martin Upton's contribution to this book in Chapter 11 (this volume) and Rich *et al.* (2005) for a review of methods. The final part of this chapter presents value chain analysis, which allows thinking on the general livestock sector, the motivations for involvement in the sector and potential changes. Value chain analysis is a useful supplementary tool to cost–benefit analysis in terms of selecting which interventions require deeper assessment, and once an intervention has been shown to be of benefit to society who needs to be targeted to ensure the intervention is successful.

Value Chain Analysis

The production economics chapter (Chapter 3, this volume) and the following information on economic assessment tools such as gross margin analysis, partial budgets and investment appraisal give the impression that all aspects of people's decisions, be they livestock producers or agrobusiness people involved in the livestock sector, are based around the rationale of costs and benefits and the free access to information. This limited model of the world is useful in examining certain market situations, but in most markets there is a need to introduce an institutional context in which that market is found. Here we can examine who are the actors in the livestock sector, what their profitabilities and opportunities are and what their constraints are in terms of regulations, investment in human

Table 10.4. Some characteristics of the methods discussed for economic impact assessment at the regional and national levels. (Modified from Rushton et al., 1999.)

	Objective	Data requirements	Outputs	Strengths	Weaknesses
Cost–benefit analysis (strict sense)	Compare programmes and interventions in terms of their societal welfare effects (including valuation of environmental effects)	Productivity impacts Costs and prices Elasticities Adoption data Discount rate Environmental valuation of impacts Productivity impacts Costs, prices	NPV IRR BCR	A framework that can combine rigour with comprehensiveness	Data requirements Analytical skills required are substantial
Economic surplus	Quantify the impacts of a shift in the supply curve and the resultant economic surplus; partition this between consumers and producers	Productivity impacts Costs and prices Elasticities Adoption data Discount rate	Economic surplus US$ NPV IRR BCR	A framework than can be extended with considerable flexibility to make it realistic at the national and international levels	Data requirements The economic surplus concept lacks intuitive appeal Analytical skills required are substantial
Mathematical programming	Maximize an objective function subject to resource and other constraints	Input–output coefficients Stakeholders' attitudes and objectives Cost–price data	Activity mixes shadow prices Depends on the objective function	A flexible framework for well-behaved and well-formulated problems	Data requirements Analytical skills required are substantial Needs a very clear understanding of stakeholders' objectives
Simulation modelling and systems analysis	Use a systems model (of some description) to carry out 'what-if' scenario analysis	Detailed understanding of the system under study	System response to particular input conditions	The ultimately flexible framework Ability to incorporate risk, uncertainty, component interactions	Analytical skills required are enormous Problem definition can be somewhat fuzzy – some models end up as tools looking for an application

capital and infrastructure. In reality, we are placing the analysis into a framework of new institutional analysis, a branch of economics that has successfully argued that markets and commercialization do not change and develop through price signals alone.

This type of analysis has been called *value chain analysis*, which covers a wide range of topics from local-level incentives to work on livestock supply and value chains to government regulations that affect how any person involved in this chain may work. The following parts of this chapter will present a limited range of methods and background theory required for a thorough value chain analysis. For those wanting more detailed information on value chain analysis they are recommended to refer to Kaplinsky and Morris (2000).

The main objectives of value chain analysis are identified to be the following:

• Identify the main actors or organizations in the livestock value chain from the input provider to the producer, trader, processor, retailer and then through to the final consumer.

• Identify the different routes to market the livestock and livestock products, which could be what currently exists and what potentially is available or could be developed.

• Assess how well the marketing chain is working.

A value chain analysis can involve different groups of people, but it is recommended that the following are contacted:

1. In the initial stages of the analysis the research should work closely with the livestock producers to identify the important input suppliers, traders and markets of livestock and livestock products. Such contact will also allow an understanding of how familiar the producers are with the final demands for a livestock product. For isolated communities this can be very important, e.g. llama producers in the Altiplano of Bolivia were not aware that consumers paid a premium for meat free of sarcocystiosis, therefore their production practices did not alter to control this disease.
2. The analysis should also work with the livestock and livestock product traders and

markets identified with the producers to determine what happens to the livestock and livestock products and who is involved. If the consumer is not reached at this stage it is recommended that work continues down the chain until the consumer is reached.
3. Once an understanding of a chain has been developed from input supplier to producer and on to the consumers, data gaps should be identified and filled with either primary or secondary data. The latter will involve contacting people and organizations who have previously collected and documented important data and information in the past.
4. The initial value chain analysis can be presented and discussed with the producers and traders, and where necessary modified and possible weaknesses identified.
5. If possible interventions are identified that are beyond the financial, human resource or logistical means of the actors in the chain, then results should be presented to government organizations, either local or national authorities for the consideration of State intervention.

A value chain analysis can be split into three basic steps:

1. Description of the value chain;
2. Identification of important routes and actors in the chain;
3. Assessing the profitability, power and institutional environment of the key actors.

Description of the value chain

A graphical representation of the livestock value chain can be developed through primary and secondary data collection. Initial results should be shared with people with knowledge of the particular livestock subsector the work is focused on to ensure that the routes for livestock marketing are accurate and well described. Such an analysis will identify the key routes of trade for the livestock and livestock products, the important actors in terms of livestock production, processing and trading and also the main consumers and who they are and where they are found. Once a description has been agreed this can be transferred to an electronic format using a program such as PowerPoint.

Some chains will be complex and involve different routes for commercialization, with consumers who have very different socio-economic status and geographic location. However, not all livestock value chains are complicated and some will be dominated by local processing and consumption.

Identifying the important routes and actors in the value chain

To identify the most important routes and actors in the livestock value chain it is recommended where possible to determine the:

1. Number of livestock producers using the different routes within a chain;
2. Volume of product that moves through the different routes of the chain;
3. Monetary value that moves through the different routes of the chain.

A combination of 2 and 3 allows an analysis of the prices paid per unit, but this information needs to be combined with quality information as some routes may pay more per unit, but demand different qualities. Figure 10.4 presents different ways of expressing the importance of the different branches of a livestock value chain.

Some of this information may be sensitive and it will not always be possible to carry out a quantitative analysis of each route in the value chain.

Assessing the profitability, power and institutional environment of the key actors

Having identified the key actors or groups of actors in the chain, where possible, enterprise budgets should be developed for their live-stock activities. In addition, these actors or groups of actors should be interviewed with regard to their input and output markets for their livestock activity, including the opportunities and constraints they perceive in terms of supply, demand and regulations of the activity. Where possible, there should also be information generated on how important each actor or group actors is in terms of their power to determine price, to set quantity and quality standards and their ability to search for, and gain entry into, new markets.

Analysis

Equitability in the chain

The market analysis presented commercialization margins and the proportion of the final product price gained by each actor. Both are possible measures of equitability along the chain but neither takes into account the costs and profits of each actor. To provide a more adequate picture of equitability, enterprise budgets should be developed for each actor or group of actors along the most important routes of the value chain. These can then be compared in terms of profit generated per unit of output, returns per unit of labour and costs per unit of key input.

Governance of the chain

The type of governance of livestock value chains can be distilled into the following categories:

1. *Markets.* There are repeated transactions among different actors but the costs of switching to new actors are low. Probably the case for low volume and infrequent sales such as the occasional sale of chickens to raise small amounts of cash.
2. *Modular value chains.* Suppliers make products to a customer's specifications. Suppliers take responsibility for competencies surrounding process technology and incur few transaction-specific investments. Some milk value chains have these kinds of characteristics where the demand for milk of a certain quality demands a premium price and the producers respond with little investment and small management changes to improve their milk quality.
3. *Relational value chains.* There is mutual dependence regulated through reputation, social and spatial proximity, family and ethnic ties, etc. For example, the speciality cheese products such as Stilton or Parmesan, or the cured ham such as Parma.

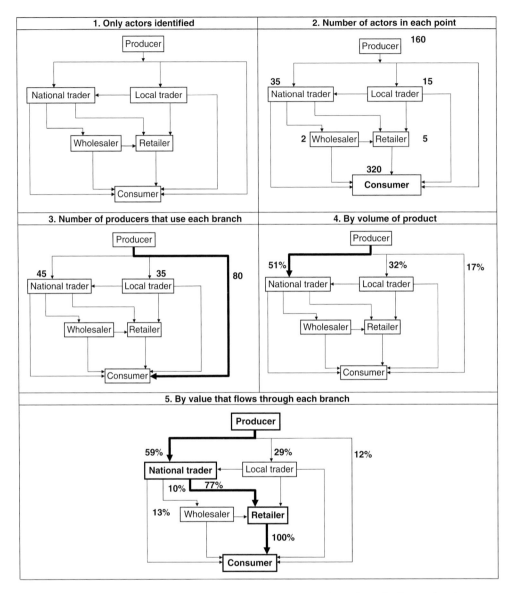

Fig. 10.4. Different ways of assessing the importance of different branches of a livestock value chain.

4. *Captive value chains.* Small suppliers depend on much larger buyers for their transactions and face significant switching costs and are, therefore, 'captive'. These networks are frequently characterized by a high degree of monitoring and control by the lead firm, creat-ing dependence on the suppliers. Many milk value chains now have this kind of structure.
5. *Hierarchy.* This implies vertical integra-tion with managerial control. The industrial chicken broiler industry has integrated value chains, often where one company owns and

manages input, production and processing units.

What type of governance develops within a chain is dependent on the following factors:

1. Complexity of the transfer of knowledge between the different actors or groups in the chain to complete a transaction;
2. The extent to which this information and knowledge can be codified and transmitted efficiently without transaction-specific investment; and
3. Capabilities of actual and potential suppliers in relation to the requirements of the transaction.

Governance of a livestock value chain is important because it can influence how the chain develops in terms of upgrading the livestock product, process and functioning of that chain or by changing to a completely new chain. Private regulation across livestock value chains is playing an increasingly important role in dictating the development of livestock production and processing standards. The enforcement mechanisms through the private sector are strong as they can be transmitted by price. This is particularly important when considering demands on the livestock sector for safer food and also for animals that have been produced in a welfare-friendly manner. The role of the private sector for animal health improvement needs to be taken into account when planning State-level interventions (Henson, 1996). Therefore, a good understanding of the governance of livestock sector chains will allow public organizations to identify the key actors in the chains and develop strategies of how they can be involved to participate in changes in animal health practices and standards.

Summary of Value Chain Analysis

The value chain analysis brings together the data and information generated and structured by gross margin and market analyses. It is a flexible tool that can be useful in identifying key constraints and opportunities within a livestock value chain. It can also be a useful means to identify possible risk areas for disease spread within a livestock sector and identify the main actors involved at these points. In turn, where the risks are deemed to be high enough, and the reduction of these risks are thought to create large impacts on society in general (termed externalities), public interventions would appear to be appropriate. Such initial 'look and see' analyses help to direct where further cost–benefit analyses are required. If these more in-depth and complex assessment methods predict that a positive return to society can be generated by a State intervention then implementation planning can begin. Value chain analysis can also be a useful tool in such planning as it directs and identifies individuals and organizations who need to be involved in order for an intervention to succeed.

Summary

This chapter has given a brief introduction into methods beyond the farm and business management tools. The next two chapters (Chapters 11 and 12, this volume) are contributions from Professors Martin Upton and David Leonard. Professor Upton makes an assessment of different economic tools available for assessing livestock markets and the livestock sector in general. Professor Leonard provides a more general overview on the use of institutional economics. This is followed by a chapter that examines the cultural aspects of livestock production and the livestock sector in general (Chapter 13, this volume). Dr Alexandra Shaw's contribution provides a very thorough overview of how to assess the costs and benefits of zoonotic diseases and their control (Chapter 14, this volume). The final chapter (Chapter 15, this volume) of this part presents an overview of general livestock systems analysis and presents examples of such analyses from around the world.

11 Tools for Assessing the Price and Market Impacts of Livestock Policies

Martin Upton

Introduction

A wide range of different qualitative and quantitative methods are available for the analysis of alternative livestock policy options. These include not only price and market analysis, but also project appraisal, risk analysis and applications of the 'new institutional economics'. All these methods are used in many different contexts, but specific issues arise in their application to livestock policy, associated with the capital investment in the animals, the rapid growth in demand, the risks of disease, and the importance of world trade.

The fact that livestock are capital assets, and that production depends upon rates of reproduction and growth, necessitates special methods of accounting, in preparing activity budgets. Allowance must be made for the appreciation of young stock and the depreciation of breeding/milking stock. These may vary from year to year, depending upon mortalities and offtake and changes in flock/herd structure. As an alternative approach, steady state herd models may be used for accounting purposes, while other herd growth models may be used to predict changes in animal numbers over time.

There is a greater need for dynamic analysis than in the case of annual crops. Thus, supply response by livestock producers is generally subject to significant time lags. These complicate the estimation of supply elasticities and may be responsible for cyclical variation in prices and quantities supplied, as occurs in the 'pig cycle'.

Price and Market Analysis

This contribution is concerned only with methods of assessing the impacts of policies on livestock prices and markets. Much emphasis was given to price analysis in the 1970s and 1980s when the international debt crisis was attributed, in part, to misguided pricing and trade policies in developing countries. The resultant distortions would, it was claimed, be corrected by privatization and market liberalization. Following structural adjustment reforms in many developing countries, price distortions have been reduced. However, tariffs and other trade barriers imposed by some developed countries affect world prices. Price and market analyses are still useful planning tools.

We deal first with partial equilibrium approaches, to assess price distortions and market impacts for a single commodity. These approaches include:

- the policy analysis matrix (PAM); and
- 'economic surplus' analysis.

Exploration of the wider market impacts of policies on prices of other commodities, and for factors of production, requires the use of larger and more complicated models. Examples include:

- social accounting matrix (SAM);
- regional- or sector-level, mathematical programming models;
- econometric multi-market models;
- computable general equilibrium (CGE) models.

The data and time requirements, for the construction of any of these multi-enterprise models, are large. They are more likely to be used as research tools rather than for more routine policy analysis. Some brief notes on their relative strengths and weaknesses follow later in these notes.

Policy analysis matrix

Purpose. The PAM is used to measure the impact of government policy on the private profitability of a specific agricultural enterprise and to assess whether there is a comparative advantage in that enterprise. The first of these aims is achieved by comparing current market prices, with the corresponding 'real', 'social'[1] or 'opportunity-cost' prices. Comparative advantage is assessed by comparing the return to domestic resources, of land, labour and capital, with the opportunity cost.

The layout of the PAM is illustrated in Table 11.1.

Data requirements. Construction of a PAM first requires the preparation of an activity budget, to estimate the average, or typical, output (A), tradable costs[2] (B) and domestic factor costs (C) per unit of production, all measured at current market prices. Note that, in the case of livestock, measurement of out-

Table 11.1. Layout for a policy analysis matrix.

| | Tradables | | Domestic | |
	Outputs	Inputs	factors	Profits
Private	A	B	C	D
Opportunity cost	E	F	G	H
Policy effects	I	J	K	L

put requires special methods to take account of multiple products and changes in capital valuations, as suggested above. Given the incomplete markets for factors of production, in developing countries, it may be very difficult to estimate a private market cost for 'domestic factors'. However, if estimation is possible then clearly the 'profit' or 'net margin' can be calculated.

These outputs and costs must then be revalued at their 'opportunity-cost' or 'real prices' for insertion at E, F and G. For outputs (E) and tradable, variable inputs (F), these values may be estimated by the 'border prices' (p^b). For the fixed costs of domestic resources, other methods must be used to estimate the opportunity costs (G), such as the gross margin or 'value added', from other activities.

The policy effects I, J, K and L are obtained by subtracting the opportunity cost from the private market price in each case.

Indices: Given p_i^d = domestic price of product, p_i^b = border price of product, p_j^d = domestic price of the jth input, p_i^b = border price of the jth input, a_{ij} = input–output coefficient

$$\text{Nominal protection coefficien } (NPC_i) = A/E = \frac{p_i^d}{p_i^b}$$

If $NPC > 1$ producers are protected and consumers or the public are taxed, but if $NPC < 1$ producers are taxed and consumers or the Government benefit.

Effective protection coefficient (EPC_i) =

$$(A-B)/(E-F) = \frac{Va_i^d}{Va_i^b} = \frac{p_i^d - \sum_j a_{ij}p_j^d}{p_i^b - \sum_j a_{ij}p_j^b}$$

---

[1] The term 'social price' is used in this sense in some of the literature. However, the term is also often applied where income distributional weightings have been used in evaluation. To avoid confusion, the term 'opportunity cost' (OC) is used in the present context.

[2] The terminology for categorizing costs differs from that used in enterprise activity budgets. However, 'tradable costs' correspond closely with 'variable costs', 'domestic factors' with 'fixed costs' and 'value added (on primary factors)' with 'gross margin'.

The same conditions apply for positive or negative protection of producers and consumers/taxpayers as for the *NPC*.

Domestic resources cost (DRC$_i$) =

$$G/(E-F) = \frac{\sum_{j=k+1}^{n} a_{ij}p_j^*}{p_i^b - \sum_{j=1}^{k} a_{ij}p_j^b}$$

This is the ratio of the opportunity cost of the domestic resources to the value-added, or gross margin, when all outputs and inputs are valued at their opportunity cost.

If *DRC* < 1, then there is a net gain to the national economy from producing the commodity. The profit or net margin (*H*) is positive.

If *DRC* > 1, then there is a net loss to the national economy from producing the commodity. The profit or net margin (*H*) is negative.

Strengths. This tool is a relatively simple and transparent approach to estimating the level of government price support provided to, or taxation (negative support) extracted from, producers. The nominal protection coefficient measures support provided through the product, while the effective protection coefficient also allows for the effects of input subsidies or taxes. Indications of both private and national economic profitability are provided, the latter being measured by the domestic resource cost.

The PAM may be used to compare levels of support and domestic resource costs before and after policy change (Rushton *et al.*, 2004; Staal *et al.*, 2004). Comparisons may also be made of support and domestic resource costs for different productive activities and possibly for different stages in the production chain, such as that for dairy products (Tulachan, 2004).

Weaknesses. The PAM is a partial analysis of one enterprise at a time, with fixed input–output coefficients. Differences between producers in scale and productive efficiency raise problems in estimating a typical, representative activity budget for the whole industry. EPCs and DRCs might differ substantially between different types of production system. The analysis is also static, referring to a single production cycle.

Measurement of the 'border parity price' raises problems of: (i) identifying an appropriate measure of the world price on international markets; (ii) deciding whether to use the official exchange rate or a shadow exchange rate; and (iii) adjustment of the border price to allow for transport to, or from, the border. Estimation of the opportunity cost of domestic resources is extremely difficult and generally requires use of an alternative planning tool such as linear programming. The classification of inputs into either 'tradables' or 'domestic factors' may raise problems of economic valuation, since 'non-tradable' items, such as electricity or local transport, do not fall into either category, yet strictly should be taken into account.

Although the impacts of government policy on product and input prices are identified, there is no clear indication of the distribution of costs and benefits between producers, consumers and government, or of the relative costs and benefits of alternative pricing policies. The PAM results provide little indication of the policy impacts on efficiency, economic welfare, the government budget or the balance of payments.

Economic surplus analysis

Purpose and method. This approach, based on estimated supply and demand schedules for a single commodity, provides estimates of the impacts of alternative price and trade policies, together with those of technological change, on producers, consumers and the Government/taxpayers. The resultant net social gain, or loss, is also identified. Generally, market margins and transaction costs are ignored.

The concept of 'economic surplus', subdivided into 'consumer surplus' and 'producer surplus', is illustrated in Fig. 11.1.

The hypothetical national supply (SS') and demand (DD') curves for milk are shown in the figure. The normal assumptions are made of a downward-sloping demand curve, reflecting diminishing marginal utility, and an upward-sloping supply curve, reflecting increasing marginal costs of production. The equilibrium, where quantity supplied equals

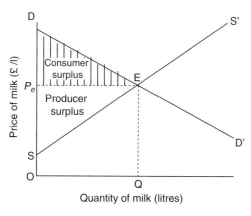

Fig. 11.1. Supply, demand and the economic surplus.

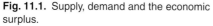

Fig. 11.2. The effect of a product subsidy in a closed economy.

the quantity demanded, occurs at point E, at an equilibrium price OP.

Given that points on the demand curve represent the price levels that consumers are willing to pay for the corresponding quantity of milk, while the price that is actually paid is only equal to OP, the difference represents a 'surplus' derived by the consumers. The total is represented by the shaded triangle, 'PED' and labelled 'consumer surplus'.[3]

Since the supply curve represents the marginal variable cost of production, the area below the supply curve (OSEQ) equals the total variable cost. However, the revenue from milk sales is equal to price times quantity, which is area OPEQ. Hence, the producer surplus, or return on fixed inputs, is equal to the difference, between total revenue and total variable cost, triangle SEP.

With this theoretical framework, a wide range of policies, for input and product pricing, international trade and technological change, can be analysed and assessed. The effect of a flat rate subsidy per litre of milk is first illustrated for a closed economy with no external trade, in Fig. 11.2.

_____

[3] Strictly speaking, as expenditure on milk is increased, the residual income of consumers is reduced. Hence the 'consumer surplus' is not an exact measure of the change in consumer welfare. However, it provides a reasonable approximation where the income effects of price changes are small.

The subsidy, per litre, is equal to OP_p minus OP_c, the difference between the producer price (P_p) and the consumer price (P_c). As a result of the subsidy, the producer price is raised from P_e to P_p while the consumer price is reduced to P_c while the quantities of milk, supplied and demanded, are increased to OQ_2.

The consumer surplus is increased by the area, 1 + 2 + 3 (1 + 2 the impact of reduced price and 3 from increased consumption).

The producer surplus is increased by 5 + 6 (due partly to increased price and partly to increased quantity sold).

However, the subsidy represents a cost to the Government or indirectly to the taxpayer. This cost equals −(1 + 2 + 3 + 4 + 5 + 6).

Thus, subtraction of the gains in consumer and producer surplus from the cost to the Government or national taxpayers leaves a net loss in social welfare, equal to area 4.

In the absence of external trade, the benefits of a subsidy are shared between both producers and consumers, the proportions depending upon the relative elasticities of supply and demand. However, for a country engaged in trade, the benefits accrue only to the producer if the local purchase price is raised above the border parity price, and only to the consumer if the local sale price is held below the border parity price. The second of these cases is illustrated in Fig. 11.3.

In this case, the border parity price is assumed to be lower than the equilibrium price with no trade. Hence, the nation benefits

140   Chapter 11

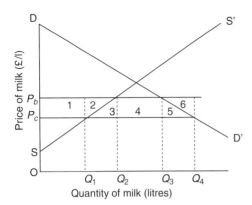

Fig. 11.3. The effect of a consumer subsidy on imported milk.

by importing milk at price P_b. The gain in consumer surplus, resulting from the lower price, is greater than the loss of producer surplus, so overall there is a net social gain. The 'small-country assumption' is also made, namely that the level of imports has no impact on the 'world price'. Hence, the border parity price is constant and can be represented by a horizontal straight line. Pre-subsidy, the domestic market price would equal the border parity price (P_b), and quantity OQ_3 would be demanded, OQ_2 supplied by domestic producers and Q_2Q_3 from imports.

A subsidy on imports reduces the consumer price to the level of P_c and increases the level of imports to Q_1Q_4. The producer price is driven down to the level of P_c, with a corresponding reduction in domestic supply. The welfare impacts are then as follows:

Increase in consumer surplus = 1 + 2 + 3 +
                               4 + 5
Loss of producer surplus = −(1 + 2)
Cost of subsidy = −(2 + 3 + 4 + 5 + 6)
Net social loss = (2 + 6).

Area 2, though part of the gain in consumer surplus, involves a cost to both producers, loss of producer surplus, and taxpayers, covered by the subsidy. Thus, a net cost is incurred. Area 6 represents a 'deadweight loss' since it is part of the cost of the subsidy but yields no benefits to society.

Data requirements. Information is needed on domestic markets, including prices, quantities and price elasticities of both supply and demand. In addition, data are needed on the levels of direct price interventions, possible shifts in the supply and possibly the demand schedule and, in the case of trade policies, levels of import and export parity prices.

Ideally the data should be accurate and complete. However, many key insights may be gained with fairly crude assessments of the market situation under different policy scenarios.

Strengths. Economic surplus analysis is a powerful theoretical and empirical tool for determining who gains and who loses from changes in public policy. Hypothetical examples, like those described above, are used to illustrate the relative impacts of a wide range of pricing, trade and technological change policies, singly or in combination. This approach forms a basis for agricultural and general economic development policy in texts by Ellis (1992), Sadoulet and de Janvry (1995) and Tweeten (1989).

In real-world situations, with reliable estimates of elasticities of supply and demand, border parity prices and supply shifts likely to result from technical change, the magnitude of changes in consumer and producer surplus may be calculated. The findings are generally useful to policy makers, even when the statistical estimates are of low accuracy.

Weaknesses. Some limitations have already been mentioned.

- This is a partial equilibrium approach, applied to a single enterprise.
- The analysis is essentially static, although time lags may be allowed for by using long-run elasticity estimates.
- Marketing margins are commonly ignored, as in the above examples. Their inclusion would be possible but would complicate the analysis.
- The consumer surplus is an inexact measure of price-induced change in consumer welfare. However, the discrepancy is small provided that either: (i) the income elasticity of demand is low; or (ii) the proportion of household income spent on the commodity is small.

In addition, there is some debate about the legitimacy of aggregating individual utilities to arrive at the consumer surplus, and individual cost curves, in estimating total variable costs for the industry and hence the producer surplus.

Finally, price elasticities of supply and demand are usually estimated from time-series data over quite a small range of price and quantity variation. Little is known about the shapes of the supply and demand functions for very small or very large quantities. No problem arises in assessing price and trade policies where relatively small changes in consumer and producer surpluses are expected. The elasticities of supply and demand may then be assumed to be constant over the expected price and quantity changes. However, for the analysis of technical change it is necessary to predict the shape of the entire supply function and the likely shift.

Multi-sectoral and Multi-market Models

The main strength of these multi-activity models, in comparison with the partial equilibrium models discussed above, is that they allow assessment of the interactions between sectors and markets. The market for a particular livestock product now forms only a small part of the whole model, but the impacts of policies for that product on markets for substitutes, complements, inputs or food processing industries may be important.

The scale and complexity of multi-sectoral and multi-market models are also a major source of weakness, in that the data, skill and time requirements are high. They are therefore costly to build. As such, model construction may involve a 2- or 3-year research effort. Unless a suitable and relevant model has already been built for other purposes, they are unlikely to be used in regular policy analysis.

Detailed description of individual methods would involve a lengthy presentation, and is unjustified given their limited regular use in policy analysis. A few brief notes follow on the distinctions between different methods.

The social accounting matrix (SAM)

The SAM provides a simple and efficient framework for organizing a complete set of accounts of transactions between sectors and agencies. It can also be used to assess the economy-wide effects of an increase in demand for one commodity, such as milk or meat, or a change in inputs to a firm or household, through what is called 'multiplier analysis'. The approach is useful in exploring links between livestock production, agriculture and the rest of the economy.

There are six types of account: activities, commodities, factors (labour and capital), institutions or agencies (farms, firms, households and government), a separate government capital account and 'the rest of the world'. The accounts are presented in a square matrix with expenditures listed in columns and receipts in rows. Since accounts must balance, the corresponding column and row totals must be equal.

Simple matrix operations allow predictions of the impacts of change, but there is no attempt to find an optimum allocation of resources.

Limitations: All relationships are assumed to be linear, with constant input–output coefficients. Hence, the analysis does not allow for price adjustments, for substitution between productive inputs or consumption goods or for changes in technology.

Mathematical programming models

These multi-enterprise models may be used to compare optimal solutions for different commodity price levels, different sets of resource and other constraints and different input–output coefficients, resulting from changes in technology. Optimization may be based on the single objective of income (gross margin) maximization, in which case shadow prices for resources may be estimated, or on multiple objectives.

Data are required on enterprise gross margins, contributions to other choice criteria, input–output coefficients, and constraint levels. Results provide indications of policy impacts on production, resource use and possibly opportunity costs, and household incomes. Applied to the agricultural sector, a single composite 'policy-maker' model may be built for the whole sector. Alternatively, separate representative farm models may be built for specific farm types. As a further step, the individual farm results may then be aggregated, as components of the whole-sector model. This last involves a further iterative process.

Limitations: All relationships are assumed to be linear, with constant coefficients. Changes in prices, constraint levels or technologies can only be introduced on a comparative static basis. No account is taken of impacts of incomes and quantities of produce generated on prices. The analysis is still only partial, dealing with a single sector, such as agriculture. The specification of the objective function is somewhat arbitrary in assuming perfect rationality and efficiency of the decision maker. Furthermore, the solution algorithm for multi-level programming is rather cumbersome. Multi-period programming is possible but greatly complicates the analysis.

Econometric multi-market models

These models differ from the previous cases in being based on non-linear equations relating to production, product demands and input supplies, together with identities for the residual impacts on the balance of trade and government revenues. They generally relate to a particular sector, such as agriculture. Producers are assumed to maximize profits, which allows optimum profit levels to be expressed as a function of input and product prices and levels of fixed factors. Time-series analysis provides estimates of the profit functions for different agricultural products and different producers, or agricultural households. Price–quantity relationships can then be derived for product supply and input demand. These together with product demand and input supply relationships allow estimation of levels of production and input use, household incomes and impacts on the government budget and the balance of trade.

These models have advantages over those discussed earlier, in taking fuller account of interactions between product markets, income effects on consumer demands and impacts on government and trade balances. Lagged variables can be incorporated

and these models may be used for forecasting. Policy analysis involves simulation of alternative scenarios. The IMPACT model used by Delgado *et al.* (1999) to review the 'Livestock Revolution' is an example applied at the global level.

Limitations: The analysis involves estimation of a large number of equations, which is costly and time-consuming. Hence, various simplifications are introduced. Although many market interactions are involved, it deals with only one sector of the economy. Many feedback linkages are ignored. The assumption of pure profit maximization, implicit in the use of indirect profit functions, is questionable in smallholder farming situations. Relationships are estimated using log-linear functions that are only valid for small deviations form the initial situation. The model is essentially static, so that dynamic changes can only be assessed using comparative statics.

Computable general equilibrium (CGE) models

This approach is based on the same comprehensive socio-economic structure as the SAM, with multi-sectoral and multi-agency disaggregation. However, it differs in that relative prices are determined, as market equilibria, while macroeconomic variables, investment and savings, balance of payments and government budgets are also included.

CGE models are of most value for analysing policies when socio-economic structure, price effects and macroeconomic impacts are expected to be important. Thus, the effects of changes in tariff policies by importing countries on the rest of the world, or of shifts in domestic social structure and income distribution may usefully be analysed using CGE models.

Limitations: A major problem is the large number of relationships to be estimated. Econometric estimation of coefficients is inevitably based on partial analysis, with risks of omitting the effects of important interactions. Some modellers adopt approximate values for the variables and calibrate them to replicate the base-year data compiled in the

SAM. The CGE model is essentially static, so is of limited value for forecasting. Because aggregation of groups of sectors and agencies is needed, CGE analysis is of limited value for detailed assessment of specific policy packages with few external impacts. Similarly, use of this tool is unnecessary for the assessment of macroeconomic policies with few micro-level impacts.

Postscript: Consistency Frameworks

A further approach to market analysis is used by FAO to identify potential gaps between agricultural production and consumption, by enterprise, for instance in the CAPPA model (FAO, 1991). Future consumer demand estimates are based on human fertility data, projected income growth and income elasticity of demand coefficients. Production growth is projected from information on land and water resources, stocks of fixed factors, expected yield gains and predicted constraints on export markets. Sensitivity analysis is used to give a range of results. The aim is to identify gaps between consumption and production, and provide a basis for planning how best to modify these gaps.

The approach must be modified in the case of livestock to account for the fixed capital stock represented by the existing animal herds or flocks. Herd growth models are used to predict future levels of production of meat and other products, and from this to estimate the demand for feeds (see Hallam *et al.*, 1983; Hallam, 1984).

Limitations. This approach takes no account of producer or consumer price response. It is inflexible in assuming fixed productivity coefficients and no scope for substitution across products.

12 The New Institutional Economics and the Assessment of Animal Disease Control

Jonathan Rushton and David K. Leonard

Introduction

During the 1980s a sea change occurred in thinking about the role of government in economic development. From the late 1940s, when 'development' came to be seen as a subject in its own right, to the 1970s most ideas about economic and agricultural development assigned an important role to State action. Most clearly this was true for the centrally planned economies such as the People's Republic of China or Cuba, but it also applied in the many other, 'mixed' economies in which private enterprise and market forces were allowed more scope. Nevertheless, by the end of the 1980s, State intervention in the economy had come to be severely questioned. Throughout the world, ideas stressing the primacy of the market as a way to organize economic activity and prescribing a small or even a minimal role for the State had come to the fore. Why the disquiet about government? Two strands of thought can be identified:

- a concern about efficiency, a managerial and economic worry;
- a desire for more direct and immediate accountability of public services to citizens, a political and social point.

In the developing world, animal health had been regarded as a predominantly public service and therefore was predominantly provided by government. However, since the 1980s the provision of animal health has been increasingly opened to market institutions, and there has been an evaluation of government services against those of the private sector. Much of the pressure for these changes came from those who simply wished to downsize the State and lessen the burden of taxes on the economy. Others assumed that the 'miracle of the market' uniformly produced unambiguous efficiency gains for society.

However, animal health (like human health) is subject to market failures and there remains a role for the State in their correction, through the provision of selected goods and services, the setting and monitoring of regulations and taxes and subsidies. In addition other policies such as education and infrastructure can have an important impact on livestock disease prevention, control and eradication. The conceptual framework of new institutional economics (NIE; Pratt and Zeckhauser, 1985; North, 1990) has been key to those who wished to take a less ideological and more analytical approach to the division of labour between private and government actors in the livestock sector (Leonard, 2004).

©CAB International 2009. *The Economics of Animal Health and Production*
(J. Rushton)

Important Concepts from New Institutional Economics

The earliest attempts to redefine appropriate roles for the private and the governmental used the distinction between 'public' and 'private' goods. *Public goods* and services, once provided to one person, are available to others at no extra cost. Pure public goods exhibit two qualities:

- that of being *non-rival* or non-subtractable in consumption, since their use or enjoyment by one person does not detract from that of another;
- that of *non-excludability*, since it is difficult or impossible to exclude other people from using or enjoying the good or service once it has been provided to anyone, whether they have paid for it or not.

An example would be a radio programme transmitting information on livestock disease control (Leonard, 2004). Pure *private goods*, on the other hand, are fully excludable and rival (Ahuja, 2004).

Private entrepreneurs are reluctant to provide public goods or services since it is difficult for them to make sure that all the beneficiaries pay for them. Therefore, they will be underprovided by private businesses, and indeed may not be provided at all. This applies irrespective of whether the benefits to society of the public good outweigh the costs of provision. When this is the case, there is a clear role for State action to provide the good or service and to finance its provision out of general taxes.

However, the public–private goods distinction is too blunt an instrument for the fine art of making veterinary policy, although it is useful in grasping the issues involved. It is more helpful to ask whether or not there are costs and benefits that are being borne by others who are not party to a private market transaction. These costs and benefits that are external to the private contract are known as *externalities*. When the externalities associated with a privately provided service are *positive* and large (as would be the case for inoculations against a feared outbreak of foot-and-mouth

disease), the market will underprovide the service. Where the externalities are *negative* (as with the pollution created by a private feedlot), the market left to itself will overprovide the service and hurt the rest of society. The externality approach first lends itself more readily to degrees of difference; the public versus private goods language is categorical and handles mixed types awkwardly. Second, the externality method leads one to do a better job in evaluating the adequacy of private demand (which sometimes, as with rinderpest inoculations, is large enough by itself to get the job done), for it quantifies rather than categorizes both the internal and external benefits (Leonard, 2000, 2004).

Where significant externalities occur, decisions left to individual producers acting in the market alone are unlikely to produce a social optimum. Governments thus have a role to correct the biases that can arise in decision making. They can do this by:

- applying taxes and subsidies to reflect the value of the externality: for example, by providing free testing, charging a handling fee (a tax) for the movement of animals through checkpoints or the provision of subsidized dips for sheep;
- supplying goods with large external benefits directly: for example, the control of the tsetse fly through aerial spraying and bush clearance;
- assigning property rights in such a way that private decision makers can no longer treat externalities as external: for example, the dairy farmer may arrange to pay the river fisherfolk compensation for loss of catch resulting from slurry disposal in the case that the fisherfolk have prior rights to the fish; or, alternatively, the fishers may have to pay the dairy farmer not to tip waste into the river in the case that the farmer has prior rights to the water;
- regulating activities, which potentially cause large external costs: for example, by decreeing the maximum amount of slurry that the pig farmer may discharge into watercourses, monitoring such pollution and taking legal action if violations occur.

Another kind of market failure concerns *transactions costs*. These are the costs of doing business, which can include those incurred:

- in gaining information prior to making deals;
- in negotiating contracts; and
- in monitoring and policing the implementation of the bargain.

Assumed to be minimal in standard microeconomic theory, in practice transactions costs can be large. Where information is difficult to obtain and where multiple parties are involved in negotiations, they become particularly large. Distance imposes a particularly heavy transaction cost on private animal health contracts in remote areas (Leonard, 2004).

In general, any restructuring of the animal health services in a particular country should pay attention to the reduction of 'deadweight losses' – places where buyers, sellers and the public at large all incur losses from transaction costs that could be eliminated for a more modest cost. There is one area therefore in which the State often has a positive role to play in reducing transaction costs – assurances of quality (Leonard, 2004).

Information costs often comprise a major part of transaction costs, and include those of *moral hazard*. This arises when the buyer in a transaction does not know if the service being provided is of the appropriate quality and the seller therefore has an incentive (particularly in the short run) to provide lower quality. (In the long run, the seller of a good-quality product also will lose from such information asymmetries, as the buyer will realize the danger and refuse to pay the price that a quality good would be worth.)

For example, the buyer of a veterinary drug paying cash incurs a moral hazard, since it may not be immediately obvious whether the drug is of the quality claimed or that the drug is actually appropriate for the treatment of the problem. Indeed, the 'drug' offered might be a fake, and this would not be clear until later when treatment has been ineffective. This particular moral hazard stems from asymmetric information, i.e. the drug seller knows what is being sold, while the buyer may have much less idea of just what is on offer or have insufficient knowledge of disease diagnosis.

Once again, there is a public role in helping to reduce transactions costs by:

- collecting and disseminating information to the public;
- establishing codes of practice;
- setting standards, including weights and measures;
- passing contract laws, including those governing descriptions in trading;
- certifying quality; and
- supervising the operation of codes, standards, laws and certification, etc.

Not mentioned in the list above, but of great importance to transaction costs, is the level of education of livestock keepers and their access to infrastructure such as roads, telephones, radio transmitters, etc. For example, if people cannot read or have difficulty understanding messages written on products then it will be difficult to disseminate information apart from direct contact. It is also likely that livestock products may be badly used. While these aspects are not directly related to the livestock sector, poor policies for education and infrastructure can have important impacts on the development of the sector.

To conclude, there are some goods and services whose provision requires some public action. The important corollary is that *all other goods and services will be provided efficiently if they are left to private enterprise to provide through the market*, unless, of course, there is some other significant market failure. Sometimes a service is provided by government not because of efficiency concerns but as a matter of welfare. This is outside of economics and could be appropriate if, but only if, goods with externalities that affect the poor are adequately provided first, for these services have a greater impact on the poor and are more efficiently provided by government. In the real world of development this condition is usually not met.

Thus, it should be noted that, if government does less than it previously did, this should allow it to do the things it does do better, since scarce administrative capacity will not have been used up in replacing private sector activities. In addition, a government that leaves the private sector to provide goods and services that have few externalities encourages the private sector to flourish as there will be no subsidized competition from the State.

To help follow how some of these concepts can be applied to animal health functions, a summary of functions, appropriate delivery channels and economic characteristics is provided in Table 12.1.

As a simple conclusion, Umali *et al.* (1992) suggest that where goods are not public, where externalities and moral hazard are small, there is no imperative for the State to act, and that, in the nearly universal conditions of budgetary scarcity, it would be better to permit private actors to supply the goods and services in question. Not only would this allow the private sector to demonstrate its potential qualities of effective and economically efficient provision, but also it would allow the State to concentrate on doing those things which the private sector cannot do, or is reluctant to do.

Conclusions

Contemporary wisdom favours less government action than has been typical in the past, on account of the record of government failure. Instead, most observers concede that private enterprise acting in the market will undertake most economic activity. However, government still has important roles in correcting market failures: by provision of public goods, correction for externalities, lowering transactions costs, providing institutions, ensuring a stable macroeconomy

Table 12.1. Suggested channels for animal health functions. (Modified from Ahuja, 2004.)

Animal health function	Appropriate delivery channel		Economic characteristic
	Public	Private	
Disease surveillance, prevention, control and eradication of			
Highly contagious disease with serious socio-economic, trade and public health consequences	✓	✓	Public good
Diseases of low contagion		✓	Private good with externalities
Quarantine and movement control	✓		Measures to correct for externalities
Emergency responses	✓		Public good
Veterinary Inspection	✓		Measures to correct for 'moral hazard'
Wildlife disease monitoring	✓		Public good
Zoonosis control	✓		Measures to correct for externalities
Disease investigation and diagnosis	✓	✓	Private good with externalities. For highly contagious diseases public and private goods
Clinical diagnosis and treatment		✓	Private good
Drug/vaccine quality control	✓		Require measures to correct for 'moral hazard'
Production and distribution of drugs and vaccines		✓	Private good
Vaccination and vector control	✓	✓	Private good with externalities
Research, extension and training	✓	✓	Public and private
Food hygiene and inspection	✓		Measures to correct for 'moral hazard'
Residue testing	✓		
Food safety tasks	✓		Public good
Compliance and monitoring	✓		Public good

and attending to social priorities. In preparing livestock disease prevention, control and eradication programmes, care needs to be taken to identify key actors in livestock product chains and examine their incentives to participate in such programmes. With good data and information on the sector, planning will help to show the importance of different government actions, and also where there are gaps that need to be filled by the government to help the livestock sector develop.

13 Social and Cultural Factors

Introduction

The book has so far concentrated on economics in the understanding of resource allocation problems within livestock systems and the livestock sector in general. However, it is true to say that economic theory and tools so far presented, while very useful, do not explain all aspects of the decision-making process of the livestock farmer or the people involved in the livestock sector. What are the reasons for this inability to explain livestock production with economic models? The following answers are suggested:

1. The decision-making process involves components that do not conform with economic theory, which can be described as social or cultural characteristics.
2. Insufficient data are available to develop a model of sufficient complexity for the decision-making process.

The lack of power to explain decision making through economic models is not a new area for economists. In the 1920s, John Roger Commons developed the idea that economic activity depended on the underlying legal and institutional relationships and that these evolved over time (Backhouse, 2002). Institutional economics as described in Chapter 12 (this volume) identified the need for transactions when

making economic decisions, and that these transactions are based on working rules which are set by the group, region or society that one is a part of, and as Leonard (2004) states decision making on allocation of resources for the reform of veterinary services is more than just a matter of money.

Others groups have also identified problems with a purely economic approach to rural development problems and have come up with a livelihoods approach (Carney, 1998) and a more general discussion can be found in Ellis (2000). This approach has similarities to the household economics framework introduced by Becker (1965). A livelihoods approach as a concept of how people operate on a day-to-day basis is very useful, but there are problems in the application of the livelihoods framework to livestock. For a discussion on this, readers are referred to Heffernan (2002).

The assumption in the current chapter is that the working rules identified by Commons are akin to the social and cultural factors that people within the livestock sector operate in. These often shape perceptions of how a problem is confronted and the type of solution that is presented and delivered. A brief description is provided of what is culture and this is followed by some examples where social and cultural factors affect decision making in animal health and production.

Culture

Culture is the man-made part of the environment, which includes all the elements that human beings have acquired from their group by conscious learning or by conditioning. There are considerable differences between countries in terms of values and cultural assumptions as the comparison between North American and Filipino culture presented in Table 13.1 shows.

Cultures can also develop around professional bodies and religious organizations. The latter will be touched upon with livestock examples later. The former will also be examined in the context of the veterinary profession providing advice for livestock farmers and also working with professionals in other disciplines.

It is suggested that the functions of culture include the following:

1. Culture unites people by means of common beliefs, attitudes, values, expectations and norms of behaviour. It is an instrument for ensuring conformity of interest.
2. Culture serves as an integrative function, by directing people's attention to matters of common interest and to problems affecting their survival as an identity group. It creates the need to develop a sense of common destiny. In pursuing that destiny and preserving its uniqueness, each culture tries to defend the values and beliefs it prizes most and to fight beliefs and values it perceives as detrimental.
3. Culture makes events both intelligible and significant to its members through certain rituals and symbolic actions. An example would be the ritual slaughtering of cattle in West Africa and Toraja, Indonesia, during celebrations.
4. Culture regulates or controls change. It is the strength of culture that determines the extent to which practices destructive to the culture are allowed to spread. Some believe that there are two kinds of forces – those seeking to promote new ideas and their adoption and those seeking to prevent them. These antagonistic forces are often described as change incentives and disincentives. One distinguishing characteristic of urban communication compared to rural is the pervasiveness of change incentives in urban areas and their corresponding scarcity in rural communities. It is sometimes difficult to overcome or circumvent these forces in development projects. Clearly it is necessary to first identify and understand them before one can attempt to circumvent them. Failure to understand the incentive forces explains the failure of many development projects.

Culture is expressed in various ways, language, attitudes, patterns of thought, which are discussed in more detail below.

Language

The sharpest distinction is the recognized languages such as English, Spanish, French, Mandarin, etc. However, it is also necessary to recognize that professional groups have their own language or 'jargon' and that this

Table 13.1. Comparison of culture between North American and Filipino culture.

North American	Filipino
Autonomy encouraged for the individual, who should solve own problems, develop own opinion	Dependence encouraged; point of reference is authority; older members of family
Clear distinction made between public and private property; materialism is a major value	Public property divertible to private hands with little guilt; spiritual, religious things are more important than material things
Competition is primary method of motivation	Communal feeling excludes the incentive to excel over others
Relations with others are informal and direct	Relations with others are more formal; social interactions more structured

can exclude people from that group either accidentally or on purpose. An awareness of the importance of language is not always well recognized in animal health planning. For example, in South America a cysticercosis control programme printed a manual for farmers with the word cysticercosis on the cover of booklet. The people in the area call this disease in pigs trichina, and they recognize that this disease is problematic to them. However, they did not use the book as they thought cysticercosis was not relevant to them. In another project, general animal health advice was first written in Spanish and then translated into Quechua, the main language in many areas of the Andes. When distributing the material to communities, families did not want the local language version because many of the older people could not read and the younger people were more comfortable reading Spanish.

These simple examples show that language can be a barrier to communication. However, if problems of language are well understood, then language becomes a very powerful tool to understand livestock sector decision making and communicating ideas to improve the livestock sector.

Attitudes

Chambers (1983) discusses how attitudes affect how people react to each other. There is a need to understand that people do not react and respond in the same way to different sets of people, and their actions may well change according to the circumstances they find themselves in. For example, a veterinarian will discuss an animal disease solution in a different way to a fellow colleague than to an economist or to a farmer.

Societies themselves can also set themselves into modes of what are believed to be measures of intelligence. Much is placed on academic intelligence (Gardner, 2004), but there are other types of intelligence from artistic, musical through to sporting intelligence. For example, one of the wisest comments made to the author has come from a cowman who worked all his life with dairy cattle. When this man was asked if he knew everything about cows, his response was that he learns something new every day and the day he stopped learning there would be no interest in his job.

Roles and role expectations

Roles and role expectations can restrict how a problem is discussed. For example, a veterinarian has a role as the expert on animal diseases and control measures. The livestock keeper is the receiver of advice, but they have something to contribute as they are the ones who know the animal and the area where it is kept. Good veterinarians are well aware of this and spend considerable time discussing with the farmer the circumstances of the animal prior to a disease problem and the possible local solutions available to a problem. In contrast, a plaque in a veterinary office that said 'Veterinarians are the cleverest doctors because they cannot ask their patients questions' would suggest that questions are not necessary in making a diagnosis. This phrase was seen in India, and was originally from the USA. Figure 13.1 presents the four squares of knowledge for veterinarians and livestock producers as a means to think about how to approach animal health problems at farm level.

Time conceptualization

People's actions and behaviour are often driven by how they perceive time. In a society where people are constantly busy with demands of work, family and pleasure activities the loss of any time becomes all important. In contrast, livestock producers who have extensive production systems and live in geographically isolated regions will probably not consider time to have as much value. In a seasonal context, people may be unwilling to carry out livestock sector interventions during periods of festivities, so in a Christian society it would be very difficult to motivate actions on Christmas Day. At an even lower level, the value of time of different people within the household may influence which

• **Veterinarians know** • **Producers know** Animals do not eat when they are ill Animals with a fever are sick	• **Veterinarians know** • **Producers do not know** Treatments for diseases Appropriate vaccines Diagnostic tests
• **Veterinarians do not know** • **Producers know** Local remedies for diseases Most important diseases in the local area Symptoms of sick animals	• **Veterinarians do not know** • **Producers do not know** Results of diagnostic tests

Fig. 13.1. The four squares of knowledge. (From Rushton and Viscarra, 2003.)

activities each individual focuses on. For example, the daily shepherding of sheep in the Bolivian Altiplano is an activity for old women or young children, which is an indication of the value of this activity (see below for an example of poultry raising). Individuals themselves will have different values of time during the day. Requesting livestock producers to carry out actions late at night could well meet with resistance.

Appreciating the cultural and economic value that societies, families and individuals place on time is a necessary component in the analysis of animal health and production, because people are the ones involved in the sector and they are the ones who will implement actions.

Pattern of thought: need for mutual understanding

The way people think and are taught to think influences how they will approach an animal health and production issue. Animal production specialists will be interested in nutritional levels of animals and how they can be modified to improve meat or milk production, a veterinarian will be interested in the diseases that affect livestock and how they can be technically diagnosed and controlled, an economists will want to place values on the interventions and the farmer will want to know how this affects their profits and their ability to support their families. All these patterns of thought have value in the aims of improving the livestock sector, but it is sometimes forgotten that other ways of thinking can add value to our own specialist area.

Most people who receive a Western-orientated education about animal science and production will be focused on commercial output from a livestock system. The list of products is obvious: meat, milk, eggs, wool and hides. This emphasis can be clearly seen by what is reported by most countries in terms of livestock production and the livestock economy. Taking a view that livestock production only concerns these commercially orientated products can create problems with an appraisal of livestock and in turn produce frustrations between technical staff and producers where there is a poor understanding of what motivates livestock keepers.

In many countries, other livestock products that have little commercial economic importance play a role that is of equal or greater importance than the list of commercial products presented above. Again the list is not that difficult products such as traction power and manure are obvious within many mixed farming systems; perhaps less obvious are the roles of livestock in terms of investments where banking services are poor and there are few alternative investment opportunities. In this way livestock can also act as means to accumulate capital, which may be used at a later date to pay for larger investments in machinery or education of the family. Livestock may also be used as a security against an informal loan, which is important in societies where land laws do not allow land to be used in this way. Animals also have cultural importance and can be an expression of wealth. Richer families may loan or gift animals to less wealthy families to create a social support network. There are also arguments that livestock provide a means for a more balanced diet, particularly for families that cannot purchase substitute protein sources due to poor market access (see below for further examples).

Levels of Cultural Rules

The cultural rules that are established can be found at different levels. The following identifies some of the critical areas.

Rule-setting at international and national level

At international animal health level, the OIE and *Codex Alimentarius* play a critical role in setting international animal health policies, a role that has been strengthened by their WTO mandate on such issues. International discussions and dispute arbitration mechanisms on animal disease control measures, particularly those linked to trade-affecting outcomes, are available through the WTO's Sanitary and Phytosanitary Committee (SPS). The benefit of these international standards and their application has been an improvement in transboundary disease control (Rushton, 2006). However, the focus on a narrow range of highly infectious diseases and the justification of large programmes for the control of these diseases have also been argued to have detrimental impacts on animal health services and livestock development in general (Scoones and Wolmer, 2006). Winter-Nelson and Rich (2008) also highlight that animal diseases that create consumer fears and have strong impacts on markets can distort allocation of resources, with perhaps little economic justification.

The development of national veterinary services in Britain was strongly influenced by the emergence of rinderpest, contagious bovine pleuropneumonia and foot-and-mouth disease as important economic diseases (Fisher,

1998). These actions occurred between 1850 and 1900 and reduced the economic impact of these diseases, supporting livestock producers and traders in the process. However, the attention of the veterinary services and animal disease control programmes did not switch to important zoonotic diseases such as tuberculosis until the 1930s even though it was known that this disease was an important cause of child mortality. The interests of meat and milk lobby groups influenced how rules of animal health were set and which actions were taken (Fisher, 1998). This relatively slow response to bovine tuberculosis has been compared to how the British government responded to bovine spongiform encephalopathy (BSE) in the 1980s (Waddington, 2002). Both examples demonstrate the power of relatively small groups to influence how rules are established at a national level.

In developing countries there were strong drives to invest in veterinary services up until the budgetary crises of the 1980s. The latter led to a reduction in money available to pay for civil servants and a massive reduction in the public veterinary services in many countries. Veterinary services were therefore influenced by an international aid agenda in their development and their demise. They were also influenced by the spending priorities of the national governments and often the inability of these governments to have a stable tax base. This demonstrates that national investments in veterinary services and programmes cannot be separated from international and national political pressures, which may well have little to do with economic profitability of livestock sector investments.

Rule-setting across livestock value chains: the importance of private regulation

Increasingly, private regulation has a powerful effect on private organizations, the institutional environment, and the behaviour of individuals (see Henson, 2006). Certainly in the case of animal health, private implementation of control strategies can be an effective way of creating cost and risk-sharing mechanisms. Good examples would be the Canadian Structured Risk Management Approach (SRMA; Burden, 2007) and the Brazilian FMD vaccination campaign (Dubois and Moura, 2004). In less industrialized countries, private regulation may be operating in a weak policy environment characterized by lack of implementation mechanisms for animal disease control.

Animal health measures are also influenced by private strategies, which are set at farm level by individual producers, at the company level by vertically integrated operations, or nationally by industry associations, which would include traders and processing companies. Their collective decisions to participate in measures such as surveillance and reporting, biosecurity and control measures, movement controls or vaccination are often the key to success in controlling disease. Producer or sector-level associations have influence based on shared vision and formal agreements or peer pressure within looser groups. The aim in such associations is to improve operations and stabilize market environment, which may incorporate some components of disease control. Across the value chain, dominant actors may set strategies that essentially govern how these chains operate. Such a situation is found in strongly integrated companies and where dominant market actors such as large supermarkets are aiming for market share and sustainable growth. Important cross-border private sector coordination is also provided by regional or international industry affiliations.

To get some benefit from such activities they will skin the carcass before burying it. If the animal has died of anthrax these people will be exposed to risk and also have an important role in reducing disease spread risks through their disposal of animals that have died of disease.

There can also be differentiation in terms of the interest in animal health and production. For example, crop farmers who keep livestock as a secondary activity are less likely to have strong experience of animal health and production; in contrast, purely livestock farmers or livestock farmer who have secondary cropping activities are likely to have both strong skills in animal health and production and strong interest in disease control. Even within specialized livestock producers, there will be different levels of knowledge and experience. Farmers familiar with local cattle breeds for draught power in India are unlikely to have knowledge of managing dairy cattle (Rushton and Ellis, 1996) and this in turn can create problems of nutrition and fertility management (Rushton, 1996). More recently, the emergence of 'hobby' livestock farmers (Rushton, 2006) in developed countries has created a group of producers who rarely see animals and this can create difficulties in disease surveillance and control (House of Commons, 2008). Therefore, identifying and understanding the motivations of livestock producers can provide explanations of poor adoption of complicated livestock packages and it can also aid the selection of people that would be appropriate to work with livestock producers.

Community or group level

If there is social differentiation within a group of livestock keepers it requires a careful examination of how this may affect access to livestock services such as feed, veterinary inputs and output markets. The Indian caste system would be a relevant example. Lower castes are rarely represented in a dairy cooperative and therefore have a restricted say in policy making. This social group can also be at more risk from a disease such as anthrax as they are asked to remove dead cattle (Rushton, 1995).

Household level

Within the household there is often gender and age differentiation on livestock activities. Some important questions on household decision making and responsibilities would be the following:

- Who owns the livestock in the household?
    - men, women or children;
    - different age groups.
- Who makes decisions on purchased inputs?
- Who makes decisions on produce sales?
    - milk, eggs, hair, wool.

- Who makes decisions on animal sales and slaughter?
- Who manages the animals?
- Who takes day-to-day care of the animals?
- Of the hierarchy of owner, decision points and animal keepers what are their general list of responsibilities?

Within poor rural households the management of rural poultry is often reported as the domain of women (Kuit *et al.*, 1986; Johnston and Cumming, 1991; P.R. Ellis, 1992; Spadbrow, 1993; Dessie, 1996). However, many rural poultry development projects are limited to technical interventions in the belief that technical problems are the principal constraints to the system. Such an approach fails to take account of the importance of women, cultural constraints and markets in the development of this sector (Rushton and Ngongi, 1998).

Examples of Social and Cultural Factors that Influence the Livestock Sector

Environmental damage

In Rajasthan, India, communal grazing access had been managed for many years by village elders. This was thought to be a restrictive practice that favoured wealthier groups, and was abolished. However, nothing was put in its place, and this laissez-faire situation on access to grazing led to the communal grazing land being over-utilized, leading to environmental damage.

In the Bolivian Altiplano, the number of livestock units per family almost doubled from 4.5 to 8.1 livestock units (LSUs) between 1976 and 2004. Initially 42% LSUs were cattle, sheep 30% and pigs and donkeys both around 11%. However, in 2004 the contribution of sheep had dropped to 20%, cattle had increased to 52% and camelids accounted for over 18%. The growth in cattle numbers relates to development projects to increase milk production and also to an increased demand for milk in nearby accessible urban areas. A reduction in the importance of sheep and increase in importance of camelids probably relates to poorer market opportunities

for sheep, particularly the crash in wool prices in the early 1990s, and better markets for camelid products. The disappearance of donkeys as an important species has two possible causes, the charging of municipality taxes for donkey ownership as they are seen as an environmental hazard and also the increased use of mechanized transport and communications infrastructure in rural areas. On the general increase in livestock units in the communities studied, apart from the attractions of livestock markets, as people become wealthier (Urioste, 2005) livestock are seen as an investment option. This is in part related to lack of trust and poor access to banking facilities and the limited ability to invest in land as current Bolivian law makes land transfers difficult.

The reasons for these changes are likely to be related to land rights, where it has been impossible to transfer land between families, plus recent land right changes have not simplified communal land management. The response by families who slowly become wealthier through rural activities and have strong links with richer urban areas through relatives who have migrated has been investment in livestock either as a simple herd increase or to provide an opportunity to exploit local milk markets. On a private individual basis this would appear positive and demonstrates the flexibility of livestock investments where other investments, particularly land, are either not available or are uncertain. However, the 'public good' implications are less favourable. Increasing livestock populations create pressures on communal pastures that appear not be managed to prevent increases beyond a sustainable capacity.

Schulte (1999) in an area further north in the Bolivian Altiplano states that, while private cultivated land is respected, the communal land particularly in agriculture-orientated communities is poorly managed. However, in livestock-orientated systems the land area management is more fluid and dependent on labour and technology. In addition, some of these areas have increasing populations of wild vicuñas whose populations are protected. The question is whether livestock product demand and livestock production technology are changing more quickly than community organization. Given that the communities are in a state of flux, with a movement of young people from the rural areas to the nearby cities and a general ageing of the rural populations, it is questionable whether the livestock changes are sustainable in the long run.

These two examples demonstrate that rules and actions outside the livestock sector have strong influences on how livestock producers behave and in turn the actions of these producers can have impacts on the environment.

Flexibility with the importance of livestock outputs and the role of livestock within a farming system

Cattle production in Zimbabwe

An analysis of Zimbabwean cattle production (Barrett, 1992) found that the common opinion was that the offtake rates from the areas were low and limiting the potential of the country to produce beef. The analysis demonstrated that the cattle keepers in the area were behaving in an economically rational manner because cattle had value in terms of the production of manure and draught power as well as live animals for sale. The draught power production is an aspect that reduces offtake rates.

Cow slaughter taboo in India

Many reports have been circulated to state that the number of cattle in India is too high that there are many useless animals. This has been brought about by the taboo of cow slaughter. However, the analysis to reach these conclusions has been done by people familiar with Western systems. In India, one of the main outputs of cattle is draught power from bullocks. These bullocks have to be produced from cows and hence there needs to be a large stock to maintain enough bullocks to provide draught power. Crotty (1980) examined the data on the Indian cattle population and production, and presented theoretical arguments about the reason for cattle being an important component of a society that

has a large cropping sector. He shows that the need for cattle to plough land has led to the beef-eating taboo and also a preference for milk, unlike the Chinese society. He uses his analysis to identify key data for livestock policy analysis and also indicate some development initiatives. Crotty demonstrates the need to examine the historical perspectives in the development of a livestock sector and how this can influence the role of livestock within a society. It also shows that livestock development is not independent and like the Barrett example is closely linked with the cropping sector.

The question remains whether the introduction of high-potential dairy cattle and the use of tractors for ploughing will change this balance and alter the cultural aspects of how cattle are perceived in India. Rushton and Ellis (1996) detail that this process is ongoing and that as cattle become less integrated into farming systems attitudes towards cattle are changing.

Non-traded goods in Nepal

Livestock are important in Nepal not just for the production of goods that can be sold in the market, but also for products that are part of the general household economy, e.g. manure and draught power for cropping etc. It is estimated that there are 2.7 million draught animals in Nepal and the majority of them are cattle bullocks (94%; Rajbhandari and Pradhan, 1991, cited by Joshi, 2002). This indicates that the majority of the Nepalese cattle population is used primarily for producing draught animals, rather than milk production. Data showing the increasing proportion of milk production from buffaloes supports this assertion (Tulachan, 2004).

Oli (1985, cited by Joshi, 2002) found that draught animals in the hills were used for an average of 62 days a year and those in the Terai for 130 days. The author estimated that the draught animals generated 1.37 million kilowatts of energy and it was worth an equivalent of NCR 1300 million at 1984 prices.

Manure from cattle and buffalo is a key component of the cropping systems in Nepal. Joshi (2002) estimated that 33 Mt of manure are generated by these species each year, which if it was all collected would have an equivalent value of US$58.75 million. However, the author stated that given the grazing systems for these animals it is unlikely that more than half the total manure produced is collected.

In addition, manure is of vital importance as a source of energy for cooking. Data from the 2001 census indicate that 10% of the households in Nepal rely on this as a source of energy and it is particularly important in the eastern and central development regions (see Table 13.2).

It is also important to emphasize that livestock are an important source of protein in the rural households of Nepal. The non-income livelihood functions that livestock keeping fulfils include:

- buffer stocks when other activities do not provide the returns required; as means of saving, accumulating assets, insurance and providing collateral for loans;
- as inputs and services for crop production;
- to capture benefits from common property rights (see later for the importance of communal forest areas), e.g. nutrients transfer through foraging on common land and forest areas and manure used on private crop land;
- for transport, fuel, food, fibre for the household; and

- to fulfil the social and cultural functions through which livestock ownership provides status and identity.

All of these functions can be identified as important for the livestock-dependent poor in Nepal. The economic value of these functions has not been estimated and, therefore, their contribution to livestock GDP is unknown yet likely to be very significant.

Social and cultural preferences for certain food types

The social and cultural preferences for livestock products can play important roles in livestock development.

Poultry

In Sri Lanka, there is a preference for eggs, in other parts of Asia it is chicken meat. In The Gambia local breed birds are sometimes quoted as being twice the price of exotic breed birds. Similarly in Taiwan, the predicted switch from local breed to exotic breed poultry has not taken place. Instead the two types of breed have an equal share in the market and the local bird fattening units have special areas for the birds to exercise so that their muscles can become more chewy and tasty.

Pig

Table 13.2. The number of households in Nepal using cow dung for cooking by development region. (Modified from Informal Sector Research and Study Centre, 2002.)

Development region	Number of households		
		Using cow dung for cooking	
	Total	Total	%
Eastern	1,012,968	175,469	17.3
Central	1,475,477	165,071	11.2
Western	863,045	65,271	7.6
Mid-western	534,310	10,010	1.9
Far-Western	367,420	201	0.1
Nepal	**4,253,220**	**416,022**	**9.8**

The Muslim and Jewish taboo against eating pork and pig products originates from the statement that the pig is an unclean animal in both the Bible and the Koran. The unclean pig can apparently be explained in part by pig behaviour in dry arid areas. The higher the temperature, the more likely that the pig will lie in its own faeces in an attempt to keep cool. It has also been suggested that as human civilizations increased in number the forest areas that were natural to pigs were destroyed (Harris, 1975). This increased the price of pigs and led to pork being an extravagance and luxury that religious groups should avoid the temptation of. However, in parts of the Pacific islands pigs are holy animals that must be sacrificed to the ancestors and eaten on all important occasions such as marriage and funerals.

Sheep

The Masai in Africa consider sheep fat important as a high-energy source for young children and pregnant women. It is possibly one reason for the rejection of breeds of sheep that do not have fatty tails. Similarly in Uganda, there is a belief that sheep fat is a preventive medicine against measles in children.

Festivals

Livestock products are often associated with festivals. Turkeys are important for Christmas in the UK, and for Thanksgiving in the USA. Beef is consumed in large quantities at the end of the period of fasting in Ethiopia. Chickens are often carried as gifts when visiting households in many parts of Africa. This may be an explanation of cyclical Newcastle disease activity.

Welfare concerns and food scares

There have been changing attitudes towards livestock production in the UK over the last 50 years. Initially there were demands for accessible and affordable meat. There was encouragement for industrial production systems of pigs, poultry and to a lesser extent ruminants. From the late 1980s onwards, there has been a growing realization of welfare concerns and health issues for the animals in these systems. In part, there has

been a separation between the general public and farming communities and practices in the UK, which, when consumers are made aware of the ways livestock are raised, leads to rapid changes in purchase of livestock products. Recent changes in demand for industrially produced chicken demonstrate how quickly the livestock producers need to adapt. Similarly, information on animal diseases can create food scares. For example, the announcement of problems of salmonella in the poultry sector of the UK in the 1980s led to a sharp reduction in egg sales.

The Changing Role of Livestock in the Mountain Regions of Nepal

There are a number of excellent studies of different parts of the mountain regions of Nepal (von Fürer-Haimendorf, 1984; Brower, 1991; Fricke, 1993; Vinding, 1998; Rogers, 2004). Brower described livestock as 'central to the Sherpa way of life in Khumbu. Not all Sherpas own cattle, and only a few families are even dominantly dependent on livestock, yet agriculture, trade and nearly every facet of both traditional and transitional Sherpa life are intimately tied up with cattle and cattle keeping'.

In a thorough study of this region, Brower (1991) identifies a number of key roles for livestock in the mountain systems (see Table 13.3).

Stevens (1996) has also carefully documented the livelihoods in the Sherpa region and provided a useful chart of the uses of different livestock in the area (see Table 13.4).

Table 13.3. Livestock roles in the Sherpa area of Nepal. (Summarized from Brower, 1991.)

Role	Species	Importance	Comments
Manure	Yak is considered to produce the most valuable manure	Seen as being very important	Manure is even collected from fields where animals graze
Stock sales	Cattle and yak crosses are sold to other areas	Stated by Brower as being the most important output	
Source of food	Yak, goats and cattle	Milk in tea, production of butter oil and churpi	Animals are not killed by the Sherpas, but they have no problem

Table 13.4. Khumbu pastoral strategies in 1990. (Taken from Stevens, 1996.)

Livestock	Herd size	Economic goals	Requirements
Yak (male)	2–6	Income from pack stock	High-altitude herding huts; hayfields
Nak (female)	15–35	Income from the sale of cross-breeds Manure Dairy products	High-altitude herding huts; hayfields
Dzopa	2–8	Income from pack stock	Winter stabling
Cows	1–6	Household dairy supplies Manure	Mid-altitude herding huts Winter stabling in village
Sheep	10–40	Wool, food, manure	None

What is important is that the livestock roles described by Brower (1991) are not static and have changed in the last 30 years due to external influences such as relations with Tibet, the development of the tourist sector, improving education and health of the local populations. In Stevens' study there is a description of changes in the region, some of which relate to government regulations and enforcement, and others are about the adoption and adaptation of technologies. What is emphasized is that this is not a static community and that experimentation is an ongoing thing for the Sherpa communities. Table 13.5 presents the changes that have taken place in this area over time.

In the lower Mustang area Vinding (1998) states that livestock are of importance to the subsistence economy. Cattle and yak and their cross-breeds are important in the production of manure, ploughing and transport. The cross-bred animal, particularly the male (dzopa), is valued as a pack animal, being able to carry up to 120 kg. The Thakali people are reported not to slaughter cattle or yak, but the demand in the area is high enough for people to bring animals from Tibet for slaughter. There is also insufficient supply of sheep and goat meat and this has to be imported from Lo and Tibet. Butter and churpi are consumed, but the latter is also in short supply and is regularly purchased from outside the area. Despite these shortcomings of the livestock system in terms of satisfying demand, it is still an important source of cash income for many households. Of the most profitable livestock activities, the mule business is stated to be the single most important source of cash income. Mules are used to transport goods along the trade routes in the area.

Rogers (2004) studied the highland communities of Manang, the district to the northeast of Mustang. His study focuses on the success of the people in this region as entrepreneurs, who are well known as traders and business people in Nepal. In his examination of why this is the case, he finds that historically this region was an important trading point bringing goods in from Tibet and exchanging them for products from the valleys and tropical areas of Nepal. In addition, the Nepali government gave the people, in this region, special rights with easy access to passports, and duty did not have to be paid on the goods imported and exported to Nepal. This encouraged further trading activities and increased awareness in business skills that have now been put to good use in the tourist trade. The role of livestock in this context was a traditional one of pack animals to transport goods and more recently pack animals for tourism.

Fricke (1993) describes a Tamang village community in the high mountain areas above the Kathmandu valley. It is an area where there are relatively few livestock per family and oxen are important particularly for draught power. Cattle make up just over 50% of the capital value of livestock holdings followed by sheep (18%) and goats (16%). Out of the total household capital including land, livestock contribute 14.5%.

Table 13.5. Changes in the use of cropping and livestock technologies by the Sherpas. (Adapted from Stevens, 1996.)

Aspect	When	Introduction	Comments
Potato production	Introduction in the early 19th century	Source unknown	It is generally thought that this has allowed the expansion of the human population
Introduction of red and yellow potato varieties	In the last 30 years	Source from individuals	
Decline in buckwheat cultivation	In the last 20 years		Change due to changing demands
Fodder crop production	In the last 20 years	Experimentation with wheat and barley as a fodder crop	Adopted to feed Dzopa
Greater use of the dzopa	In the last 20 years	Existed previously	Has become important as a pack animal, but requires more fodder than the yak
Animal herding	Constantly changing	Internal	Dependent on labour demands and labour costs

In summary, the impression from literature is that the well-studied mountain regions of Nepal have active and innovative people who adopt and adapt technologies according to their socio-economic reality. These communities are very dynamic and have undergone considerable changes since the late 1970s. Some of these changes have been stimulated by government with regard to access to common property resources and enforcement of restrictions on the slaughter of female animals.

Summary

It is recommended that there should be a greater recognition of the context in which livestock production, animal health actions and the general livestock sector operate in order to improve how the sector works. This requires a flexibility of mind, an openness to learn and an ability to see other people's point of view. The message from this is that everyone has something to offer, and openness to receive information and data from different people with different skills and experience can enhance and improve abilities to assess animal health and production problems. This need for openness in assessing animal health and production is further explored in the chapter that looks at livestock populations and production systems (Chapter 15, this volume).

14 The Economics of Zoonoses and Their Control

Alexandra P.M. Shaw

Prevalent but Neglected

Veterinarians are very much accustomed to dealing with pathogens which affect several species of livestock as well as companion animals and wildlife. Their work encompasses veterinary public health activities – from meat inspection to rabies vaccination – but these activities are usually undertaken independent of work by the human health authorities. While animal health economists are used to tackling the difficulties of quantifying the impact of disease on livestock production, their work only occasionally extends to putting monetary values on losses to wildlife and companion animals and rarely trying to estimate the burden of these diseases in humans alongside that in animals. Yet some 60% of human pathogens are zoonotic in the sense that they are 'a species infectious to and capable of causing disease in humans under natural transmission conditions' (Woolhouse and Gowtage-Sequeria, 2005). The authors conclude that of 1407 human pathogens, 886 (58%) are zoonotic. Zoonoses are even more important among emerging and re-emerging diseases; of 177 such pathogens listed by Woolhouse and Gowtage, nearly three-quarters (130 or 73%) are zoonoses. These range from emerging diseases which have hit the headlines such as avian influenza, severe acute respiratory syndrome (SARS), West Nile virus, Nipah virus and, of course, BSE, to ancient diseases which are re-emerging as public health problems for a number of reasons. These include the most feared of all zoonoses, rabies, as well as anthrax, brucellosis, bovine tuberculosis, zoonotic trypanosomiasis and conditions associated with tapeworm infections such as cysticercosis and hydatid disease (cystic echinococcosis). Food-borne zoonoses are of particular concern, with *Salmonella*, *Campylobacter* and *Escherichia coli* infections of animal origin affecting millions of people annually. Both brucellosis and bovine tuberculosis are usually contracted by people drinking unpasteurized milk.

Despite their ubiquitousness, the control of many zoonotic diseases is grossly neglected when set against the magnitude of the dual burden which they impose on human and animal health (Zinsstag *et al.*, 2007). There are a number of reasons for this. First, the control of many zoonoses is most effectively undertaken via their animal, often livestock, reservoir. Control is thus considered to be the responsibility of the veterinary services; however, these diseases are not necessarily among the major causes of mortality and lowered productivity in livestock, the main benefits being to human health. Thus, where veterinary services are overstretched or underfunded, zoonoses control can be neglected in favour of activities which directly benefit livestock and agriculture.

Second, as Schwabe (1984) stated in his seminal work on human health and veterinary medicine, 'zoonoses are amongst the most under-diagnosed diseases of man in most countries'. The symptoms of zoonoses are often confused with other diseases, e.g. the intermittent fever characteristic of brucellosis is assumed to be due to some virus or misdiagnosed as malaria in the tropics, and few of the diarrhoeas associated with food-borne infections are investigated. In addition, the diagnosis of some zoonoses is inherently difficult, with few cheap and reliable bedside or penside tests available. Thus, in Africa sleeping sickness is misdiagnosed as acquired immunodeficiency syndrome (AIDS) and few laboratories are equipped to differentiate between bovine and human tuberculosis.

Third, zoonoses primarily affect farmers and farm families, who, to quote again from Schwabe, 'often live in very intimate contact not only with domesticated, but also with wild vertebrate animals and invertebrate vectors, are also the proportion of the population with least access to primary health care and competent diagnostic services' so that 'the actual burden of zoonoses upon them has been very poorly estimated and reported in most countries'. This not only exacerbates the problem of under-diagnosis, but also means that these diseases tend to affect those people with the least access to health care, particularly poor and marginalized populations – so that the control of these diseases is further neglected (WHO/DfID, 2006).

Lastly, in the case of food-borne diseases, particularly in the developing world, the challenges of health education, tracing outbreaks and supporting the setting up of food outlets and the encouragement of food processing and preparation practices which will minimize these disease problems are very great.

Evaluating the Burden of Zoonotic Disease

As has been discussed in previous chapters of this part, analysing the costs or burden of disease involves looking at:

- the way in which morbidity and mortality affect infected individuals and populations;
- the accompanying ongoing expenditure in time and money for treatment and preventive measures.

The same two components have to be analysed in the case of zoonoses, but the analysis becomes far more complex because:

- impact on both humans and animals has to be analysed;
- putting a monetary value on human health is both ethically questionable and technically complex;
- several animal species are often affected and these may include companion animals and wildlife as well as livestock.

The burden in humans

In human health economics, the difficulties of placing a monetary value on human life and ill health have led to the development of a number of indicators, collectively referred to as health-adjusted life years (HALYs). These make it possible to compare the burden of diseases with very different effects on health and longevity, between countries and for both economically active and inactive groups. The most widely used measure currently is the disability-adjusted life year (DALY), whose use is laid out in Murray (1994) and is discussed, in the context of zoonoses by Coleman (2002) and cysticercosis and echinococcosis in Carabin et al. (2005). The World Health Organization (WHO) publishes annual tables showing how many DALYs a year different diseases are estimated to cost. However, the zoonotic component of infectious diseases is largely missing from the league tables (Coleman, 2002). This reflects both a lack of knowledge and the under-reporting of these diseases. Estimates of the global burden of some zoonoses have been published (Knobel et al., 2005; Budke et al., 2006). These tend to be low in the global league tables, but very high in affected localities. This is because their occurrence depends on the close coexistence of people and animals, usually in a particular livestock production system. Furthermore, while some zoonoses are debilitating, many zoonoses have high case-fatality rates – notoriously so in the case of avian influenza and rabies, but also in less well-known diseases. Human African try-panosomiasis, also called sleeping sickness, has a zoonotic form and is fatal in untreated individuals. A recent analysis (Fèvre *et al.*, 2008) shows how in an area of eastern Uganda, although the ratio of reported cases of malaria to reported cases of sleeping sickness was 133:1, the ratio of the DALYs, measuring the burden of disease, was only 3:1.

Nevertheless, despite their usefulness in facilitating comparisons, especially across countries and social groups, DALYs and other similar non-monetary measures all have strengths and weaknesses: disability levels have to be estimated; the rationale for age-weighting is debatable (Table 14.1). These and other issues have received much discussion in the literature.

It is, of course, perfectly possible to try and estimate the cost of illness and the value of life by looking at the cost of diseases in terms of days of work lost due to illness and future incomes sacrificed due to premature death, as is indicated in the second column of Table 14.1. Such estimates are frequently made in developed countries, when arguing for safety at work or allocation of resources to health care and preventive medicine. When valuing the direct losses due to people's ill health, the DALYs are usually used as the basic figure. Estimates of the income losses are given as additional information or as sub-stituting for the DALY value, as it is generally thought that including both involves an element of double-counting, hence the 'and/or' between the headings of the first two columns in Table 14.1.

The second two columns of Table 14.1 deal with the more easily calculated compo-nent of the burden of disease – expenditure on treatment and prevention. From the econo-mist's point of view, the important thing is to be aware that a full assessment of these costs has to include both public and private compo-nents. Thus, the costs incurred by households,

Table 14.1. Components of the burden of zoonotic disease in humans.

Direct losses due to ill health or death			Costs of treating and caring for those affected and costs of prevention		
Non-monetary	*and/or*	Monetary	Households	*plus*	Medical service
DALY, the most widely used to measure, which includes two components: • YLD: years of life lived with disability, both during illness and after recovery, if there are lasting after-effects – 'sequelae' • YLL: years of life lost due to disease if it leads to premature death Age-weighting can be applied, whereby economically active adults' years receive a higher weighting		A proportion of patients' earned income or the value (opportunity cost) of their contribution to the running of their household is lost during illness Premature death leads to the loss of patients' whole future income and contribution to their household	At the household level, patients and their families incur costs • while seeking treatment and correct diagnosis • during the course of illness and follow-up These costs may be financial (transport to health facilities, cost of medicines, medical care) or they may be opportunity costs in terms of time spent by family members accompanying and caring for the patient. Households often also bear some of the costs of prevention (usually travel costs and time)		Medical service costs can usually be estimated relatively straightforwardly in terms of medical practitioners' time, costs of medicines, diagnostics, hospital days, etc. Often it is necessary to work out the share of resources going to a particular group of patients for a particular disease. Costs of routine prevention (e.g. immunization) can also be calculated

including a value for the time spent by family members looking after sick relatives, and financial costs need to be included alongside those of the public health services. Because of the difficulty in diagnosing some of these diseases, patients often spend much time and money before they actually begin the right treatment (see e.g. Odiit *et al.*, 2004; Kunda *et al.*, 2007). Methods for calculating these costs – and for evaluating the other components of the burden of disease in humans are given in Drummond *et al.* (2005) and a very useful introduction can be found in Meltzer (2001).

The burden in animals

In animals, calculating the burden of disease is both more straightforward (most of the direct losses due to ill health or death have obvious monetary values, especially in livestock) and more complex (so many species, with so many roles in human society). Table 14.2 sets out the options, making the important economic distinction between livestock, companion animals and wildlife. The importance of zoonotic disease in wildlife can often be forgotten; however, some of

Table 14.2. Components of the burden of zoonotic disease in animals.

Affected animals	Direct losses due to ill health or death			Costs of treating and caring for affected animals and costs of prevention	
	Non- monetary	*and/ or*	Monetary	Animal keepers *plus*	Veterinary services
Livestock	Society values farming and the presence of livestock, particularly breed and species diversity		The steps involved in calculating the losses due to disease in livestock (valuing mortality and the components of morbidity) are discussed in detail in Chapter 10 (this volume)	Livestock keepers' costs consist of expenditure on veterinary pharmaceuticals, veterinary care and of, often very substantial, investments of livestock keepers' time	Veterinary public health services are involved in diagnosis, treatment, prevention (e.g. vaccination) and in food hygiene (e.g. abattoir inspections). Such costs are usually recorded
Companion animals	People derive psychological and health benefits from keeping companion animals, some of which could be quantified in DALYs		• Some companion animals, such as guard dogs, actually fulfil an economic role which could be quantified. • Companion animals are bought and sold and so have an economic price	In affluent countries substantial sums are spent on caring for companion animals. Owners' time and costs could thus be estimated	Public services are involved in dealing with zoonoses in companion animals. Such costs are usually recorded
Wildlife	Society values wildlife and places a particularly high value on rare and endangered species		There is a growing literature on how to value wildlife. Approaches used include estimating their value to tourism and 'contingent valuation' whereby members of society are asked what value they place on defined wildlife resources or what they would be prepared to pay to conserve them	Wildlife parks and game reserves will devote some of their resources to caring for sick animals	Veterinary services will be called in to deal with zoonotic disease outbreaks in wildlife

the world's rarest animals are menaced by zoonoses (Cleaveland *et al.*, 2006; Haydon *et al.*, 2006). In Tanzania's Serengeti, the population of African wild dogs is threatened by rabies, as is that of the Ethiopian wolf, the world's rarest canid. Valuing companion animals and wildlife poses challenges of its own, as outlined in Table 14.2. Although there are non-monetary values to be considered, in most cases methods for monetary valuation of the direct losses exist. In parallel with disease in humans, the costs of treating and preventing these diseases also need to be quantified in animals – and again it is important to include not just veterinary service costs but also the money and time invested by the animal keepers themselves.

Assessing incidence or prevalence

It is generally the case that the incidence of disease in both people and animals is under-reported, but as explained above in the introduction to this chapter, such under-reporting is particularly severe in the case of zoonotic diseases in people. A major task for epidemiologists in this field is to find ways of estimating what the level of under-reporting for these diseases is likely to be. Some studies have tackled this. For rabies in Tanzania, Cleaveland *et al.* (2002) developed a model based on local data on the frequency of dog bites and the proportion of these that were likely to be from rabid dogs. This indicated that the actual number of human deaths from rabies was likely to be over 100 times that reported. This model was later used by Knobel *et al.* (2005) to estimate the total burden of rabies in Africa and Asia. For the acute form of sleeping sickness, the rate of under-reporting was estimated by Odiit *et al.* (2005) by analysing the stage of infection in patients presenting with the disease. They estimated that, for every ten reported cases, seven cases were unreported. Because these individuals were untreated they would have died, so that for every reported death from the disease, 12 further unreported deaths occurred. For hydatidosis, Serra *et al.* (1999) combined information on

mortality, hospital discharges and surgery with the reported incidence to estimate four unreported cases of cystic echinococcosis for every reported case. Thus, individual zoonoses require individual methods for assessing under-reporting and finding ways of estimating this is essential to understanding what the true human health burden of these diseases is.

In animals there is likely to be a parallel problem of under-reporting. Since the animal reservoir is usually greater than the human reservoir, for chronic diseases this can usually be determined by conducting cross-sectional surveys of at-risk animal populations. For diseases such as anthrax or rabies where sporadic outbreaks occur, surveys and interviews with animal health authorities and animal keepers in affected regions can help improve estimates of their real incidence.

The total societal burden

To an economist it seems self-evident that decisions on resource allocation for controlling animal disease need to be made on the basis of their total socio-economic cost – often described in the medical field as the 'total societal burden'. The total societal burden includes all the components outlined in Tables 14.1 and 14.2. Conventionally, the direct burden of disease in people is measured in DALYs, and all the other components (direct losses in animals and costs of prevention and treatment in people and animals) are measured in monetary terms.

Increasingly studies are trying to include most of these components, as was shown in the review by Schelling *et al.* (2007). Thus, for cystic echinococcosis, Budke *et al.* (2006) estimate the annual global DALY burden at 285,000 from reported cases, rising to 1,010,000 if under-reporting is taken into account. Similarly, the monetary losses, in terms of lost incomes and associated costs, are estimated at US$193 million, rising to US$764 million if under-reporting is included. On the livestock side losses for liver condemnations alone were estimated at US$141 million annually, rising to US$1250 million if other losses were included, and nearly doubling to US$2190 million if under-reporting was taken into account. A different picture is presented by rabies, where Knobel *et al.* (2005) estimated that some 55,000 people a year die of the disease, representing a burden of 1.8 million DALYs. The monetary losses were estimated at US$584 million a year, of which only US$12 million were losses in livestock, US$87 million were for controlling dog rabies and the remaining US$485 million for human post-exposure treatments. For brucellosis in Mongolia, Roth *et al.* (2003) analysed the potential benefits of mass vaccination of livestock over 10 years. For a scenario of a 52% reduction in brucellosis transmission, these came to 49,000 DALYs averted. The potential monetary benefits were estimated at US$26.7 million, of which US$15.4 million went to the agricultural sector, US$3.0 million to the public health system, US$5.0 million in patients' out-of-pocket costs and increased incomes of US$3.3 million.

Thus, while the relative weights of the burden on human health, livestock sector losses, the ongoing cost of controlling these diseases in people and in animals vary, in all cases, the total societal burden is substantially greater than the burden to one sector (human or animal health) alone.

The Economics of Controlling Zoonoses: the Analytical Challenges

Having examined the components of the burden of these diseases, the task is to compare the costs of control programmes, which for zoonoses often involve tackling the animal reservoir, with the benefits, in terms of a reduction in the burden of disease.

In health economics the comparison is either in terms of:

- cost per non-monetary unit (which could be per life saved or per person treated, but usually cost per HALY, and most often cost per DALY averted) called cost-effectiveness or, in some cases, cost-utility analysis (Meltzer, 2001; Drummond *et al.*, 2005); or
- cost per monetary unit (where the cost is compared with a monetary benefit) fol-

lowing the standard rules of cost–benefit analysis (see Chapter 10, this volume) and in which case the direct costs to human health are usually valued in terms of income lost.

The principle of discounting (Gittinger, 1982; Drummond *et al.*, 2005) is applied in the same way as in livestock projects, with the possible exception that lower discount rates (3–5%) tend to be used.

In order to find an economic solution to the problem of the burden of control falling on the veterinary sector while the bulk of benefits accrue to the human health sector, the 'separable costs' method has been adapted to find a method of equitably sharing costs. Gittinger (1982), in his classic text, sets out how costs should be shared in proportion to benefits. Roth *et al.* (2003) applied this to their benefit calculations for brucellosis in Mongolia, so that the health sector's share of costs would be equivalent to its proportion of the monetary benefits. The health sector would then compare this cost to the DALYs gained. This thus provides a basis both for cost-sharing and for estimating cost-effectiveness.

From the point of view of advocacy, in the health sector and in terms of persuading governments to support the allocation of funds to the veterinary sector for controlling the animal reservoir, the classic cost-effectiveness measure of US$/DALY averted is the most persuasive. WHO considers disease control investments which cost less than US$25 per DALY averted as its most cost-effective band. Roth *et al.*'s (2003) study of the benefits of mass vaccination of cattle, sheep and goats to control brucellosis in Mongolia came to US$19 per DALY averted and Carabin *et al.* (2005) cite US$10–12 for controlling echinococcosis in China, both using the separable costs method. Unpublished calculations by A. Shaw and S. Cleaveland (unpublished data, 2006, Tanzania) indicated that dog vaccination undertaken in Tanzania could cost as little as US$10 per DALY averted, rising to US$26 if the full research component of the work were included in the costs. For zoonotic sleeping sickness, estimates by A. Shaw and P. Coleman indicated that treating the cattle reservoir plus limited vector control could cost as little as

US$9–18 per DALY averted. If the full benefits to cattle production were evaluated, it is possible that the monetary benefits would equal or outweigh the monetary costs, so that the cost per DALY averted would fall to zero, or conceivably be negative. More research into these types of scenarios is needed, so that veterinary and medical sectors have clear evidence on which to base cooperation, cost-sharing and, most importantly, resource allocation.

Conclusion

Economics has a vital role to play in finding and analysing evidence so as to show how important zoonoses are and in demonstrating how cost-effective their control can be. This involves, first, calculating the total societal cost of these diseases, i.e. not just the direct impact on human health in terms of DALYs as is usually done by medical organizations, but also the ongoing monetary costs of treating people and animals as well as the income losses in affected families. Second, the cost of controlling the diseases both in humans and, often more importantly, in their livestock reservoir needs to be accurately assessed. The third and most important step is comparing these control costs with their potential benefits in terms of reducing the various components of the burden of disease. When this comparison is extended to include costs and benefits to both the medical and veterinary sectors, it becomes evident that dealing with these diseases ranks among the most cost-effective health control measures. Looking at both sectors also offers the opportunity of introducing cost-sharing options which reflect the distribution of benefits.

Such economic analyses could thus help to argue for a better and more equitable allocation of resources to the control of these diseases and thus help to mitigate the under-reporting, neglect and high burden these diseases place on poor and marginalized populations. They would also bring us closer to the ideal of 'one medicine', the concept which the late Calvin Schwabe developed in the 1960s, advocating an approach where diseases in people and animals are considered together and veterinary and medical groups work together to control diseases of affected populations, irrespective of species.

Acknowledgements

The author would like to thank the doctors, veterinarians and scientists with whom she has worked who have provided the information and ideas about how these diseases can be controlled and how they affect people and their livestock. These underpin her analysis of the economics of dealing with them. Her particular thanks go to Eric Fèvre, Sarah Cleaveland, Paul Coleman, Ian Maudlin, François Meslin, Martin Odiit, Sue Welburn, Lee Willingham and Jakob Zinsstag, whose enthusiasm and interest have inspired her to work in this field.

15 Livestock Populations and Production Systems

Introduction

There are no hard and fast rules of how to present data on livestock populations or how to analyse the livestock systems and the livestock sector in general. The initial part of this chapter will provide information on classification systems and then present examples of the analysis of livestock systems at regional level (Latin America), at national level (Nepal) and at local level (a southern region of Bolivia). These examples demonstrate that different tools can be applied, and much can be gained through combining qualitative judgement and observation with quantitative analysis.

Farming Systems and Theories of Their Evolution

A number of authors have attempted to classify farming systems (Grigg, 1974; Ruthenberg, 1980; Mortimore and Turner, 1993) and some have tried to classify livestock systems (Jahnke, 1982; Wilson, 1995; Peeler, 1996). Classification systems have value in terms of reducing the number of farming systems for analysis, and also for targeting research findings (Collinson, 1981; Jolly, 1988; Williams, 1994). They also provide indications of the critical information required for each system.

Ruthenberg (1980) classifies farming systems 'according to type and intensity of land use'. He makes a specific distinction between cultivation and grassland systems, the latter being important for livestock rearing. For each farming system identified, he discusses the importance of the animal production systems and analyses their value to the household. Ruthenberg concludes that 'various farming systems described are all subject to change'. He proceeds to discuss these changes in terms of trends in cropping, livestock, chemical inputs and the labour economy. For the livestock trends, he highlights the greater integration of livestock activities within the household when the agricultural system is intensified.

Grigg (1974) presents a historical perspective of agricultural evolution, and describes the farming systems identified by Whittlesey (1936). Grigg argues that the systems identified by this classification occupy the majority 'of the earth's agricultural area and employ most of the world's agricultural population'. He relates the development of the major agricultural systems to human population increase, the speed of technology and economic development.

Mortimore and Turner (1993) use intensification and crop–livestock integration as a basis for classifying crop–livestock systems in semi-arid Africa. They argue that such a classification system is useful for 'understanding the time-trajectories of farming systems along degradational or conservationary pathways'. Mortimore and Turner (1993) state that the household/farm unit is inappropriate for the assessment of environmental changes caused by farming practices, and that it is necessary to look either at the village, communal or territorial level. They measure livestock integration in terms of crop residue use, fodder production, traction and transport use and cattle movement. Their hypotheses are tested with data from the literature on crop–livestock systems in semi-arid Africa. Mortimore and Turner (1993) conclude that 'crop–livestock integration, agricultural intensity and population intensity are found to correlate in practice'.

Jahnke (1982) attempts to classify the livestock systems found in Africa. He identifies five basic systems: pastoral range, lowland crop–livestock, highland crop–livestock, ranching and landless. The purpose of the classification is to identify critical constraints and develop appropriate solutions.

Steinfeld and Mäki-Hokkonen (1995) and Wilson (1995) both provide a worldwide classification of livestock systems. The former use their classification system to determine the relative importance of the identified systems in terms of meat and milk production. The production systems identified by Steinfeld and Mäki-Hokkonen (1995) are:

- solely livestock systems:
  landless livestock systems;
  grassland-based systems.
- mixed farming systems:
  rain-fed mixed farming systems;
  irrigated mixed farming systems.

Using data on livestock numbers and production parameters of each system, Steinfeld and Mäki-Hokkonen (1995) found that mixed farming systems keep the largest number of livestock and produce the majority of the world's meat and milk.

Peeler (1996) classifies the livestock systems of Kenya, and provides a database of livestock production parameters for the identified systems. The database is provided to assist future livestock planning and policy making. Peeler's classification makes no reference to the farming system in which

livestock are maintained, and ignores non-commercial livestock products such as draught power and manure.

Most methods of classifying farming or livestock systems attempt to identify critical constraints to those systems. They also generally agree that farming systems are not static, but are constantly evolving. This evolutionary process is influenced by many factors such as climate and resource availability. A number of general theories of farming systems evolution have been proposed.

A traditional view of farming systems evolution argued that the evolution was related to the resource endowment, climate and agricultural technology. Resource endowment could not be influenced by man, and subsequent agricultural technology advancements were related to the physical factors of the area. The production level from a farming system is, therefore, restricted by physical resources. Thus, there is a limit to the number of people any area can support.

Boserup (1965) questioned the whole basis of this argument in her thesis on 'The conditions for agricultural growth'. She argued that human population growth triggered farming system change and evolution. Increasing population pressures affected the resource pricing of land and labour. At low population pressure, land has a low value relative to labour. For these areas, land use is extensive and agricultural technology is primitive or, in some cases such as hunting and gathering, non-existent. At high population pressures, land becomes more expensive relative to labour. In this scenario land use intensifies, and the search for improved agricultural technology increases as human population rises. Higher levels of intensification lead to the integration of crop and livestock activities, in order to capture enterprise synergy. Some of the technology changes affect the resource availability in an area, and the implication is that the original resource endowment may not ultimately determine the number of people an area can support.

Boserup's conceptual methodology is the basis of Pingali et al.'s (1987) book on livestock mechanization and McIntire et al.'s (1992) book on crop–livestock integration. Both books detail empirical evidence for the

Boserup view of farming system evolution and McIntire *et al.* (1992) explain livestock integration in terms of human population density and agro-climate. While Pingali *et al.* (1987) and McIntire *et al.* (1992) provide interesting insights into farming systems evolution and the role of livestock, neither presents an adequate framework for farming systems evaluation.

Farming system classification and evolution summary

The literature on farming systems classification and evolution is clear; farming system change is occurring, and in some instances it is possible to classify systems that appear through the evolution process. But these theories do not provide quantitative structures to assess change, or to examine the advantages of one type of system compared with another. As Mortimore and Turner (1993) state: '[W]hat is beyond dispute (in our view) is that the crop and livestock sectors are interactive components of rainfed farming systems, and that understanding the dynamics of these interactions is important if degradation, sustainability and productivity trends in farming systems operated by smallholders are to be correctly interpreted.'

Livestock production system classification and livestock disease impact assessments

When estimating livestock disease losses or returns to livestock disease control programmes, it is often necessary to classify the production systems and define the populations in each system. The reason is obvious in that some systems have higher levels of inputs and outputs than others and, consequently, the impact of a disease will be different. Also the control of a disease may be different and possibly the number of animals affected, i.e. the epidemiology of a disease usually reflects the management system that the animals are under.

Some country classification systems exist such as in Kenya, but they are usually poorly supported by information on livestock numbers and livestock parameters.

Seré and Steinfeld (1995) produced a classification of livestock systems in the world, with estimates of the population in each system and the level of production. Their classification includes the following systems:

1. Grassland-based systems:
    (a) temperate zones and tropical highlands;
    (b) humid and sub-humid tropics and subtropics;
    (c) arid and semi-arid tropics and subtropics.
2. Mixed rain-fed systems:
    (a) temperate zones and tropical highlands;
    (b) humid and sub-humid tropics and subtropics;
    (c) arid and semi-arid tropics and subtropics.
3. Mixed irrigated systems:
    (a) temperate zones and tropical highlands;
    (b) humid and sub-humid tropics and subtropics;
    (c) arid and semi-arid tropics and subtropics.
4. Landless systems:
    (a) monogastric production system;
    (b) ruminant production system.

This is not the only classification of livestock systems at world level, but it is the only one available that is supported by quantitative information on livestock populations and production in the different systems identified. At present, the quantitative analysis is based on the FAO statistics for populations and production. These statistics are generated from national statistics, which in some country are not very reliable, but they are the best available.

Therefore, there exists a classification system for livestock systems in the world with estimates of populations and production, but there is no corresponding information on the diseases in each system, their prevalence levels or their impact on production parameters. Work is currently being carried out to address this gap and the system that Seré and Steinfeld have devised is the basis for FAO work on the impact of livestock diseases.

Production parameters

To carry out an economic assessment of a livestock disease the following parameters are necessary for an animal or herd with and without the disease:

- age at first calving, lambing;
- inter-calving period;
- mortality rate in different age groups and sexes;
- offtake rate in different age groups and sexes;
- for milk production systems, lactation yields.

This list is the very bare minimum to obtain approximate estimates of disease losses in terms of production. Additional information such as growth rates and feed conversion rates are recommended particularly in more intensive systems.

Regional Example: Ruminant Livestock Systems in Mountainous Regions of Latin America

Mountainous regions (as defined by FAO, 2002) are those either above 2500 m or lying between 300 and 2500 m that have either steep slopes or a wide range of elevation within a small area. For this particular study, a focus will be made on the Andes, the Central American Highlands and the Sierra Madre and Mexican Highlands but it will not include the Brazilian Highlands. FAO (2002) estimated that 112 million people live in these mountainous regions in Latin America, which is around a fifth of the total population. Within these regions over half the people are in areas below 1500 m with steep slopes, 40% live between 1500 and 3500 m and the remainder in the areas above 3500 m. While 25 million of these people are classified as being vulnerable to food insecurity, this may be as high as 45 million (FAO, 2002). However, in comparison with other developing country regions, these regions have a lower prevalence of food insecurity, in part explained by the greater urbanization, with major urban centres being found in the Andes, Central America and Mexican Highlands. Therefore, while these mountainous regions have a relatively high level of urbanization, many people are vulnerable to food insecurity.

To facilitate the analysis of the livestock systems the mountainous areas of Latin America will be examined as the following regions: (i) the Southern Andes and Patagonia (Chile and Argentina); (ii) the Central Andes (Bolivia, Peru and Ecuador); (iii) the Northern Andes (Colombia and Venezuela); and (iv) the Central American Highlands (El Salvador, Guatemala, Honduras and Nicaragua), the Sierra Madre and the Mexican Highlands (see Fig. 15.1).

Southern Andes and Patagonia

Argentina

With about 8.5 million head, over 60% of the national flock (SAGPyA, 1996), sheep production is the most important activity in Patagonia. In the northern part (in the provinces of Neuquen and Río Negro) the flocks (mainly Australian Merino) have a high proportion of castrated males as wool is the main output. In southern Patagonia, in the provinces of Chubut, Santa Cruz and Tierra del Fuego, the Corriedale dominates with the focus again on wool, with meat being a secondary product except in Tierra del Fuego and southern Santa Cruz, where lambs are important. Extensive grazing systems predominate, with farm size dictating flock numbers. In Neuquen, Río Negro and Chubut flock size varies between 2500 and 4500 head, while in Santa Cruz and Tierra del Fuego flocks average 7000 head. There is also some goat production in this region, mainly for mohair using Angora breeds.

Cattle production in the mountainous regions is of little importance at national level, with only about 3% of the national herd (SENASA, 2002). In Patagonia, there are 0.88 million head, with production concentrated in Monte Oriental (north-east Río Negro). Productivity is low, with animals grazed extensively, in part because an irrigation infrastructure has not been developed to exploit the Río Negro valleys. Further north, the Cuyo region has less than 1% of the national herd (SENASA, 2002). In San Luis and western La Pampa sufficient beef is produced to supply local demand. The cattle are

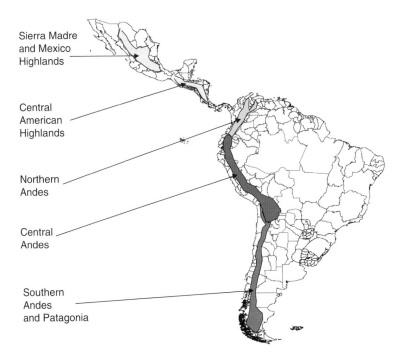

Sierra Madre
and Mexico
Highlands

Central
American
Highlands

Northern
Andes

Central
Andes

Southern
Andes
and Patagonia

Fig. 15.1. Mountainous regions of Latin America.

again extensively grazed on natural pastures with an annual production of 5–30 kg forage/ ha. Sheep production is of little importance (<1% of the national flock, INDEC, 1999), while goat production (meat and hides) is concentrated in the provinces of Mendoza and San Juan and based on extensive grazing and browsing systems.

The provinces of Jujuy, Catamarca, La Rioja and the western part of the province of Salta in northern Argentina have fragile eco-systems with little available water for animal production. Despite these difficulties, cattle and goat production, based on the extensive grazing of natural pastures (there is little improved pasture), are the mainstays of the economy. The cattle are mainly local 'criollo', although some British cattle breeds and zebu have been introduced. It is estimated that 20–30% of the properties, comprising up to 80% of the cattle population, are under commercial management. The remainder are found in family systems with little infrastruc-ture and communally grazed. While this region has <1% of the national herd supplying

only local requirements (SENASA, 2002), it has 1.22 million goats (mainly criollo), approximately one-third of the Argentinean goat population. Meat production dominates, although secondary products such as hides, manure and cheese are also important. The animals are kept in extensive grazing systems based on natural pasture and shrubs. In La Rioja goat production is common, kidding occurs in spring and winter, with the main output as 'cabrito mamón' – young kids between 30 and 50 days old. Sheep produc-tion is of lesser importance than cattle or goats and the area has around 0.93 million animals (about 7% of the national flock, INDEC, 1999). The sheep, usually criollo, which are often extensively grazed alongside goats and cam-elids, are mainly kept by families in semi-subsistence systems.

Chile

Southern Chile is typified by low tempera-tures and strong winds, with precipitation up to 600 mm annually, occurring throughout the year. Sheep production is the most important livestock activity, with the Austral region having very few cattle or goats. Region XII, with 1.9 million head, has just over half the Chilean sheep flock. These, generally Corriedales, are kept in extensive grazing systems as small family-run flocks in the north of Region XII. The Reino Nevado has both low rainfall and low temperatures. Here cattle production is relatively important as the region has 20% of the national herd (INE, 1997, 2002) and produces 14% of the national milk supply (Anrique, 1999, cited by Hargraves and Adasme, 2001). The main dairy breeds are American Holstein, the dual-purpose European Friesian and crosses. The dual-purpose Brown Swiss and Jersey have recently been introduced, with the main beef breeds Hereford, Aberdeen Angus plus the above dual-purpose breeds. Sheep and goat production is also practised in Reino Nevado, generally in extensive systems with goats mainly in marginal areas of poor fertility.

Neither cattle nor sheep production is of any importance in northern Chile, with 46,000 cattle and 95,000 sheep, respectively. Production is for the local market with sheep grazing confined to areas which cannot be exploited by cattle. However, in Regions III and IV goat production is of importance, with Region IV having 0.306 million goats, about 40% of the Chilean herd (INE, 2002). Criollo breeds dominate, and are kept for milk and meat production in extensive grazing systems that are highly dependent on unpredictable rainfall. Not only does the population vary with this rainfall but transhumance systems are typical. Recently, Cashmere breeds have been introduced to this region.

Summary

The mountainous regions of the southern Andes and Patagonia are largely dominated by sheep production although cattle and goats exploit important niches. Wild camelid species (guanaco to the south and vicuña in the north) are kept in extensive grazing systems, largely at the individual household level to supply local market requirements. A degree of transhumance where cattle are moved according to seasonal fluctuations in
pasture availability occurs, plus there is some trading associated with beef demand on the Chilean–Argentinean border.

Central Andes

The majority of the 7–8 million sheep found in Bolivia are criollo breed (small, producing poor-quality wool). While about 25% are found in the valleys, 70% are in the Altiplano or high Andes. Camelids are also concentrated in the Altiplano, with 2.4 million llamas and 0.4 million alpacas managed on 53,000 holdings (UNEPCA, 1997). The majority of alpacas are found in the wetter northern areas around Lake Titicaca and where the departments of La Paz and Oruro abut the Chilean frontier.

Llamas, alpacas and sheep in the Bolivian Altiplano are important in meat and wool production for home consumption and income generation in areas that have few possibilities for crop production. During the rainy seasons sheep are also milked, with the majority used to make cheese. In the recent past, llamas were also important pack animals, being used to carry salt from the high Andes to the valleys to exchange for maize. Sheep and camelids are kept in extensive grazing systems. In the areas of the Altiplano with higher rainfall and warmer temperatures, important cattle populations are found, especially to the east of the Bolivian high Andes, around Lake Titicaca and close to the cities of La Paz and Oruro. These cattle are kept for milk production, traction power or are fattened for sale. Most of the cattle are found in mixed farming systems, being grazed on communal pasture, stubble or crop residues. Dairy cattle receive limited amounts of concentrate feed.

In the Bolivian valleys, cattle are an important source of traction power and this is reflected in the high proportion of adult males in the herd (Rushton et al., 2001a). There are also an important dairy area close to the city of Cochabamba and two smaller dairy areas close to the cities of Tarija and Sucre. Sheep production in the valley is closely linked with cereal production (grazing stubble and being fed crop residues, with their manure used to maintain soil fertility). Goats in specific valley regions are reared in production systems based on browsing communal areas. The main goat populations are found in the south where the departments of Chuquisaca, Potosi and Tarija meet and on the border of the department of Chuquisaca and Cochabamba. The goats are raised for their milk, used in cheese production, and meat. Another important output is manure, which is greatly valued in potato cultivation.

The Sierra region of Peru has two-thirds of the national cattle and goat populations, and about 80% and 85% of the sheep and camelid populations, respectively (Rushton and Viscarra, forthcoming). The majority of these livestock are found in extensive grazing systems which are poorly integrated with cropping systems. About half the sheep population is criollo breed raised by smallholder farmers; however, a high proportion of improved breeds occur that are important in wool production. A third of the goat population is found in the poorest parts of the country – the departments of Huancavelica, Ayacucho and Lima. The camelid population is concentrated in the departments of Puno, Cusco, Huancavelica, Arequipia, Ayacucho and Apurimac with fibre production, the main output. Within the valley farming systems, cattle are closely associated with crop production (draught power and manure; Lescano Rivero, 1988; Fernández Baca and Bojorquez, 1994). Dairy cattle are an important component of the rural economy throughout the Peruvian Highlands and particularly in Cajamarca (Bernet, 2000).

In Ecuador half the cattle population, all the sheep population and 85% of the goat population are found in the Sierra region of the country (INEC-MAG-SICA, 2002). This region has important crop production systems into which the cattle are well integrated, again providing draught power and manure (Bernard et al., 1992; Meininger, 1997). It is estimated that 60% of all farms have cattle and a third sheep. The departments of Chimborazo, Cotopaxi and Tungarahua have important sheep populations and two-thirds of the small goat population is found in the department of Loja in the south of the country. The small camelid population is concentrated in the departments of Cotopaxi, Tunguruhua, Bolivar and Chimborazo. Sheep, goats and camelids are all kept in extensive grazing systems.

Northern Andes

There are estimated to be 6.88 million cattle in the Andean region of Colombia (DANE, 2002; Rushton and Viscarra, forthcoming). Of note in this area are the intensive dairy systems close to the cities of Bogotá and Cali with a high investment in infrastructure and management. These areas also have a large number of dual-purpose systems within the general farming system. The Andean region of Columbia also has small populations of sheep and goats (DANE, 2002; Rushton and Viscarra, forthcoming). In the Venezuelan states of Trujillo, Mérida and Táchira there are significant numbers of smallholder dairy farms with mainly dual-purpose systems. In these higher zones, there are also family farms that are dedicated to sheep production focused on wool (Rushton and Viscarra, forthcoming).

Central American Highlands, the Sierra Madre and the Mexican Highlands

In the Central American Highlands, the Sierra Madre and the Mexican Highlands cattle dominate and are mainly found in dual-purpose systems (Rushton, 2004; Rushton et al., 2006b,d). While goats and sheep are of little importance in Central America (Rushton et al., 2006b,d), small ruminants occupy important niches in Mexico, although they are relatively insignificant in terms of total livestock units (Rushton et al., 2006b). There are no wild ruminant species of importance.

Similar patterns of livestock production systems to those found in the northern Andes occur, ranging from intensive and semi-intensive dairy systems, dual-purpose cattle systems and livestock systems integrated into crop systems to extensive grazing systems. Smallholder livestock producers are the most important numerically, with many Central American smallholders farming poor-quality land on steep slopes.

Espinoza-Ortega and Arriaga-Jordan (2005a) make important distinctions between the different dairy systems in the Mexican Highlands, identifying large-scale industrial dairying, tropical and small-scale dairy production. The latter has been linked to maize production, which is in crisis, and recently dairy production has become a main source of income (Espinoza-Ortega and Arriaga-Jordan, 2005b). This useful classification is unfortunately not adopted at national level in the presentation of population statistics, where cattle are placed in either beef or dairy systems, with the use of the dual-purpose category having been dropped in the 1990s (SIAP, 2003). Arriaga-Jordan and Pearson (2004) describe the importance of livestock to the economy of households in different areas of the Central Mexican Highlands, with cattle being the most important source of income and dairy production in particular. These livestock systems are generally well integrated into cropping activities (Gonzalez *et al.*, 1996; Arriaga-Jordan and Pearson, 2004), but with some potential to increase more specialized forage and feeding strategies in dairy cattle systems (Arriaga-Jordan *et al.*, 2005) and in sheep systems the use of extensive grazing systems on native pasture (Aviléz-Nova *et al.*, 2005).

Overview

Sheep are an important domestic species throughout the Andes and Patagonia, but are of little importance in Central America and occupy niche systems in the Mexican Highlands. In many cases they are integrated into cropping systems, where they are an important source of protein for households, utilizing crop residues and producing valuable manure. In the extensive grazing systems of the high Andes, the utilization of poor-quality pastures by sheep concentrates organic matter in the form of manure which is used for limited cropping activities. The products from this species (meat and wool and the seasonal production of milk for cheese production) are poorly integrated into markets, and the integration became far less with the crash in wool prices in the late 1980s and early 1990s. It is also noted that this species has a strong gender bias, with women being important in their management, particularly pasture management.

Cattle, which have a variety of roles within farming systems, are important in regions close to urban areas and where climate is less harsh. In smallholder farming systems with a focus on cropping, such as in the lower valley regions of Bolivia, Peru and Ecuador and in the highlands of Central America and Mexico, cattle provide vital draught power. In peri-urban areas dairy production is important and ranges from intensive units to smallholder dual-purpose systems. Evidence from Bolivia would suggest that dairy production is becoming increasingly important in smallholder systems and this will be discussed later. Animals are also kept for fattening to sell, while in many areas ownership is closely linked with status or collateral.

Llamas and alpacas are concentrated in Bolivia and Peru with small populations also found in Ecuador, Chile and Argentina. In the southern parts of this region, llamas are used as pack animals, but with improved road networks and alternative transport means this role is disappearing. So far there has been little use of llamas as pack animals in tourist treks. In these areas llamas are also an important source of meat for local consumption, and also in areas with good links to towns and processing facilities, for external markets. Meat is sold either fresh, partially dried (challona) or dried (charque). Fibre is the most important output from the alpacas and these activities are concentrated in the regions around Lake Titicaca. There is also some fibre production from llamas, but prices for llama fibre are about a half of those for alpaca fibre. Recent export and promotion of products in global markets have stimulated the use of camelids for fibre, but camelid fibre is still only a small part of the world fibre markets (Delgado Santivañez, 2003). In some areas with poor soils, camelid manure is used to maintain small cropping areas and, similar to cattle, camelid ownership has an important social status. A small market that has been exploited by the Chileans is the export of live animals. This market requires a high level of animal disease control and animal health status that neighbouring countries have been unable to comply with.

The wild ruminant species of importance in the mountainous regions of Latin America are also camelids, the vicuña and guanaco

(Benito Gonzalez *et al.*, 2000). These species have been used for centuries, particularly the vicuña, which was a source of meat and fibre in Inca systems (Rabinovich *et al.*, 1991). Currently, wild camelids are protected, but are of importance to the livestock producers in central and southern Andes and Patagonia as their populations are expanding, such that competition for pasture with domestic species is increasing (Aguilar and Rushton, 2005). To overcome the conflicts between conservationist strategies and people's livelihoods, there has been a relaxation of laws governing their use which allows them to be used for fibre harvesting (Sahley *et al.*, 2006). However, the potential for these wild camelid species to provide a profitable livelihood has to be tempered by the harsh environment and limited potential to improve productivity from such activities.

While the above description of the mountainous regions of Latin America has focused on ruminants, it would be amiss not to mention the importance of non-ruminant species in this region. Pigs and poultry are found in areas with grain production, particularly maize, while guinea pigs are of importance in the high Andes of Bolivia, Peru and Ecuador. These species are normally found in smallholder farming systems providing household protein and acting as an emergency cash source.

To summarize, there are differences across the mountainous regions of Latin America. In the southern and central parts of the general region, sheep are important and so are the domestic and wild species of camelid. Going further north, cattle become increasingly dominant as the main ruminant species, with small ruminants becoming almost irrelevant in the highlands of Central America and with only niche importance in the Mexican Highlands. Cattle are also important in the southern areas, but are less dominant in terms of their contributions to ruminant livestock units.

National Example: Nepali Livestock Sector

Nepal is one of the poorest countries in the world, with an annual per capita income of US$200 in 1998 and an estimated population of 23 million people (2001 census). It also has a low human development index (ranked 144 out of 174 countries). Poverty levels are high throughout the country, but are particularly marked in the rural areas. In addition, the inequality in society is high with the top 10% of the population earning the equivalent of the bottom 50%. In many areas this poverty is deep-rooted, often leading to food insecurity for part of the year.

Economy and human population

It is estimated that 86% of the Nepalese population live in the rural areas and that most of this population is supported by agricultural activities that account for around 40% of the GDP. The proportion of the GDP contributed by the agricultural sector fell slowly during the late 1990s in response to improved economic growth (see Fig. 15.2).

Political problems due to the Maoist insurgency at the end of the 1990s and in the early part of the current decade, plus a poor monsoon in 2002, have had negative impacts on the economy. The economy shrank in 2002, in part because of difficulties in the tourist sector.

The country can be divided into three main regions: mountains, hills and Terai. The majority of the human population is found in the hills and Terai. For development purposes the country is further divided into five regions: Eastern, Central, Western, Mid-western and Far-western. Just over three-quarters of the population (77%) are found in the Eastern, Central and Western Development Regions (see Table 15.1).

Very little of the land area in the mountain agroecological zone is suitable for cultivation (4.6%) and although this region has a low population density per total land area it has a high human population density per cultivated land area. Nearly a quarter of the land area (23.8%) in the hill agroecological zone is cultivated land and the human population density per square kilometre of cultivated land is similar to the mountain region. Just over a third of the land area (36.5%) is cultivated in the Terai agroecological zone, but this region has a high population density per total land area and per unit of cultivated land (see Table 15.2). The high population density in this area has to be put into the

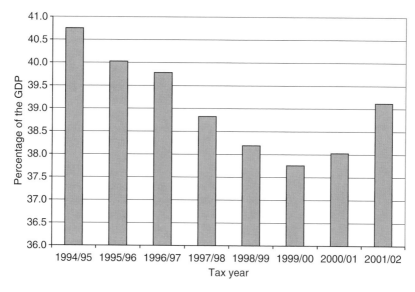

Fig. 15.2. Percentage of the GDP derived from the agricultural sector. (Modified from Central Bureau of Statistics, 2002.)

context that some of this land is irrigated and that the climate would allow double- and in some cases triple-cropping (Koirala, 1998).

Just over a quarter of the Nepalese economy is in the hill zone of the Central Development Region where Kathmandu is found. A further 21% of the economy is concentrated in the Terai zone of the Central Development Region. These are the only two areas where the percentage of GDP is greater than the percentage of the population and together they account for nearly half the Nepalese economy (see Table 15.3).

Human development index data show that the development is concentrated in the south-eastern area of the country (see Table 15.4).

Table 15.1. Human population by agroecological zone and by development region.

| Agroeco-logical zone | Number of | | | Population per development region | | | | |
	People	Households	Household size	Eastern	Central	Western	Mid-western	Far-western
Mountains	1,687,859	319,887	5.3	401,587	554,817	24,568	309,084	397,803
Hills	10,251,111	1,982,753	5.2	1,643,246	3,542,732	2,793,180	1,473,022	798,931
Terai	11,212,453	1,950,580	5.7	3,299,643	3,934,080	1,753,265	1,230,869	994,596
Total	**23,151,423**	**4,253,220**	**5.4**	**5,344,476**	**8,031,629**	**4,571,013**	**3,012,975**	**2,191,330**

Table 15.2. Land area (km^2) and human population density (people/km^2) by agroecological zone.

| Agroecological zone | Total land area | Cultivated land | Forest | Unproductive land | Population density by | | |
					Total land	Cultivated land	Cultivated and forest
Mountains	51,513	2,355			33	717	
Hills	61,816	14,718			166	696	
Terai	33,852	12,363			331	907	
Nepal	**147,181**	**29,436**	**57,401**	**60,344**	**157**	**786**	**267**

Table 15.3. The Nepalese economy (PPP US$1999) by development region and agroecological zone. (Modified from Informal Sector Research and Study Centre, 2002.)

Agroecological zone	Development regions					Nepal
	Eastern	Central	Western	Mid-western	Far-western	
GDP per capita (PPP US$1999)						
Mountains	1,003	1,023	731	731	629	898
Hills	1,012	2,059	858	741	744	1,262
Terai	1,109	1,520	1,276	1,040	1,144	1,267
Total	**1,073**	**1,713**	**1,022**	**861**	**899**	**1,237**
GDP ('000 PPP US$1999)						
Mountains	402,792	567,578	17,959	225,940	250,218	1,464,487
Hills	1,662,965	7,294,485	2,396,548	1,091,509	594,405	13,039,913
Terai	3,659,304	5,979,802	2,237,166	1,280,104	1,137,818	14,294,193
Total	**5,734,623**	**13,758,180**	**4,671,575**	**2,594,171**	**1,970,006**	**28,728,556**
Percentage of GDP						
Mountains	1.4	2.0	0.1	0.8	0.9	5.1
Hills	5.8	25.4	8.3	3.8	2.1	45.4
Terai	12.7	20.8	7.8	4.5	4.0	49.8
Total	**20.0**	**47.9**	**16.3**	**9.0**	**6.9**	**100.0**
Percentage of the population						
Mountains	1.7	2.4	0.1	1.3	1.7	7.3
Hills	7.1	15.3	12.1	6.4	3.5	44.3
Terai	14.3	17.0	7.6	5.3	4.3	48.4
Total	**23.1**	**34.7**	**19.7**	**13.0**	**9.5**	**100.0**

Therefore, the most developed part of the country is the hill zones of the Eastern, Central and Western Development Regions and the Terai zones of the Eastern and Central Development Regions. The poorest and most underdeveloped parts of the country are found in the south and to the west (see Map 1).

Livestock and their importance for the Nepalese people

The livestock sector is estimated to contribute 34% of the agricultural GDP in Nepal and had a growth rate in the late 1990s of 3.6%. Within the livestock sector the most important

Table 15.4. Human development index in Nepal by development region and agroecological zone. (Modified from Informal Sector Research and Study Centre, 2002.)

Agroecological zone	Development regions					Nepal
	Eastern	Central	Western	Mid-western	Far-western	
Human Development Index (HDI)						
Mountains	0.424	0.437	0.414	0.322	0.286	0.378
Hills	0.513	0.510	0.487	0.433	0.393	0.510
Terai	0.488	0.462	0.435	0.458	0.425	0.474
Total	**0.484**	**0.493**	**0.479**	**0.402**	**0.385**	**0.466**
Percentage of National HDI						
Mountains	91.0	93.8	88.8	69.1	61.4	81.1
Hills	110.1	109.4	104.5	92.9	84.3	109.4
Terai	104.7	99.1	93.3	98.3	91.2	101.7
Total	**103.9**	**105.8**	**102.8**	**86.3**	**82.6**	**100.0**

Proportion of Nepal HDI

■	>100%
■	95–100%
□	90–95%
■	80–90%
■	60–70%

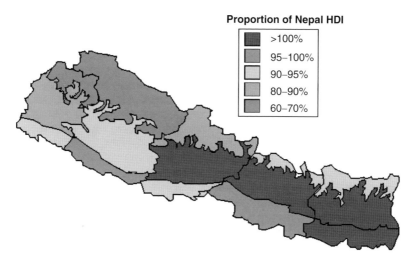

Map 1. Human development index map for Nepal as a proportion of the national HDI.

products are milk (62.6% of livestock GDP), meat (32.4%) and eggs (5.0%; Mandip *et al.*, 2004). It is noted that livestock products such as manure and draught power are not included in the estimates of livestock GDP. These are intermediary products used in crop and other production systems. Due to this omission the proportion of agricultural GDP from livestock is actually higher than the estimated figure stated above.

Livestock populations

The hill agroecological zone has just over half the total livestock population, the Terai just over a third and the remainder are found in the mountain zone. However, there are more livestock per household, per person and per hectare of cultivated land in the mountain region than in the hills or the Terai. The hills have greater densities of livestock per person, per household and per hectare of cultivated land than the Terai (see Table 15.5).

Approximately half of the livestock units are cattle. Cattle and buffalo contribute approximately 80% of the total livestock units. This pattern does not vary very strongly between development regions. Goats are the third most important species in terms of livestock units, contributing 10% of the total. In the Eastern Development Region, pigs are the fourth most important species and this region

has almost half the pig population of the country. In the Central Development Region poultry are the fourth most important species and this region has half the national poultry flock (see Table 15.6). This is a reflection of the development of intensive and semi-intensive poultry systems in this region.

The Central Development Region has the lowest number of livestock units per household and per person and the Midwestern and Far-western Development Regions have the highest number of livestock units per household and per person (see Table 15.6).

There are more cattle in the east and central parts of the country, with the Terai in the Eastern Development Region and the hill zone of the Western Development Region having the largest cattle herds. Just over a fifth of the national buffalo herd is found in the hill zone of the Western Development Region and the hill zone of the Central Development Region has 13% of the national herd. Approximately half of the national sheep population (53%) is found in the hill zones of the Western and Mid-western Development Regions and the mountain zone of the latter development region. The national goat herd is concentrated (71%) in the Terai zones of the Eastern and Central Development Regions and the hill zones of the Eastern, Central, Western and Mid-western Development Regions. A quarter of

Table 15.5. Livestock population and the number of livestock units by agroecological zone. (Modified from Mandip *et al.*, 2004.)

Zone	Cattle	Buffaloes	Sheep	Goat	Pig	Chicken	Total
Livestock population ('000)							
Mountain	821	358	352	904	98	1,454	
Hill	3,394	2,052	389	3,544	535	11,177	
Terai	2,764	1,291	99	2,158	301	8,740	
Nepal	**6,979**	**3,701**	**840**	**6,606**	**934**	**21,371**	
Livestock units ('000)							
Mountain	411	179	35	90	25	15	**754**
Hill	1,697	1,026	39	354	134	112	**3,362**
Terai	1,382	646	10	216	75	87	**2,416**
Nepal	**3,490**	**1,851**	**84**	**661**	**234**	**214**	**6,532**
Percentage LSUs contributed by each species in each ecological zone							
Mountain	54.4	23.7	4.7	12.0	3.2	1.9	**100.0**
Hill	50.5	30.5	1.2	10.5	4.0	3.3	**100.0**
Terai	57.2	26.7	0.4	8.9	3.1	3.6	**100.0**
Nepal	**53.4**	**28.3**	**1.3**	**10.1**	**3.6**	**3.3**	100.0
Percentage LSUs contributed for each species by ecological zone							
Mountain	11.8	9.7	41.9	13.7	10.5	6.8	**11.5**
Hill	48.6	55.4	46.3	53.6	57.3	52.3	**51.5**
Terai	39.6	34.9	11.8	32.7	32.2	40.9	**37.0**
Nepal	**100.0**	**100.0**	**100.0**	**100.0**	**100.0**	**100.0**	100.0
LSUs per household							
Mountain	1.28	0.56	0.11	0.28	0.08	0.05	2.36
Hill	0.86	0.52	0.02	0.18	0.07	0.06	1.70
Terai	0.71	0.33	0.01	0.11	0.04	0.04	1.24
Nepal	**0.82**	**0.44**	**0.02**	**0.16**	**0.05**	**0.05**	**1.54**
LSUs per person							
Mountain	0.24	0.11	0.02	0.05	0.01	0.01	0.45
Hill	0.17	0.10	0.00	0.03	0.01	0.01	0.33
Terai	0.12	0.06	0.00	0.02	0.01	0.01	0.22
Nepal	**0.15**	**0.08**	**0.00**	**0.03**	**0.01**	**0.01**	**0.28**
LSUs per hectare of cultivated land							
Mountain	1.74	0.76	0.15	0.38	0.10	0.06	3.20
Hill	1.15	0.70	0.03	0.24	0.09	0.08	2.28
Terai	1.12	0.52	0.01	0.17	0.06	0.07	1.95
Nepal	**1.19**	**0.63**	**0.03**	**0.22**	**0.08**	**0.07**	**2.22**

the national pig herd is found in the hill zone of the Eastern Development Region. Just over a quarter of the national poultry flock is found in the hill zone of the Central Development Region.

Nepalese livestock are concentrated (67.5% of the LSUs) in the Terai zones of the Eastern and Central Development Regions and the hill zones of the Eastern, Central, Western and Mid-western Development Regions. It is the hill zone of the Western Development Region that has the largest amount of livestock, which is in large part explained by its large cattle and buffalo population (see Table 15.6). Even though livestock are concentrated in these areas of Nepal, with the exception of the hill zones of the Eastern and Mid-western Development Regions, there are relatively few livestock per household or per person in this area in comparison to other parts of the country (see Table 15.7).

Table 15.6. Livestock population and the number of livestock units by agroecological zone. (Modified from Mandip *et al.*, 2004.)

Region	Cattle	Buffaloes	Sheep	Goat	Pig	Chicken	Total
Livestock population ('000 heads)							
Eastern	1,851	769	121	1,760	427	3,972	
Central	1,461	907	96	1,764	196	10,543	
Western	1,344	1,008	186	1,291	123	3,070	
Mid-western	1,346	538	349	1,199	132	2,881	
Far-western	976	479	87	593	57	904	
Nepal	**6,978**	**3,701**	**839**	**6,607**	**935**	**21,370**	
Livestock units							
Eastern	926	385	12	176	107	40	**1,645**
Central	731	454	10	176	49	105	**1,524**
Western	672	504	19	129	31	31	**1,385**
Mid-western	673	269	35	120	33	29	**1,159**
Far-western	488	240	9	59	14	9	**819**
Nepal	**3,489**	**1,851**	**84**	**661**	**234**	**214**	**6,532**
Percentage LSUs contributed by each species in each development region							
Eastern	56.3	23.4	0.7	10.7	6.5	2.4	**100.0**
Central	47.9	29.7	0.6	11.6	3.2	6.9	**100.0**
Western	48.5	36.4	1.3	9.3	2.2	2.2	**100.0**
Mid-western	58.1	23.2	3.0	10.3	2.8	2.5	**100.0**
Far-western	59.6	29.3	1.1	7.2	1.7	1.1	**100.0**
Nepal	**53.4**	**28.3**	**1.3**	**10.1**	**3.6**	**3.3**	100.0
Percentage LSUs contributed for each species by development region							
Eastern	26.5	20.8	14.4	26.6	45.7	18.6	**25.2**
Central	20.9	24.5	11.4	26.7	21.0	49.3	**23.3**
Western	19.3	27.2	22.2	19.5	13.2	14.4	**21.2**
Mid-western	19.3	14.5	41.6	18.1	14.1	13.5	**17.7**
Far-western	14.0	12.9	10.4	9.0	6.1	4.2	**12.5**
Nepal	**100.0**	**100.0**	**100.0**	**100.0**	**100.0**	**100.0**	100.0
LSUs per household							
Eastern	0.91	0.38	0.01	0.17	0.11	0.04	1.62
Central	0.50	0.31	0.01	0.12	0.03	0.07	1.03
Western	0.78	0.58	0.02	0.15	0.04	0.04	1.60
Mid-western	1.26	0.50	0.07	0.22	0.06	0.05	2.17
Far-western	1.33	0.65	0.02	0.16	0.04	0.02	2.23
Nepal	**0.82**	**0.44**	**0.02**	**0.16**	**0.05**	**0.05**	**1.54**
LSUs per person							
Eastern	0.17	0.07	0.00	0.03	0.02	0.01	0.31
Central	0.09	0.06	0.00	0.02	0.01	0.01	0.19
Western	0.15	0.11	0.00	0.03	0.01	0.01	0.30
Mid-western	0.22	0.09	0.01	0.04	0.01	0.01	0.38
Far-western	0.22	0.11	0.00	0.03	0.01	0.00	0.37
Nepal	**0.15**	**0.08**	**0.00**	**0.03**	**0.01**	**0.01**	**0.28**

In conclusion, it would appear that the livestock economy is concentrated in the Terai zones of the Eastern and Central Development Regions and the hill zones of the Eastern, Central, Western and Mid-western Development Regions (see Map 2).

However, animals play a more important role in the livelihoods of the families in the mountain region than in the hills or the Terai and in the Far-western and Mid-western Development Regions where there are more livestock units per household and per person (see Map 3).

Table 15.7. The number of livestock units in Nepal by agroecological zone and development region. (Modified from Informal Sector Research and Study Centre, 2002; Mandip *et al.*, 2004.)

Agroeco-logical zone	Development region					
	Eastern	Central	Western	Mid-western	Far-western	Nepal
LSUs ('000 units)						
Mountain	220	174	11	154	196	754
Hill	672	746	1016	617	311	3362
Terai	753	604	359	389	312	2416
Total	**1644**	**1524**	**1385**	**1160**	**819**	**6532**
Proportion of the national total of LSUs						
Mountain	3.4	2.7	0.2	2.4	3.0	11.5
Hill	10.3	11.4	15.5	9.4	4.8	51.5
Terai	11.5	9.2	5.5	6.0	4.8	37.0
Total	**25.2**	**23.3**	**21.2**	**17.8**	**12.5**	**100.0**
LSUs per household						
Mountain	2.85	1.55	2.14	2.77	2.80	2.36
Hill	2.17	1.08	1.79	2.29	2.18	1.70
Terai	1.20	0.90	1.24	1.86	2.02	1.24
Total	**1.62**	**1.03**	**1.60**	**2.17**	**2.23**	**1.54**
LSUs per person						
Mountain	0.55	0.31	0.44	0.50	0.49	0.45
Hill	0.41	0.21	0.36	0.42	0.39	0.33
Terai	0.23	0.15	0.20	0.32	0.31	0.22
Total	**0.31**	**0.19**	**0.30**	**0.38**	**0.37**	**0.28**

Summary

Therefore, livestock are probably a more important entry point in the mountains than in the other agroecological zones, and in the Far-western and Mid-western Development Regions because these geographical regions probably have fewer economic alternatives and have greater investments in livestock per person and per family than the other regions of the country.

The cash livestock economy is dominated by milk and milk products produced from buffalo and cattle. However, the key output from cattle in Nepal appears to be draught power. This explains why cattle are not highly regarded as milk-producing animals. In addition, livestock produce manure critical for cropping activities throughout the country and are important as a source of energy for cooking in the Eastern and Central Development Regions. Livestock also provide important sources of protein for rural households.

The livestock sector and economy is concentrated in the hills of the Western, Central and Eastern Development Regions and the Terai of the Central and Eastern Development Regions. This geographical area is the most developed part of Nepal. However, the area, with the exception of the eastern hills, has less dependency on livestock per family and per person than other areas of Nepal. The pattern would suggest that the more economically developed parts of the country have a larger and more active livestock economy, but the families in these areas are less dependent on livestock to maintain their livelihoods, i.e. the economy is more diverse. In the less economically developed and poorer parts of Nepal, the livestock economy is smaller, but the families are more dependent on animals. From the macro-level data, it would appear that livestock dependency is associated with poverty and underdevelopment.

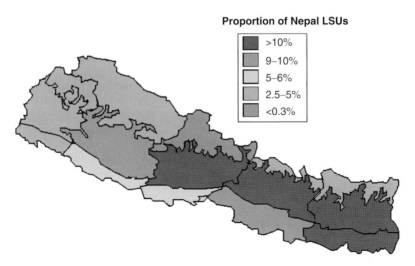

Proportion of Nepal LSUs

■	>10%
■	9–10%
□	5–6%
■	2.5–5%
■	<0.3%

Map 2. Proportion of LSUs in Nepal per geographical area in terms of development regions and agroecological zones.

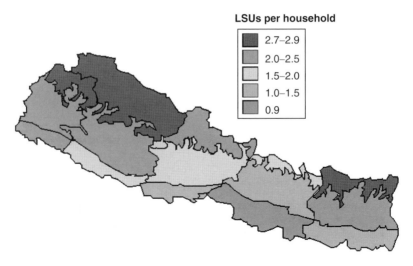

LSUs per household

■	2.7–2.9
■	2.0–2.5
□	1.5–2.0
■	1.0–1.5
■	0.9

Map 3. The number of livestock units per household in the development regions and agroecological zones of Nepal.

Local Example: Livestock Population and Livestock Income Estimations in the Cintis Region of Bolivia

Bolivia has many different estimates of livestock populations from different institutions and these have varying strengths and weaknesses (see Table 15.7). As can be seen the last agricultural census was carried out in 1984 and only the National Institute for Statistics (INE)

and the Ministry of Agriculture (MAGDR) have made projections for the livestock populations since that date. These estimates differ and neither organization covers all species. The differences are largely due to INE using the 1984 census as its baseline and MAGDR using a population baseline from 1978. Both organizations have assumed straight-line increases in livestock populations and did not seem to have a mechanism to check whether

Table 15.8. The Bolivian livestock population estimates and their strengths and weaknesses. (From Rushton *et al.*, 2001a.)

Source	Strengths	Weaknesses
Census (1984) of cattle, pigs and sheep held by the Instituto Nacional de Estadistica (INE)	Populations available to third political level and there is information on herd or flock age structure	For the La Paz and Cochabamba Department there is an incomplete census. The census was carried out during a period of hyperinflation
INE's estimates of cattle, pigs, sheep and goat populations	The estimations are regularly updated	The estimates are not linked to livestock production system or sector changes
The Ministry of Agriculture's estimates of cattle, pigs, sheep, llamas and alpacas	The estimations are regularly updated	The estimates are not linked to livestock production system or sector changes
Santa Cruz Cattlemen's Federation (FEGASACRUZ) estimates of cattle for Santa Cruz department	The Federation has strong links with producers	How the estimates are made is unknown
Beni Cattlemen's Federation (FEGABENI) estimates of cattle for Beni department	The Federation has strong links with producers	How the estimates are made is unknown
Estimates from the municipality plans of all parts of the livestock species	There are estimates for all species	Not all municipalities have plans, and not all plans have livestock sector estimates

these increases change over time (see Table 15.8). Other organizations also keep figures on livestock populations, but they tend to reflect the geographical and species interests of the organization.

Table 15.9 shows the livestock population estimates produced by the two national organizations INE and MAGDR.

The differences between the estimates of the two organizations are large for pigs, quite significant for sheep and very small for cattle. However, the cattle estimates are very different for the Department of Chuquisaca, a department with limited grazing land. What is difficult to say is whether changes over time predicted by the organizations are actually real. The lack of good population data creates difficulties for the following reasons:

- Livestock economy estimates are based on livestock populations.
- Livestock sector planning needs information on the economic importance of the sector.
- Planning activities within the livestock sector such as vaccination campaigns require population estimates.

- Without good estimates of the livestock population and livestock economy there is a strong risk that resources allocated to, and within, the sector will be poor.

Therefore, it is of no surprise that in Bolivia there was a strong discussion on the need for a new livestock census. However, no action was taken and the cost and complication of a census put decision makers off. Given this situation, it is important to consider alternative methodologies that are not so costly, but could provide reasonable population estimates. At this point, it is worth returning to the economic principles outlined in the production economics chapter (Chapter 3, this volume). A better estimate may cost more money and time to implement, but may generate additional benefits in terms of planning and support to the livestock sector. A comparison of the marginal costs and benefits for such a data collection and analysis exercise is needed. It is also worth mentioning that a livestock census is also an estimate with errors and will not generate an exact figure. A badly implemented census will also generate bad population estimates.

Three alternatives for generating population estimates are considered: population

Table 15.9. Livestock population estimates for the Departments of Bolivia by INE and MAGDR.

Department	Cattle		Pigs		Sheep		Goats[a]
	MAGDR	INE	MAGDR	INE	MAGDR	INE	INE
Beni	2,813,711	2,772,550	120,539	89,492	8,338	9,006	449,858
Chuquisaca	568,647	387,532	621,937	302,346	557,059	654,818	33,937
Cochabamba	279,128	304,276	292,410	116,732	1,224,049	980,823	174,604
La Paz	357,328	369,308	259,783	347,092	2,658,855	2,792,579	1,034
Oruro	48,142	45,580	33,267	18,471	1,653,529	1,045,553	660,258
Pando	20,545	18,287	29,764	28,718	3,989	2,719	209,072
Potosí	130,953	129,418	111,051	130,105	1,438,272	1,243,430	48,521
Santa Cruz	1,549,130	1,387,773	712,262	315,503	178,742	59,672	8,262
Tarija	350,102	315,301	300,917	175,771	316,100	279,139	180
Total	6,117,686	5,730,025	2,481,930	1,524,230	8,038,933	7,067,739	1,585,726

[a]MAGDR did not have an estimate for the goat population.

models to generate office-based estimates; a new census or a livestock survey supported with analysis. The advantages and disadvantages of each method are outlined in Table 15.10.

From the brief analysis presented in Table 15.10, it could be concluded that a livestock survey well used and analysed could produce a similar quality of population estimates to a census. Wint and Robinson (2007) demonstrate that mixing methods of GIS, vegetation cover and ground truthing through cluster samples are good ways of making population estimates. The question that was examined was whether a similar process could be applied in Bolivia.

To test this idea, data were collected during an epidemiology study in North and South Cinti, two Provinces of the Department of Chuquisaca in the south of Bolivia. The following

Table 15.10. Advantages and disadvantages for different methods of updating livestock population estimates.

Methodology	Advantages	Disadvantages
1. Livestock models based on previous census data	Low cost	Often little confidence in the estimates, if badly done Low quality of livestock economy estimates Low quality of estimates of the importance of the livestock sector Difficulties in planning and allocating resources for the livestock sector
2. New census	Should provide better population estimates if well done, and hence will give a better basis for estimating the livestock economy, its importance and need for resources	High financial and human resource cost A badly implemented census does not generate better estimations Long to plan and analyse, and complicated to implement
3. A livestock sector survey combined with data from the 2001 census	Should provide better population estimates if well done, and hence will give a better basis for estimating the livestock economy, its importance and need for resources	Average cost in terms of financial and human resources

presents the methodology to estimate livestock populations at a local level and how this was then used to estimate the livestock economy. The latter draws on work that was developed in the late 1990s and early 2000s at national level for Bolivia (Rushton *et al.*, 2001a).

Materials and methods

In May 2001, an epidemiology and livestock sector study was implemented in the Cintis of Chuquisaca. This region is one of the poorest of Bolivia, with a population of a little under hundred thousand people (Table 15.11).

Official estimates of livestock populations in the area were last updated in 1993. These data indicate that the region has important populations of sheep and goats (see Table 15.12).

The study collected blood and faecal samples from cattle, sheep, goats and pigs from the six muncipalities in the region. During the survey, data were collected on species and numbers of animals kept by each family. A total of 341 families took part in the survey. Tables 15.13–15.16 summarize the data on the livestock data by species.

Livestock population estimates

Livestock population estimates were made using the data generated from the livestock survey, secondary data on the number of households and observations made during the data collection. The following formula was used to make the estimates:

$$P_n = f_n * nh * a_n * hp_n$$

where P_n = Population estimate for species n

f_n = Correction factor for the species (see below)

nh = Number of households in the municipality (Ministerio de Desarrollo Humano, 1993)

a_n = Percentage of the producers that have species n based on the livestock sector survey

hp_n = Average flock or herd size for species n.

A correction factor was felt necessary as the survey had sought families that kept livestock in order to collect blood and faecal samples. These factors are subjective and based on the experiences and observations of the field teams. For the estimates made below, the correction factors were 0.67 for cattle and sheep,

Table 15.11. Human population and number of households in the Cinitis of Chuquisaca. (From INE, 2002.)

Province	Municipality	Number of communities	Population	Average household size	Number of families
South Cinti	Las Carreras	20	3,336	4.2	791
	Villa Abecia	10	3,160	5.4	588
	Culpina	57	18,793	4.9	3,844
North Cinti	Camargo	21	13,749	4.5	3,059
	Incahuasi	49	20,309	5.0	4,046
	San Lucas	102	31,808	3.3	9,644
Total		259	91,155	4.2	21,972

Table 15.12. Livestock populations in the Cintis of Chuquisaca. (From MACA and SNAG for cattle and INE for sheep, goats and pigs.)

	Cattle		Sheep		Goats		Pigs	
Province	Number	%	Number	%	Number	%	Number	%
North Cinti	51,986	9.40	179,375	33.90	103,624	27.00	72,228	13.30
South Cinti	25,440	4.60	48,680	9.20	53,731	14.00	33,670	6.20
Chuquisaca	553,043	100.00	529,130	100.00	383,788	100.00	543,079	100.00

Table 15.13. Number of cattle surveyed and an estimate of average herd size.

	Number of interviews	Cattle producers		Total cattle	Average herd size
		Number	Percentage		
North Cinti					
Camargo	53	11	21	114	10.36
San Lucas	106	68	64	451	6.63
Incahuasi	74	49	66	167	3.41
Total	233	128	55	732	5.72
South Cinti					
Villa Abecia	40	11	28	91	8.27
Culpina	43	26	60	650	25.00
Las Carreras	28	14	50	142	10.14
Total	111	51	46	883	17.31

Table 15.14. Number of sheep surveyed and an estimate of average herd size.

	Number of interviews	Sheep producers		Total sheep	Average flock size
		Number	Percentage		
North Cinti					
Camargo	53	17	32	142	8.35
San Lucas	106	71	67	3,092	43.55
Incahuasi	74	42	57	1,577	37.55
Total	233	130	56	4,811	37.01
South Cinti					
Villa Abecia	40	14	35	157	11.21
Culpina	43	28	65	1,302	46.50
Las Carreras	28	22	79	316	14.36
Total	111	64	58	1,775	27.73

Table 15.15. Number of goats surveyed and an estimate of average herd size.

	Number of interviews	Goat producers		Total goat	Average herd size
		Number	Percentage		
North Cinti					
Camargo	53	15	28	1,006	67.07
San Lucas	106	60	57	2,122	35.37
Incahuasi	74	9	12	90	10.00
Total	233	84	36	3,218	38.31
South Cinti					
Villa Abecia	40	11	28	915	83.18
Culpina	43	25	58	980	39.20
Las Carreras	28	20	71	953	47.65
Total	111	56	50	2,848	50.86

Table 15.16. Number of pigs surveyed and an estimate of average herd size.

	Number of interviews	Pig producers		Total pigs	Average herd size
		Number	Percentage		
North Cinti					
Camargo	53	27	51	117	4.33
San Lucas	106	56	53	215	3.84
Incahuasi	74	44	59	363	8.25
Total	233	127	55	695	5.47
South Cinti					
Villa Abecia	40	34	85	170	5.00
Culpina	43	28	65	482	17.21
Las Carreras	28	23	82	110	4.78
Total	111	85	77	762	8.96

0.5 for goats and 0.75 for pigs. These reflect the opinions of the ability of the families to keep these different species

Table 15.17 presents the estimates for the cattle populations in the Cintis; the crude estimate does not use the correction factor presented above. For comparison the population estimates from INE and MACA-SNAG for 1993 are also provided.

Similar estimates were made for sheep, goats and pigs, and they show much larger differences than for cattle (see Tables 15.18–15.20).

The results of the analysis indicate that the new estimates are different from the official estimates of 1993. The new population estimates derived using the correction factor were used as a basis to estimate the income generated by the different livestock species kept in the Cintis. This is summarized in Table 15.21.

As can be seen the estimated monetary values of output were combined with estimates of per capita income to provide some indication of the importance of livestock in the different zones of the Cintis and also to indicate the importance of individual species. In addition, estimates were made on the importance of different species according to the percentage of households that keep the species and the level of income generated by those species for families that keep them. A summary of this socio-economic analysis is presented in Table 15.22 and Fig. 15.3.

In the North Cinti province there were fewer cattle and pigs and more sheep and

Table 15.17. Cattle population estimates, number of households (Ministerio de Desarrollo Humano, 1993) and 1993 official population estimates (MACA-SNAG) for North and South Cinti.

	Number of households	Population estimate		Population 1993
		Crude	Modified	
North Cinti				
Camargo	3,059	6,580	4,386	
San Lucas	9,644	41,032	27,355	
Incahuasi	4,046	9,131	6,087	
Total	16,749	56,743	37,829	51,986
South Cinti				
Villa Abecia	588	1,338	892	
Culpina	3,844	58,107	38,738	
Las Carreras	791	4,012	2,674	
Total	5,223	63,456	42,304	25,440

Table 15.18. Sheep population estimates, number of households (Ministerio de Desarrollo Humano, 1993) and 1993 official population estimates (MACA-SNAG) for North and South Cinti.

	Number of households	Population estimate		Population 1993
		Crude	Modified	
North Cinti				
Camargo	3,059	8,196	5,464	
San Lucas	9,644	281,314	187,542	
Incahuasi	4,046	86,224	57,482	
Total	16,749	375,733	250,489	179,375
South Cinti				
Villa Abecia	588	2,308	1,539	
Culpina	3,844	116,393	77,595	
Las Carreras	791	8,927	5,951	
Total	5,223	127,628	85,085	48,680

Table 15.19. Goat population estimates, number of households (Ministerio de Desarrollo Humano, 1993) and 1993 official population estimates (INE) for North and South Cinti.

	Number of households	Population estimate		Population 1993
		Crude	Modified	
North Cinti				
Camargo	3,059	58,063	29,032	
San Lucas	9,644	193,062	96,531	
Incahuasi	4,046	4,921	2,460	
Total	16,749	256,046	128,023	103,624
South Cinti				
Villa Abecia	588	13,451	6,725	
Culpina	3,844	87,607	43,804	
Las Carreras	791	26,922	13,461	
Total	5,223	127,980	63,990	53,731

Table 15.20. Pig population estimates, number of households (Ministerio de Desarrollo Humano, 1993) and 1993 official population estimates (MACA-SNAG) for North and South Cinti.

	Number of households	Population estimate		Population 1993
		Crude	Modified	
North Cinti				
Camargo	3,059	6,753	5,065	
San Lucas	9,644	19,561	14,671	
Incahuasi	4,046	19,847	14,885	
Total	16,749	46,161	34,621	72,228
South Cinti				
Villa Abecia	588	2,499	1,874	
Culpina	3,844	43,089	32,316	
Las Carreras	791	3,108	2,331	
Total	5,223	48,695	36,521	33,670

Table 15.21. Population estimates for cattle, sheep, goats and pigs with the estimate of the income generated by each species in total and per household in the Cintis, Chuquisaca, Bolivia.

	North Cinti				South Cinti				Total
	Camargo	San Lucas	Incahuasi	Total	Villa Abecia	Culpina	Las Carreras	Total	
Population									
Cattle	4,386	27,355	6,087	37,829	892	38,738	2,674	42,304	80,133
Sheep	5,464	187,542	57,482	250,489	1,539	77,595	5,951	85,085	335,574
Goats	29,032	96,531	4,921	130,483	6,725	43,804	13,461	63,990	194,474
Pigs	5,065	14,671	14,885	34,621	1,874	32,316	2,331	36,521	71,142
Chickens	15,295	48,220	20,230	83,745	2,940	19,220	3,955	26,115	109,860
Livestock income generation (US$)									
Cattle	131,202	1,052,555	234,222	1,417,979	26,674	1,490,545	79,991	1,597,210	3,015,188
Sheep	39,409	1,352,685	621,903	2,013,997	11,097	559,670	42,925	613,692	2,627,690
Goats	304,182	1,011,414	51,558	1,367,155	70,465	458,958	141,040	670,463	2,037,618
Pigs	95,246	275,897	373,247	744,390	35,247	607,742	43,830	686,818	1,431,208
Chickens	154,091	485,799	203,810	843,700	29,619	193,634	39,845	263,099	1,106,799
Total	724,131	4,178,349	1,484,740	6,387,220	173,103	3,310,549	347,631	3,831,283	10,218,503
Estimated number of households with animals									
Cattle	423	4,124	1,786	6,334	108	1,550	264	1,921	8,255
Sheep	654	4,306	1,531	6,491	137	1,669	414	2,220	8,712
Goats	433	2,729	246	3,408	81	1,117	283	1,481	4,889
Pigs	779	3,821	1,804	6,405	375	1,877	487	2,739	9,144
Chickens	3,059	9,644	4,046	16,749	588	3,844	791	5,223	21,972
Estimated percentage of households with animals									
Cattle	13.8	42.8	44.1	36.6	18.3	40.3	33.3	30.6	37.6
Sheep	21.4	44.7	37.8	37.2	23.3	43.4	52.4	38.4	39.6
Goats	14.2	28.3	6.1	18.0	13.8	29.1	35.7	25.2	22.3
Pigs	25.5	39.6	44.6	40.9	63.8	48.8	61.6	57.4	41.6
Chickens	100.0	100.0	100.0	100.0	100.0	100.0	100.0	100.0	100.0
Livestock income generated per household per year									
Cattle	310	255	131	224	247	962	303	831	365
Sheep	60	314	406	310	81	335	104	276	302
Goats	703	371	210	401	872	411	499	453	417
Pigs	122	72	207	116	94	324	90	251	157
Chickens	50	50	50	50	50	50	50	50	50

Table 15.22. Summary of the socio-economic analysis of livestock in the region using secondary data and data generated during participatory workshops.

Province	Estimation of the percentage of income from animals per household	Importance of the species by the percentage of households that keep these animals	Importance of the species by income generated by the animals per household
North Cinti			
Camargo	16	Pigs, sheep and goats	Goats, cattle and pigs
Incahuasi	25	Pigs, sheep and cattle	Sheep, pigs and cattle
San Lucas	50	Sheep, cattle and pigs	Goats, sheep and cattle
South Cinti			
Las Carreras	38	Pigs, sheep and goats	Goats, cattle and sheep
Villa Abecia	19	Pigs, sheep and cattle	Goats, cattle and pigs
Culpina	65	Pigs, sheep and cattle	Cattle, goats and sheep/pigs

goats. In this province, it is predicted that sheep are the most economically important species overall, but that more families keep pigs. Combining data with the proportion of families with a species and the income generated by a livestock species within these families, it is possible to say that in the Municipality of Camargo a group of families has goats and they provide a sig-

nificant source of income. In the Municipality of Incahuasi pigs were an important activitiy.

For South Cinti, the population estimates are greater than the official livestock population data for all species in 1993, and these differences were large for cattle, sheep and goats. More than half the households had pigs, but only in Culpina is this livestock enterprise a

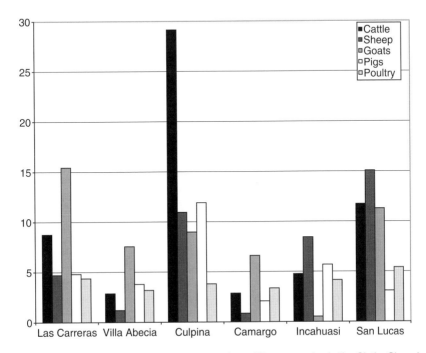

Fig. 15.3. Estimation of the proportion of rural income from different species in the Cintis, Chuquisaca, Bolivia. (From Rushton *et al.*, 2001b.)

significant economic activity. In Culpina and Las Carreras, sheep and goats are important in terms of the number of families who have them and the income these species generate. In Villa Abecia, the income generated by goats per family is high, but very few families keep goats. In Culpina, cattle were estimated to generate important sources of income.

The data collection and analysis were used in helping plan further investments for the livestock sector of the Cintis. In particular, there were no projects to support goat development and the analysis helped to identify the need to direct resources to families with goats (Rushton *et al.*, 2001b). The methodology was also further refined and combined with the animal disease data and this can be found in Rushton (2003).

Summary of Livestock Population Data and Livestock Systems

The final chapter of the Economic Theory and Tools (Part I, this volume) has presented a brief review of the work that has been ongoing in the classification of farming systems and more recently livestock systems. This work continues with important studies on the environment (Steinfeld *et al.*, 2006) and applications of GIS methods and statistical analyses for various livestock initiatives (see Shaw *et al.*, 2006; Wint and Robinson, 2007). Readers are recommended to look at these new works, particularly the pioneering work on GIS and livestock disease risk assessment (Wint and Robinson, 2007) and the spatial mapping of economic impact (Shaw *et al.*, 2006).

Looking back Putt *et al.* (1988) provide a list of general points when analysing epidemiological data, which is also a useful checklist for livestock data in general. The list is as follows (p. 49):

- Look at the data to gain an insight into the problem being studied.
- If data generated by other investigators are being used, find out as much as possible about how the data were generated. This may reveal significant omissions or biases in the data, which may influence the analysis.

- Do not ignore anomalies in the data; investigate them. Often such anomalies provide valuable clues to a deeper understanding of the problem being investigated.
- Avoid the temptation to use complicated statistical techniques if the quality of the data does not warrant it. Above all, avoid using such techniques to try and establish relationships between variables unless you can satisfy yourself that there are valid biological reasons for such relationships.
- Be cautious about making inferences from sampled to target populations. Your own experience should normally tell you whether such inferences are valid or not. If any inference is made, the populations involved should be clearly defined and the fact that an inference is being made clearly stated.
- When setting out findings, display the data used and the analyses undertaken in a simple, clear and concise form. A series of simple tables or graphs is preferable to one complicated table or graph. Long, complicated data sets should be placed in the appendix. Any limitations in the data presented should be clearly stated.
- Look at the data during the study, not just when it has been completed. This may enable the study design to be modified so as to include lines of inquiry which appear promising and to disregard those which do not.
- Finally remember that a 'negative' result, i.e. one that does not prove the hypothesis, is often as valuable as a 'positive' one. Do not be afraid to record negative findings.

One of the common errors when beginning to analyse data is having a fixed mind on the analytical structure or the importance of livestock products. While it has been argued above that analytical structures are important for directing data collection and structuring analysis, it is not recommended that the theory and tools presented in this section are the only ones that should be used or available. As Putt *et al.* (1988) mention, if interesting patterns occur in the data, investigate them and this may need other types of analytical structures.

Part II

A Review of the Application
of Economics to Animal Diseases
and Health Problems

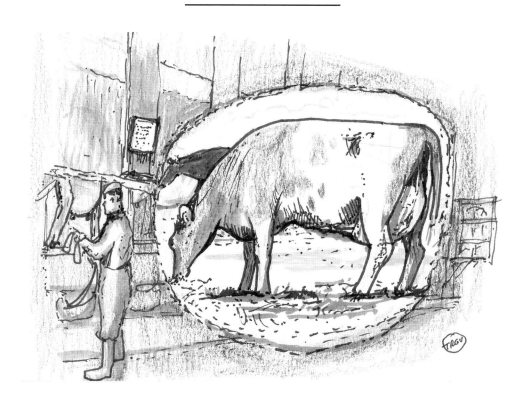

Introduction

Chapter 1 and Part I of this book have covered the history of animal health economics and introduced economic theory and tools, respectively. Part II will provide a wide-ranging literature review of the application of economics to animal diseases and health problems. Part II is divided into four chapters that cover reported studies on diseases that affect:

- a range of livestock species;
- large ruminants;
- small ruminants;
- pigs;
- poultry.

The structure follows the system developed for CABI's *Animal Health and Production Compendium* (Rushton, 2002). This part draws heavily on the material developed for the Compendium and below is a short explanation of what were the objectives of this work, and what became the final output.

Economic Assessment of Livestock Diseases

The initial terms of reference for the section on the economic assessment of livestock diseases within CABI's *Animal Health and Production Compendium* were to estimate the global costs of disease in different regions of the world and in different production systems. This was based on the format presented with the *Crop Protection Compendium* produced by CABI. However, this aim proved to be impossible because data are not available to provide estimates that have any validity. There are also a number of issues that the reader should be aware of with global estimates of disease:

- The impact of disease is not the same in all places because:
  - Different systems will have different impacts. For example, mastitis in a cow giving 30 l a day has been predicted to reduce milk yield by 6.2 l (Yalcin *et al.*, 2000), but a cow giving 5 l a day, which is the average in most double-purpose systems around the world, would lose between 0.5 and 1 l a day.
  - The impact of a disease will be different for systems with different disease status. For example, a herd of cattle that has endemically stable infection with piroplasmosis and babesiosis will have few clinically sick animals, but a herd that is endemically unstable for these diseases may suffer losses of animals with the entry of infected animals.
  - Value of animals and livestock products is different in different places. For example, beef prices in February 2001 in the UK were approximately US$2.32/kg deadweight; the equivalent price in Santa Cruz, Bolivia, on this date was US$1.17. The reasons for these differences are due to access to markets and subsidies in the different places, but the fact that these differences exist means that the impact of a

disease that reduces the weight of an animal, such as FMD, will be different in Bolivia and the UK. This in turn means that the response to the control to that disease should be different.
- Costs of medicines and vaccines to control disease will be different in different places. Production systems that have access to good communication structures and well-trained veterinary support services will probably pay less for medicines and veterinary services than production systems that are isolated from centres of economic activity.
- Costs of control of a disease will be different at different times, because previous actions and controls will change disease status, and investments in drug and vaccine development will alter costs of disease control. For example, Dufour and Moutou (1994) estimated that the policy of controlling FMD with annual vaccine was 13 times more expensive than the policy of extra surveillance and no vaccine that was adopted in 1991 in France. With the same disease the development of the oil adjuvant vaccine increased the duration of protection and hence reduced the number of vaccines needed per year.

In addition to the comments made above, the reader should be aware that the majority of the livestock in the world (see below) are found in systems that are extensive. The data on livestock populations in these systems are usually unreliable and information on the production parameters for these systems is not generally available. Work continues to address this (J. Otte and FAO, personal communication, Rome, 2002), but the reality is that good data on livestock populations and livestock production parameters generally only exist in the more intensive livestock systems of the world. Therefore, there are good reasons that many of the advances in the subject of livestock disease economics have taken place in Europe and the USA.

Despite the words of caution above, it is important to say that estimates of the economic impact of diseases and their control are necessary to guide resource allocation at farm, national and regional level. Many decisions are made on 'gut feelings' about the importance of disease, but since the late 1970s much more attention has been paid to justifying investments in animal disease research and control through the use of cost–benefit analysis techniques (see Chapter 1, this volume). These investments have made a significant contribution to the increased world production of livestock, which Delgado *et al.* (2001) have likened to the green revolution. They argue that the 'Livestock Revolution' has been propelled by demand, but the supply has been supported by major advances in the control of contagious disease, namely FMD, CSF, rinderpest and Newcastle disease, which have allowed farmers to adopt more intensive production systems in areas that were previously too hostile to keep animals.

Therefore, the following section will present a framework for the economic assessment of livestock disease and comment on the work currently being developed by FAO in the area of global estimates of livestock disease impact.

Framework

To begin this discussion, it is necessary to make clear what can be analysed for the economic assessment of livestock diseases:

1. It is possible to estimate the losses caused by disease and make no reference to the potential costs of eliminating the disease. This may be valid if there is interest in researching a new vaccine or drug to control or eradicate that disease, but the estimates of losses need to examine if a change in disease status will affect markets and prices. These types of estimates are the most common in the literature and their value is dubious as it assumes that the base situation is zero disease and generally there is no comment about the potential cost reaching this zero disease status.
2. The second type of assessment is the value of a disease control and/or eradication programme. This requires much more information on the technical, epidemiological and economic situation of disease control and is effectively looking at productivity changes within disease control.

These two points are important in the review of information on the economic impact of diseases in the following sections.

The framework presented in this section follows that by Rushton *et al.* (1999). This is based on the concept of productivity changes with disease control and not simply on the idea of global disease losses. Productivity is a measure of efficiency of the production system and is represented as a quantitative term of the output(s) divided by the input(s).

$$\text{Productivity} = \frac{\begin{array}{c}\text{Total value of}\\\text{outputs per unit of time}\end{array}}{\begin{array}{c}\text{Total value of inputs}\\\text{per unit of time}\end{array}}$$

Changes in disease status that lead to productivity increases are favourable and encourage investment. This can be compared to changes that increase production, but at a cost that is greater than the benefits, i.e. it lowers productivity. There is much confusion in the literature about these two terms and many authors use the word productivity where they actually mean production. This confusion can lead to frustrations with the different actors involved in disease control programmes, namely farmers and veterinary staff. The latter can demonstrate that disease control will increase production, which they believe is good, the former is aware that to achieve this increased production requires extra inputs and work which have to be balanced against the greater return, i.e. the farmer is interested in productivity increases. This simple scenario can be applied to larger-scale investments where governments and international agencies have contemplated where best to use their resources. It is necessary with diseases to determine the losses caused by a disease, but this in itself is not sufficient. Beyond this, there is need to determine the costs of reaching a new disease status and then comparing this with the estimates of loss. When this information is available the farmer, government or international agency has a basis to judge whether an investment in animal disease control or eradication is appropriate. The latter is an application of the principles of rational economic judgement explained in Chapter 3 (this volume).

With this in mind, the following will detail some of the important processes in the economic assessment of livestock diseases.

Losses caused by livestock disease can be classified into the following categories:

1. Direct losses:
   (a) visible losses, e.g. deaths and stunting;
   (b) invisible losses, e.g. reduced fertility, change in herd structure
2. Indirect losses:
   (a) additional costs, e.g. drugs, vaccines;
   (b) revenue forgone, e.g. denied access to better markets, use of suboptimal production technology.

Many of these losses cannot be calculated directly, because the impact of a disease may not be fully understood until some time after an outbreak. For example, FMD in an extensive beef system causes some losses at the time of the outbreak, but the most important impact is reduced number of animals available for sale between 3 and 4 years after the outbreak occurrs. To fully understand this impact requires models (see Chapters 7 and 8, this volume) that simulate a healthy herd or flock and a herd or flock affected by disease. Such models in turn require information on:

- production parameters, such as mortality rate, fertility rate, age at first calving, milk production levels, growth rates, of the healthy and infected herd; and
- the number of animals in the affected population.

With this information the output and productivity of the two herds, healthy and infected, can be compared.

The added complication of some livestock diseases is that they can also cause disease in humans, e.g. trypanosomiasis (sleeping sickness), rabies, cysticercosis. Other diseases may not cause disease in humans, but may produce economic hardship. This further complicates the analysis by adding a dimension of human welfare and, as mentioned in Chapters 10 and 14 (this volume), this can be calculated as DALYs saved.

Once an understanding of the losses caused by a disease has been obtained, the question that decision makers have to make, be they farmers, government officials or international agency bureaucrats, is what should be done about the disease. In some situations, it may be acceptable to do nothing, because, although the disease causes losses, the cost of eradicating the disease and eliminating these losses may be too high. This type of analysis at farm level is relatively straightforward, because the impact of a change in healthy status at individual farm level is unlikely to have an impact on livestock and livestock product markets. However, large-scale programmes at national or regional level are likely to change the amount of product produced and in turn change the prices that the producers receive and the consumers pay for that product. This requires analysis to determine changes in consumer and producer surplus, which in turn requires information on the market for products and impact of production changes.

In summary the following information is required to carry out the economic assessment of disease:

1. Population affected;
2. If it is a large population or a population with very different types of animal management (e.g. a farm with beef and dairy systems), a classification of the livestock production systems with an estimate of the population in each system;
3. Production parameters of each livestock system with and without disease;
4. Estimation of the percentage of animals affected in each production system each year;
5. Costs of current disease control methods in each system;
6. A model to simulate the herd or flock with and without disease for each production system;
7. Costs of changing the disease status, be it reducing the prevalence of the disease or eradicating the disease;
8. The impact of the change in disease status in quantity of produce and market prices for the product; and
9. Comparison between costs and benefits of a change in disease status.

Points 1–6 are sufficient to obtain information on disease losses, but points 7–9 are required to make decisions on disease control strategies for the future. The following section will detail some of the information available for the economic assessment of livestock diseases.

Summary

Returning to the history of the application of economics to animal diseases and health the following periods are identified:

- Period prior to the 1960s involved pro-grammes of control and eradication of contagious diseases that were known to cause serious production losses and in some cases human health problems. These programmes were implemented without analysis of the costs and benefits, i.e. it was assumed to be a good thing.
- From the early 1970s, there was growing interest in making economic analyses of livestock diseases and their control. The diseases of greatest interest have been those where people were not sure if con-trol or eradication would give positive returns, e.g. there are a number of stud-ies on the control of helminths.
- From the mid-1980s, there was a growing interest in public health. This perhaps began with *Salmonella*, but more recently has focused on *Escherichia coli* H157 and bovine spongiform encephalopathy (BSE). The issues here are not about pro-duction losses, but human health risks and the subsequent costs if a disease from animals is transmitted to humans via animal protein. It is suggested that the growing interest in this subject is related to the costs of such problems. Outbreaks of food poisoning in a rich country quickly translated into high medical bills and large amounts of lost work and leisure time that is valued highly. In the case of BSE, the costs could be even more serious if a large epidemic occurs in the economically active popu-lation of the UK. These impacts make some of the production-level losses look small and it is likely that particularly in rich industrialized nations livestock dis-ease prioritization will have to take these impacts more seriously. This will need new skills in animal health economics to translate human health needs into ani-mal health decisions and policy making.

Accurate assessments of the economic impact of livestock diseases are rare and at global level not available. The reasons presented above indicate that the difficulties of devel-oping global estimates, the assumptions required and the data constraints would make such estimates superficial. However, there has been some ranking of the world's livestock diseases by national and global vet-erinary services around the world in order to prioritize the allocation of resources on disease control efforts. In recent times, these assessments have been supported by eco-nomic analyses and the following chapters detail the main studies in this field.

16 The Main Livestock Diseases

The Office International des Épizooties (OIE) is the international organization for animal health. In 1929, a group of ten experts generated a list of livestock diseases on the basis of 'the degree of seriousness' of the contagious diseases (OIE, 2001a). This list has not remained static because as production systems change the importance of diseases change and in some cases new diseases emerge (OIE, 2001b). For a long period, the OIE had two distinct classes of disease:

1. List A diseases, which are 'transmissible diseases that have the potential for very serious and rapid spread, irrespective of national borders, that are of serious socio-economic or public health consequence and that are of major importance in the international trade of animals and animal products'.
2. List B diseases, which are 'transmissible diseases that are considered to be of socioeconomic and/or public health importance within countries and that are significant in the international trade of animals and animal products'.

The interesting thing about these statements is that they are largely founded on 'gut feelings' rather than quantitative analysis. For example, the 2001 foot-and-mouth disease (FMD) outbreak in the UK had veterinarians and economists searching for information about the economic impact of the disease. What was discovered is that estimates of production losses caused by FMD are based on expert opinion of the impact and not on scientific investigations. Note that many of the losses caused by this disease are related to human actions such as animal movement restrictions.

The OIE list has great importance with relation to international trade. Diseases such as FMD are effective barriers to the trade of livestock and livestock products, but can also have an impact on the trade of fresh fruit and vegetables.

The following section will detail information available on the economic impact of the major world livestock diseases that affect a range of species.

Foot-and-mouth Disease (FMD)

FMD is probably the most important disease in the world in terms of economic impact. The reasons for this are not only about its ability to cause losses in terms of production, but are also related to the reaction of the veterinary profession to its presence and the restrictions on the trade of animals both locally and internationally. It should also be made clear that FMD is capable of infecting cattle, sheep, goats, pigs and humans. It is a disease that has high morbidity, but low mortality, and is highly contagious.

The main impacts of FMD in terms of animal production are the following:

- Causes abortions in pregnant animals.
- Causes reductions in milk yields and increases the probability of mastitis due to damage to the teats.
- Causes lameness in animals, which reduces their ability to work in terms of ploughing fields and transporting goods.
- Causes losses in weight due to animals being unable to eat while they are sick.
- Increases mortality in young animals.

These losses are more pronounced in cattle and pig systems; the impact in goat and sheep systems is generally low. The effects are also much more dramatic in intensive systems of cattle and pigs; in particular FMD can cause devastating losses in dairy systems and in intensive pig systems. However, the impact of the disease in extensive cattle systems is small and the incentives to control the disease are also small. Oleksiewicz *et al.* (2001) report that pigs are difficult to immunize against FMD and that their response to the disease is variable, but they stress the need for rapid and effective control of this disease in areas with high pig densities. One of the important issues with pigs and pork products is that these animals are rapid multipliers of virus and pork products have been shown to be a potential risk of disease in countries with FMD-free status (Farez and Morley, 1997).

Given that Europe, the USA and other developed countries have concentrated areas of intensive animal production, there is a great need to protect these areas from this disease. Therefore, the impact of FMD is much greater when it is considered that:

- Live animal trade cannot take place between a FMD-infected country and FMD-free country.
- There are heavy restrictions on the trade of livestock products from FMD-infected countries to FMD-free countries. In the worst scenario only meat that has been processed and tinned can be exported, which would be the case for a country regularly reporting outbreaks of the disease. In the best situation meat can be exported deboned, but there need to be active vaccination campaigns and an official veterinary service capable of reacting to outbreaks.
- The presence of FMD can affect the export of fresh fruit and vegetables to FMD-free countries.
- In countries with active veterinary services local trade is affected when outbreaks occur. Animal movement restrictions are put in place, making it difficult to buy and sell animals, and in some countries there are restrictions on the movement of people. The latter are particularly important in countries where the rural economy is dedicated to tourism and not to animal production.

It is important to note that countries with the highest prices for livestock products such as Japan, the USA and the European Union are the strictest in terms of applying trade restrictions for livestock and livestock products. The incentives to achieve FMD-free status for countries with the potential to export meat are therefore high.

Finally, FMD has a list of costs related to its control, which are different depending on the disease status of the countries concerned:

- Countries with the disease usually have vaccination campaigns in attempts to control outbreaks and in some cases in a plan to eradicate the disease.
- Countries close to the eradication of FMD usually adopt a slaughter policy for animals detected with the disease. This policy is normally for animals infected and contact animals. The carcasses of these animals are either buried or burnt.
- Countries that are free dedicate resources in border controls, checking the veterinary services and slaughterhouses of exporting countries with FMD.
- Countries that are free maintain active surveillance systems for FMD. (Note: In 1991, the European Union changed its policy for control of FMD from annual vaccination to surveillance and slaughter of animals involved in outbreaks.)
- Countries that are free but experience occasional outbreaks normally react by

adopting a slaughter policy to eliminate infected animals and animals in contact.

- Most countries maintain laboratory services that are capable of diagnosing whether animals have FMD.
- Countries that are free maintain stocks of vaccine for the possibility of outbreaks within their country.

The list of impacts of FMD is long and complicated, but different in different countries. For example, countries with one or all of the following characteristics:

- do not have the capacity to export livestock and livestock products;
- import livestock and livestock products from countries with FMD;
- the majority of their production systems are extensive;

are unlikely to have much incentive to run eradication campaigns. The reasons for this are that the returns to a change in disease status are small and possibly negative.

However, countries with the following characteristics:

- export livestock and livestock products; (Note: this can include semen and embryos.)
- the majority of their production systems are intensive;

have large incentives to control and eradicate FMD and in the case of countries free of FMD to invest resources to maintain this status. The pattern of eradication of FMD follows closely these characteristics, with the USA being one of the first to eliminate the disease followed by European countries and some Latin American countries such as Uruguay in more recent times.

Given the importance of this disease at local and regional level, it is of no surprise that there are many references on the economic impact of its control. However, as mentioned above, the estimates for losses in production are based on expert opinion, not on scientific findings. The following section provides a summary of available literature.

Table 16.1 provides a brief summary of some of the articles published on FMD economics considered to be important in the economic assessment of this disease.

Table 16.1. Major studies on the economics of FMD.

Country	Major findings	Comments	Authors
UK	Compares two control strategies, stamping out policy and vaccination to control FMD. This is based on the 1967–1968 FMD outbreak in the UK. It finds that both policies are positive, but the stamping out policy is favourable if no account is taken of unquantifiable benefits	Thorough study, one of the first to be done at country level. The findings are now not so relevant in the UK where the rural economy has changed and the importance of tourism is so high	Power and Harris (1973)
General	Lists the major losses caused by FMD	The information is generally based on expert opinion, but the layout is a useful starting point for the economic assessment of FMD	James and Ellis (1978)
South-east Asia	Presents a combined epidemiology and economic model to assess the profitability of FMD eradication in South-east Asia. The analysis would suggest that eradication is attractive, but in some countries is dependent on the export of pig products. However, in Thailand eradication gives good returns without exports	The article reviews estimates of returns to FMD found in consultancy reports and stresses the need for systems analysis in assessing disease control campaigns (cf. Obiaga *et al.* (1979) in Latin America)	Perry *et al.* (1999)

Europe

Europe was considered to be an endemic zone for FMD up until the late 1980s. In Italy, where there were regular outbreaks, it was estimated that the benefits from FMD control were 42,855 million Italian lire (Caporale *et al.*, 1980) and that the costs of this programme were 5316 million Italian lire (Ghilardi *et al.*, 1981). Stougaard (1984) estimated the costs of different strategies of controlling FMD in Denmark. The author found that an annual vaccination policy was the most expensive in comparison to policies of ring vaccination and slaughter and control with no vaccination. However, Stougaard is clear that prevention is better than cure and that a livestock exporting country such as Denmark should not take risks of losing valuable export markets by dropping its vaccination policy. However, during the late 1980s and early 1990s much research was carried out with regard to the change in policy on control of FMD in Europe due to a change in its FMD status.

Mainland Europe had a policy up until 1991 to control FMD with annual vaccination; this was changed to increased surveillance and a stamping out policy in the case of outbreaks. Dufour and Moutou (1994) estimated that the new policy cost 13 times less than the vaccination policy, and the burden of costs had shifted from the farmer to the State. They make the comment that their analysis did not include any estimation on the risks of reinfection with the two policies. In The Netherlands, Dijkhuizen (1989b) showed that a change in policy would be favourable, and an analysis by Berentsen *et al.* (1990a) calculated that there would have to be four outbreaks every 10 years to make the annual vaccination policy more attractive than the surveillance and slaughter policy. The latter authors also reported that the change in European policy was positive for The Netherlands even taking into account the increased risks of reinfection and the impact of export bans, provided that outbreaks were controlled with a ring vaccination and slaughter policy (Berentsen *et al.* 1990b, 1992). In Italy, the change in policy was also found to be positive even taking into account risks of outbreaks in the Po valley, which is a zone with intensive livestock pro-

duction (Amadori *et al.*, 1991). In Germany, Lorenz (1988) estimated that the surveillance and stamping out policy was in the long term more profitable than an annual vaccination with a stamping out policy. His research examined the different risks involved of outbreaks with the two policies. Davies (1988) in a slightly different analysis found that the costs of annual vaccination in seven European Union countries were equivalent to the direct cost of 200 outbreaks of FMD in these countries.

Mahul and Durand (2000) suggest that for countries with FMD-free status, a policy of stamping out outbreaks was economically optimum, and they stress the importance of minimizing the period when a country cannot export livestock and livestock products as being the key to high returns.

Latin America

Latin America has a long history of control and eradication campaigns against FMD, which are based on vaccination. The regional institution for these campaigns is over 25 years old and its successes have been limited to countries with serious intentions to export agricultural products. Information in the literature on the economics of these control campaigns is scarce, but Carpenter and Thieme (1980) developed a model to assess the control of FMD in Brazil, which was part of the programme by the Inter-American Development Bank to review investments in animal health at a time when a number of Latin American countries were investing in FMD eradication campaigns. In addition, there are some studies on the importance of a change in vaccine technology, the importance of livestock systems analysis in FMD campaigns and the economic impact of FMD at farm level.

- Astudillo and Auge de Mello (1980) report the advantages of a change in vaccine technology, with the oil adjuvant vaccine being more cost-effective in a South America scenario than a vaccine with aluminium hydroxide adjuvant. They noted the difficulties at the time of adopting this technology due to a lack of a commercially available product, but this vaccine technology has since been widely adopted.

- Obiaga *et al.* (1979) analysed the importance of livestock production systems as determinants of FMD epidemiology and argued that control campaigns need to recognize and classify systems before beginning campaigns. The methodology outlined was the basis for future FMD campaigns in Latin America.

- In Paraguay, it was reported that farmers were unwilling and hostile to vaccinating all their animals against FMD each year (Mendoza *et al.*, 1978). The authors present the importance of this campaign for the national economy, but make no mention of the farm-level incentives.

- In Colombia, returns to farm-level controls of FMD in dairy farms were found to be positive (Cardona *et al.*, 1982). They report that, in a dairy farm that experienced FMD with 280 cattle, 74% of the animals were affected, leading to a 26% drop in milk production, an increase in mortality (0.7% died) and an average loss in weight of 23 kg. Losses per sick animal were estimated at 12,900 Colombian pesos.

- In Bolivia, Bulman and Terrazas (1976) reported an outbreak on a dairy farm in Cochabamba where 45% of the cows were affected even though the herd had been vaccinated 2 months previously. During the outbreak milk production was reduced by 15%, two cows died and four lost one or more quarters.

India

India has nearly 15% of the world cattle population that are dedicated to draught power and milk production. It is also a country with FMD disease. Ellis and James (1978) found that there were positive returns to a campaign to eradicate the disease.

A socio-economic study in the Indian Punjab found that the education level of the farmers was related to the likelihood of FMD outbreaks and it was suggested that this was related to educated farmers being more likely to seek professional advice and to vaccinate their animals regularly (Saini *et al.*, 1992). Saxena (1994a) used a survey within India to estimate losses caused by FMD in terms of production of milk and abortion. He estimated that in India the losses per year were 3508 million l of milk, which is approximately 6.5% of total annual national milk output. In terms of value at 1990 prices, the annual loss of milk was Rs 12,520 million in terms of lost foreign exchange, and between Rs 16,500 million and Rs 18,730 million in terms of lost domestic economic surplus. In a further study, Saxena (1994b) estimated the losses relating to lost draught power, animal deaths and costs of treatment as being Rs 18,130 million. On average there were Rs 125 losses per head of cattle and buffalo in the country.

Australia and the USA

Australia and the USA are countries free without vaccination who are aggressive exporters of livestock products. Both have active surveillance systems for FMD and their interest is to remain free. Garner and Lack (1995) estimated the consequences of an outbreak of FMD if it was to occur in Australia. It was found that the impact would be greater where the production systems were not diversified, but the authors believed that the impact in terms of trade would be less due to the possibility of zoning a country. In a very early study McCauley *et al.* (1978) looked at the costs of FMD if the USA was endemic. It is of interest in that it examines costs with different control strategies.

Other countries

A range of other studies have been carried out in other countries:

- Ertan and Nazlioglu (1981) estimated that losses due to FMD in Turkey were 141 million Turkish lire. The disease infected 57,000 cattle and 76,000 sheep.
- In Israel, losses in a non-vaccinated dairy herd were US$231,000 and in a partially

immune herd were US$65,700 (van Ham and Zur, 1994). On average the national losses per year were US$289,900 with costs in terms of vaccination of US$1.47 million. However, the authors indicate that without vaccination the losses would increase to US$68.09 million and the returns to the present policy were positive.

- Farag *et al.* (1998) found that sheep and goats were infected throughout Saudi Arabia, but clinical FMD in these species was not common. Controlling FMD in a country like Saudi Arabia is difficult as it imports large numbers of live animals from endemic countries and these animals have been reported to have been exposed to FMD, but do not appear to be carriers (Hafez *et al.*, 1994).
- Leabad (1981) reports that the stamping out of a FMD outbreak in Morocco cost US$3.3 million. This country had been free for 20 years and it was suspected that the outbreak came from meat imported from Latin America.
- A study of an outbreak of FMD in Ethiopia indicated that cattle, sheep and goats were affected by the disease. In cattle the disease caused mortality in calves (6%) and 64% of the farmers reported FMD as a harmful disease. Of these farmers the majority reported losses in milk production and loss in draught power production of approximately 20 days.
- Analysis of data from a FMD disease outbreak in Sahiwal cattle indicated that 70% were affected in the herd even though it had been vaccinated previously. Of the cows affected 69% had reduced milk yields (74l) and 74% lost weight (average 18 kg). It is also reported that this herd had experienced six outbreaks of FMD in a 14-year period (Kazimi and Shah, 1980).

Summary for foot-and-mouth disease

FMD is probably the most important economic disease in the world. It is a disease that affects large and small ruminants, pigs and humans. It causes greatest production losses in cattle and pigs and in particular in intensive dairy and pig systems. FMD disease status is an important determinant of international trade in livestock products and the existence of FMD is an effective barrier from the markets with the highest prices for these products. Therefore, many resources have and are dedicated to the surveillance, control and eradication of this disease. This input has paid off in that many areas of the world are now either free from FMD or have the disease under control. The incentives of these control activities are dependent on the export potential of countries and types of livestock systems that are found within the countries.

Anthrax

Anthrax is a disease that can affect large and small ruminants, pigs, poultry and humans. The disease kills animals quickly and can rarely be cured. It is not infectious and the spread of the disease depends on how the carcasses of the infected animals are handled. Grazing animals are most susceptible to the disease. Barnes (1997) states that, although birds can be infected by anthrax, chickens are highly resistant, but ducks and ostrich have been reported to be affected. It is of greatest importance in cattle and buffalo, but this may be related to reporting bias as it is more likely that farmers will report the loss of a big animal.

Anthrax is found throughout the world and, where it is reported in the developed world, the number of outbreaks is usually small and well controlled. Most European veterinary services report one or two cases a year, but a report in Italy in 1979 indicated that there were 50 outbreaks in that year (Mattioli and Gagliardi, 1980). The impact of this disease is:

- Cost of annual vaccination in endemic areas. (Note: the bacterial spores can survive for 50 years, making it necessary to vaccinate animals.)
- Occasional outbreaks which cause animal death.
- Disposal of carcasses affected by the disease either by burial or by being burnt.

- Costs of treatment with antibiotics during outbreaks with valuable animals. Gill (1982) reports that antibiotic treatment of cattle at risk can be worthwhile if the value of the animals is high.
- Impacts on human health, where particularly slaughterhouse workers may be affected by pulmonary or skin forms of anthrax.
- In poorer countries and regions of the world, there are reports of people consuming carcasses with anthrax and dying. A report from the Department of Veterinary Services, Kenya (1972) states that cattle and pigs died due to anthrax and people eating the carcasses were also affected. PROMED reports have also indicated human deaths in Zimbabwe and Kenya.

In Indonesia, Ronohardjo *et al.* (1986) state that anthrax is one of the major diseases in the country but they do not list it in the top five diseases that affect large ruminants. In Nigeria, Akerejola *et al.* (1979) list anthrax as a disease that affects sheep and goats, but indicate that it is not that important. Nurul Islam (1984) in a study of livestock keeping in smallholder farms indicates that heavy losses of cattle were suffered in Bangladesh. Rushton (1995) reports an anthrax outbreak where many cattle were lost over a period of a year, mainly because of poor disposal of affected carcasses.

In summary, anthrax is a disease that occurs sporadically in all parts of the world. Its main economic significance is that it kills large and small ruminants and its presence requires control processes such as effective disposal of affected carcasses and possibly annual vaccination in areas known to be endemic. It is also known to be a problem in areas with poor knowledge of the dangers of eating carcasses with anthrax and a number of countries have reported human deaths because of this disease.

Tuberculosis

Tuberculosis is a disease that affects humans, large and small ruminants, pigs and poultry. Its impact in terms of livestock disease is related to its potential threat to human health. There are losses in production due to:

- Condemnation of carcasses and organs of animals affected by the disease. This seems to be a problem associated more with cattle and pigs and to some extent poultry.
- Some losses are associated with milk production, some animals suffer mastitis.

However, many of the costs associated with the control and eradication of the disease are often far greater than the losses caused by the disease. These are as follows:

- testing of animals, which requires two visits of trained staff;
- slaughter of positive animals, which becomes more expensive the lower the prevalence, because there are a higher percentage of false positives;
- control of wildlife populations that act as reservoirs of tuberculosis;
- trade with countries.

The justification for the control of tuberculosis is usually the public health concerns, which are related to:

- Human tuberculosis caused by the ingestion of milk from tuberculous cows. Normally, this produces bone and intestinal tuberculosis and this form of the disease was one of the main causes of infant mortality in the UK at the beginning of the 20th century.
- Human tuberculosis due to contact with animals with tuberculosis.

Both these possible routes of infection have increased in importance in Africa, where a high percentage of the human population has AIDS, making them more susceptible to tuberculosis infections. However, in developed countries, where eradication campaigns have reduced prevalences of tuberculosis to very low levels and milk is almost invariably pasteurized, the risks of contracting tuberculosis from animals is small. Attention has often turned to why this disease cannot be completely eradicated in these countries and it has been found that wildlife reservoirs exist that make it difficult to achieve full eradication. Much time, money and energy has been dedicated to this subject and there is a cor-responding literature on the economics of the control of tuberculosis through wildlife control.

With regard to the literature on the con-trol of wildlife reservoirs the following is available:

- Kao and Roberts (1999) compared the control of bovine tuberculosis using cat-tle vaccination or culling of possum, which are a wildlife reservoir for this dis-ease in countries such as New Zealand. They found that the returns depended on the density of the cattle population, with higher densities favouring a strategy of culling the wildlife reservoir.
- Eves (1999) reported that the removal of badgers in County Offaly in Ireland led to a reduction in the number of positives per 1000 animal tests and in the reactor rate from 3.72 to 0.45 in a period of 6 years.
- Tuyttens and Macdonald (1998) suggest a sterilization of badgers rather than a cull to reduce the wildlife threat, but they men-tion public concerns over such actions.
- McInerney (1986) found that there was no economic justification of the badger culling in south-west England and he states that the control of bovine tuber-culosis through badge control is a politi-cal problem.
- Power and Watts (1987) found that this control method had lost several millions of pounds sterling and they state that future benefits are unlikely to accrue as the control method did not appear to be very effective.

Information on production losses due to tuberculosis is as follows:

- Cuban data found that an eradication programme in six dairy farms increased milk production (Vera et al., 1984).
- In Mauritius, Jaumally and Sibartie (1983) estimated that losses caused by bovine tuberculosis were Rs 800,000 a year, with a reactor rate on the island between 0.07% and 0.57%. They do not mention the costs of eradicating the dis-ease and eliminating these costs.

- In Mexico, Valdespino Ortega (1993) found that the depreciation costs associated with animals detected and culled due to tuber-culosis were higher than the general aver-age indicating the costs of such a test and slaughter policy at farm level.
- In Nigeria, Alonge and Ayanwale (1984) reported that 0.2% of cattle have tuber-culosis and within this infected popula-tion 1% die of the disease. They estimated that at that time the losses due to bovine tuberculosis were 14.24 million naira in a population of 9.3 million head of cattle.
- Zhilinskii et al. (1986) in Belorussia report that losses due to bovine tuberculosis were between four and nine times the costs in lost production which was due to lower productivity and poorer-quality products.
- Smolyaninov and Martynov (1982) found reductions in milk and meat production and fertility in herds that retained posi-tive tuberculin reactors; these losses were reduced by the slaughter of positive ani-mals and repopulation of the herds. However, there is no reference to the prevalence of tuberculosis within these herds.

Carcass and organ condemnation is an import-ant cost in an area with tuberculosis:

- Bolitho (1978) estimated that in the UK 0.42% of pig meat was condemned and a third of this was condemned due to tuberculosis lesions. The author requested that the dangers of eating meat from a tuberculous animal should be reassessed.
- In Cameroon, Nfi and Alonge (1987) found that 0.2% of carcasses were totally condemned because of tuberculosis, with a higher percentage of organs and parts being condemned. This would indicate the presence of the disease, but its eco-nomic impact is not that high. In the same country, Awa et al. (1999) report that 33% of pigs inspected at slaughter had tuberculosis lesions.
- Zorawski et al. (1982) report that between 7% and 8% of the pigs slaughtered in a re-gion of Poland had tuberculosis lesions.

- In Germany, Texdorf (1981) reported that approximately 0.25% of pigs slaughtered in the Marburg abattoir were condemned with tuberculosis lesions.
- In the USA, Berthelsen (1974) estimated that a pig passed for cooking due to tuberculosis lesions incurred losses of US$61.93, which was approximately US$5933 per hundred thousand pigs slaughtered. Dey and Parham (1993) analysed the changes in the regulations with regard to tuberculosis lesions in pigs in the USA. They estimated that between 1975 and 1988 a lower proportion of pigs had been condemned or passed for cooking and losses due to condemnation had reduced from US$2.3 to US$0.97 million/year between this period. This loss is only 0.01% of the animal value of this industry.

Returns to control or eradication campaigns of tuberculosis vary:

- Bernues *et al.* (1997) report that returns to the eradication campaign in a mountain area of Spain are not positive due to the high compensation costs paid for positive reactor animals.
- Andrews *et al.* (1980) examined the use of different methods to eradicate tuberculosis in the tropical zone of Australia and suggested that measures such as the separation of young stock from older animals were effective. However, not all farmers were willing or able to implement these measures and this could have a serious impact on the control of this disease. Later, Stoneham and Johnston (1987) report that tuberculosis had not been eradicated from northern Australia and they evaluated the tuberculosis campaign to find the most cost-effective method of eradication of this disease.
- Denes (1983) reports on the tuberculosis eradication programme in Hungary between 1963 and 1981, which reduced the prevalence of bovine tuberculosis from 30% to 0.2%. The author states that the campaign, although costly in terms of compensation payments for replacement animals, had saved the country nearly 17 times the cost of the campaign.

- Caporale *et al.* (1980) found that the Italian tuberculosis campaign between 1965 and 1978 (reducing prevalence from 12.1% to 0.78% in a herd of 6.6 million cattle) produced gross benefits of 63,500 million Italian lire and cost 8436 million Italian lire (Ghilardi *et al.*, 1981).

Tuberculosis exists in poultry at a worldwide level at prevalences that range between 1% and 26%. As in pigs, this can lead to the condemnation of birds at slaughter and it is reported that birds with the disease suffer listlessness and are generally unproductive. *Mycobacterium avium* causes tuberculosis in poultry and is the source of tuberculosis infection in pigs and has also been reported to cause tuberculosis in humans (Thoen, 1997).

Summary for tuberculosis

Tuberculosis was a very important zoonosis in European countries during the 19th century. However, eradication campaigns in these countries have reduced the prevalence of this disease to very low levels. The main costs in these industrialized countries now relate to testing of animals and also culling of wildlife reservoirs. In developing countries, prevalences are generally low, but the importance of the disease particularly in African countries may be increasing due to a high percentage of the human population having AIDS and being more susceptible to tuberculosis infections. Control and eradication campaigns of tuberculosis can rarely be justified on the basis of production losses.

Salmonella

Salmonella is not one disease or one causal agent. This is a key point in the economics of salmonella, because what is conjured up by this word is food-borne diseases. However, some *Salmonella* subspecies such as *S. pullorum* rarely cause public health problems and are specific to one species and in this case cause serious losses in poultry production systems. Other *Salmonella* such as *S. typhimurium* can affect a number of different species and is a serious threat to human health. Therefore, two issues are identified in this section:

- the production losses caused by *Salmonella* species; and
- costs to human health associated with the contamination of food products with *Salmonella* species.

It appears that in most situations the former has reduced in importance as veterinarians and producers have successfully controlled many of the *Salmonella* that cause serious losses. However, attention has focused on the public health issues, with an increasing number of human cases of salmonellosis, which occurs in countries with high incomes and expensive medical services.

The following two sections will outline some of the critical issues when assessing the economic impact of salmonella on livestock.

Production losses or problems due to salmonella

The production losses or problems due to salmonella can be divided into:

- Abortions in large and small ruminants, but the percentage of abortions caused by *Salmonella* species is normally low.
- Diarrhoea-associated mortality of the young animals of large and small ruminants and pigs. An outbreak kills young animals and requires treatment of those sick; however, survivors, although they lose weight, usually regain this weight at a later stage. Pigs do not appear to be very susceptible and the production losses in this species are probably very low.
- Losses of young chicks and poults.
- Lower egg production.
- In the case of *S. pullorum* and *S. gallinarum* in hens and *S. arizona* in turkeys, adult mortality.

Costs associated with these disease problems are:

- treatment of sick animals;
- destocking of farms;

- higher feed costs due to poor feed conversion;
- testing of breeding flocks for the presence of *S. pullorum* and *S. gallinarum*.

The following information is available in the literature on production losses reported due to salmonellosis in large and small ruminants, pigs and poultry:

- Bilbao and Spath (1997) studied the losses due to salmonellosis in dairy calves in Argentina. They reported a morbidity rate of 6.8% and mortality rate of 3.4%. Losses for calves that died were US$77 for male calves and US$127 for female calves. In animals that survived, the losses in terms of weight loss were estimated to be US$7.70. In addition, there were costs of treatment that totalled to US$3.36 per sick calf. The major proportion of the costs was dead calves and the authors suggest that early treatment would help to reduce the economic impact of this disease.
- Sharp and Kay (1988) estimated that an outbreak of *S. typhimurium* in a group of 48 calves reduced the gross margin per calf from £31.95 to £10.95. They reported that the outbreak killed eight calves and required that 17 were treated. The affected calves that survived had a lower body weight at weaning but had no difference in weight at 168 days.
- Peters (1985) reported an outbreak of salmonellosis in calves due to *S. dublin*. There were morbidity of 62% and mortality of 13.5%. The affected calves were treated and found to have a lower weight at between 77 and 118 days of age, but no difference in weight at 477 days of age. It was estimated that the outbreak cost £25.36 per surviving calf and 70% of these losses were due to the loss of dead calves.
- Schulz et al. (1975) found that *S. dublin* caused between 2.7% and 3.7% of abortions in two regions in Germany and was diagnosed in between 18% and 19% of post-mortem examinations. The prevalence of this pathogen in calves was between 7.65% and 11.7% and 1.17% in adult animals. Between 1965 and 1973,

they believed that 1161 cattle died from salmonellosis and of these a third were between 5 and 8 weeks old.

- Froyd and McWilliam (1975) report that *Fasciola*-infected herds have increased prevalence of *Salmonella* carriers, increasing the losses caused by this parasite.
- In the USA, Blackburn *et al.* (1980) describe the spread of *S. dublin* and raise concerns about the economic impact of the spread of this bacterium.
- Tenk *et al.* (2000) in an experiment with vaccination against *S. enteritidis* found that, after vaccination, salmonella-associated losses and condemnations were reduced to one-third of the level observed before vaccination, the hatching performance improved, the quality of the day-old poults was better and performance figures were higher.
- Anderson (1992) reports that a *S. pullorum* outbreak in five states of the USA during 1990 and 1991 caused more than a million dollars worth of losses.
- Luthgen (1979) reported an outbreak of *S. pullorum* in a laying flock in Germany. The outbreak initially reduced egg production by a half and then killed half the flock. The disease was controlled by the destruction of the remaining birds.
- Lowry *et al.* (1999) state that *S. arizonae* and *S. gallinarum* are important in poultry production because of the losses they cause in young poultry during the first week after hatching.
- Minev *et al.* (1983) describe an outbreak of fowl typhoid (*S. gallinarum*) in which the major cost was the closure of the hatchery for 3 months and the other costs related to lost production, death and slaughter of infected birds.
- In Egypt, Shahata *et al.* (1983) report the impact of duck flocks infected with *S. typhimurium, S. enteritidis, S. paratyphi* C and *S. thompson*. In these flocks, there was a 66% fertility rate, 52.3% hatchability rate and a mortality rate of newly hatched ducklings of 7.8%.
- Ding ChangChun and Li LiHu (1998) suggest than one of the causes of rectal prolapse, which is a major cause of bird mortality in laying hens, is *Salmonella*.

- In Denmark, Bisgaard *et al.* (1981) observed that compulsory salmonella control had reduced the percentage of condemnations due to arthritis in ducks from 0.4% to 0.12%. They estimate that losses due to this type of condemnation between 1959 and 1968 were 207,579 Danish crowns, but these losses were only a third of the sum for the next 10 years which corresponds to the salmonella control programme.
- Curtin (1984) estimated that the production losses due to salmonella disease in the Canadian poultry industry were US$2.8 million a year.

Food-borne problems

This section is divided into four parts in an attempt to separate some of the issues with regard to the costs of salmonella and its control. These are:

- animal feed;
- animal carriers and contamination of food products during the production phase;
- food processing;
- impact of salmonellosis in humans.

Food for animals

One of the potential sources of infection of animals with *Salmonella* is from food. Concerns have been voiced about the:

- use of poultry litter in the feeding of large and small ruminants;
- use of poultry litter as fertilizer for pastures; and
- susceptibility of certain foodstuffs to *Salmonella* contamination.

Nursey (1997) suggests that a possible control of *Salmonella* food contamination is to add organic acids to foodstuffs. This lowers the pH and reduces the risk of *Salmonella* contamination in feed, but the author does not provide information on cost or the effectiveness of this measure.

Carriers

Sero-surveys and tests for positive animals in slaughterhouses would suggest that salmonella

is at low prevalence in large and small ruminants and in pigs. In poultry, the prevalence
ranges depending on the region. The following
information was collected on animal carriers
and products contaminated with *Salmonella*:

- Sawicka-Wrzosek *et al.* (1997) report
  approximately 6% prevalence of salmonella in pigs and very low prevalences in
  cattle and sheep.
- In Papua New Guinea, Caley (1972) found
  that pigs in rural systems had a salmonella
  prevalence of 9%, whereas those in intensive piggeries had a prevalence of 54%.
- In Iran, Tadjbakhch *et al.* (1992) found that
  2.6% of sheep slaughtered were *Salmonella*
  carriers. Bernardo and Machado (1990)
  found much higher levels of infection in
  slaughtered animals in Portugal, with
  20.3% of the cattle, 7.3% of the sheep, and
  25.4% of the pigs being reported to have
  Salmonella infections.
- Otaru *et al.* (1990) reported low prevalences of *Salmonella* carrier status in cattle
  (1.7%) and goats (4.8%) in Tanzania.
- The Scottish Centre for Infection and
  Environmental Health (1997) reported
  a 21% increase in the number of reports
  of salmonella in animals between 1996
  and 1997.
- Radkowski (2001) did not find *Salmonella*
  on the shells of or inside the eggs sold in
  a market in Poland.
- In Bangladesh, Ali *et al.* (1987) found that
  4.3% of duck eggs were infected with
  Salmonella, but none of the hen eggs they
  tested were infected.
- An analysis of screening for *S. enteritidis* in
  laying hens reduced the proportion of contaminated eggs by 43.7% with one screen
  and 65.4% with two screenings (Ament
  et al., 1993). The returns on this process are
  dependent on the costs of the screening but
  the analysis indicates that there are positive returns to culling of infected flocks.
- Leslie (1996) modelled *S. enteritidis* in
  laying flocks and predicted that between
  0.42% and 2.24% of eggs could be infected
  with this pathogen.
- Little and de Louvois (1999) did not find
  Salmonella in unpasteurized goat and
  sheep milk in the UK.

- Wray (1985) documents the changing of
  Salmonella isolates in England and Wales
  between 1975 and 1983. The serotypes
  over this period changed in the different
  species.

Food processing

Food processing has been found to be important in the dissemination of contamination
and also in the multiplication of *Salmonella*.
The following information has been collected
on this aspect of salmonellosis:

- Swanenburg *et al.* (2001) indicated that a
  major source of contamination of pigs
  with *Salmonella* is during the waiting to
  be slaughtered in the lairage of abattoirs.
- Davies *et al.* (1999) found that 7.0% of
  carcasses had *Salmonella* contamination
  and 11.6% of the gut contents were contaminated. However, these authors found
  that pigs that were held overnight before
  slaughtering had lower levels of contamination than pigs that were held for 2 or
  3h before slaughter.
- Carraminana *et al.* (1994) found that
  Salmonella contamination increased significantly after the chlorinated baths of
  the processed birds.
- Yule *et al.* (1988) analysed the returns to
  irradiation of poultry meat to eliminate
  salmonellosis risks. They found that this
  change in food processing had positive
  returns, but they add a word of caution
  about the assumptions made on the costs
  of unreported salmonellosis cases.
- Whiting and Buchanan (1997) developed
  a risk assessment model for the pasteurization of liquid eggs, which showed that
  this form of treatment was adequate to
  protect consumers. However, if badly
  managed this treatment method can produce a hazardous product.
- In an analysis of the cost and benefits of
  banning the sale of unpasteurized milk
  in Scotland, it was found that the returns
  were high when based on an outbreak of
  human salmonellosis due to the consumption of unpasteurized milk. The
  analysis took account of the costs of
  investment of pasteurization equipment,

compared to the costs of treating sick people for salmonellosis and the loss of time and life. Even under the most pessimistic assumptions this change in milk processing proved positive.

- Nauta *et al.* (2000) developed a model to test strategies for reducing salmonella problems in the poultry meat chains in Holland.
- Caswell (1991) presents an outline of how to make an economic assessment of food-borne pathogens with an analysis of the control of salmonella in poultry in Canada.

Impact of salmonellosis in the human population

If a food product contaminated with a pathogenic *Salmonella* reaches a consumer, then the consequences at best can be diarrhoea, at worst hospitalization and possibly death. The concern about food-borne diseases and in particular *Salmonella*-contaminated products has increased since the late 1980s to a point where some governments are passing laws banning the consumption of animals infected with *Salmonella* species that are non-pathogenic to humans (Valheim and Hofshagen, 1998). Other reactions have been more understandable, in that plans have been put in place to reduce prevalence of disease in animals and improve food processing measures. However, these actions have costs and impacts in the livestock sector. The following information has been collected on this aspect of salmonella:

- Bender and Ebel (1992) analysed the impact of *S. enteritidis* in poultry firms. They found that the presence of this pathogen could reduce income by a half, if the firm was not allowed to sell to the table egg market. The chapters explore options of depopulating within the regulations that applied at that time.
- Sander (1993) reports an increasing rate of *Salmonella* infections in humans between 1970 and 1990 with a decrease in *S. typhimurium*-related infections and an increase in *S. enteritidis* infections. The author states that chicken and eggs are a frequent source of *Salmonella* infections in humans.

- Brede (1992) found that numbers of human *Salmonella* infections between 1989 and 1991 were increasing rapidly and suggest that the reasons are low hygienic quality of animal feeds, intensive rearing systems and poor food preparation.
- Cohen and Tauxe (1986) report that in the USA there are 40,000 cases of salmonellosis, with 500 deaths each year. The financial costs associated with this food-borne disease problem are estimated to be US$50 million.
- In Canada, Curtin (1984) estimated that the annual losses due to salmonellosis in humans were US$84 million/year, of which US$21 million were due to the consumption of contaminated poultry products. The study then examines the costs of control of this disease by examining the poultry sector, from the feed manufacturers through to the processing of poultry products in the home. It looks at costs of education at the household level.
- Todd (1992) analysed data between 1975 and 1984 in Canada and found that on average there were 5.6 deaths/year caused by food-borne disease and that salmonella was one of the main causes of these problems. The author states that most of the problems came from food service establishments.
- Steinbach and Hartung (1999) found that, in 1996 and 1997, 20% of human salmonellosis originated from pigs in Germany.
- In Holland, Bunte *et al.* (2001) state that there are 20,000 human salmonellosis cases each year, costing between 1.8 and 5.6 million Dutch florins/year.
- Buzby *et al.* (1998) examined the issue of food safety in a different manner from other researchers. They compared estimates of the costs of illness in terms of loss of days' work, cost of treatment and suffering, with experiments to estimate willingness to pay for a safe food product.
- Noordhuizen and Frankena (1994) identify that *S. enteritidis* is a major concern in poultry, with prevalence levels in pigs and veal calves being low. They call for concerted efforts of control and prevention in response to the fears for public health.

- Ortenberg (1998) writes that the aim of the salmonella programme in Sweden is to ensure that all food is free from *Salmonella* contamination.
- Laegaard and Hedetoft (1999) calculated that in Denmark the voluntary salmonella control programme was more expensive and had less impact than the government programme that began in 1996.
- Branscheid (1993) reports that salmonella scares have had an impact on the consumption of eggs in Germany, where consumption has fallen. However, poultry meat consumption has increased and there are a range of other factors associated with the fall in egg consumption such as concerns about cholesterol levels.
- Borger (1985) suggests that measures should be taken to reduce the risks of food being contaminated by pathogenic *Salmonella*, but these measures should be assessed using cost–benefit analysis techniques.
- Lindgren *et al.* (1980) evaluated the Swedish salmonella control campaign and found that it had been effective in reducing the number of outbreaks reported, but the costs had increased from 1.655 million Kr in 1974 to 6.35 million Kr in 1978. The authors do not mention if these prices have been adjusted for inflation, which was high during this period in Europe.

Summary and general impact of salmonellosis

In general, the *Salmonella* species cause a range of disease problems in livestock. In large and small ruminants they are responsible for a small percentage of abortions and can also cause high rates of mortality in young animals. In pigs, the impact of salmonella on production is less pronounced. However, in poultry a number of *Salmonella* subspecies cause specific disease problems such as pullorum disease and fowl typhoid. It is in poultry that the major impact on production is found with salmonella.

In addition to production losses, the last 30 years have seen an ever-increasing interest in the impact of salmonella due to food-borne disease. The impact of human salmonellosis is far greater than the production losses, because many of the officially reported cases occur in the developed countries where salaries and medical costs are high. This has prompted much research into how to reduce risks of food poisoning through control and eradication campaigns at farm level, improved food processing and education campaigns for households. Again the most important group of livestock in human salmonellosis is poultry.

Finally, this section concludes with information from Roberts (1988), who quotes that the estimated costs of *Salmonella* infections in the USA in 1987 were US$1000 million in terms of medical costs and productivity losses. However, according to this author the cost estimates should also include:

- pain and suffering, lost leisure time and chronic disease costs;
- reduced feed efficiency at farm level;
- reduced weight gain at farm level;
- deaths because of chronic salmonellosis at farm level;
- costs of food safety regulatory programmes;
- costs to the industry for product recalls; and
- plant closures due to food-borne salmonellosis outbreaks.

Obviously, this list provides ample justification, particularly in the industrialized countries, to dedicate resources to reduce the economic impact of salmonella.

Brucellosis

Brucellosis is a disease that affects humans, large and small ruminants and pigs. It is an important reproductive disease causing abortions in the last third of pregnancy. The main losses are:

- abortions;
- loss of milk production;
- weak calves.

It is spread from livestock to humans by the consumption of untreated milk or milk products.

Control costs include:

- diagnostic tests;
- vaccination;
- the slaughter of positive animals, which can be high where there are large differences between the value of replacements and the meat value of the animal;
- incentives to encourage farmers to eradicate brucellosis at herd level.

Other costs include:

- public health costs;
- trade issues.

Brucellosis in cattle has been controlled and in many countries eradicated in large and long campaigns since the late 1970s. These countries are the industrialized or developed countries, which have the majority of the intensive dairy systems of the world. The importance of the disease in terms of production losses in cattle has therefore reduced, as have the investments in control. Attention has changed to maintaining free status and controlling trade of live animals to stop reinfection.

In other regions of the world brucellosis in cattle is usually seen at low prevalences. Although still capable of causing losses in terms of production, efforts to eradicate brucellosis often fail due to a lack of government resources and a lack of incentive at farm level.

Brucellosis in sheep and goats is of importance again because of production losses, but also because these species are important in the production of soft cheeses from unpasteurized milk. Therefore, the disease in small ruminants has a considerable public health risk. However, most information on brucellosis in sheep and goats seems to indicate that it is at low prevalences. Please note that further details of brucellosis in small ruminants are found in the reproductive diseases of small ruminants in Chapter 18 (this volume).

Brucellosis in pigs also carries a public health risk and causes losses in production. Prevalence levels appear to be higher than in cattle, but information on the economic impact of this disease in pigs was not found in this review.

Information available

This section is divided into:

- information on the prevalence of brucellosis in different regions of the world and different species;
- production losses caused by brucellosis;
- general study on brucellosis including epidemiology and economics of the disease;
- public health impact of brucellosis;
- cost–benefit analyses of control campaigns.

Prevalence

The following information was found on prevalence of brucellosis in different species:

- In the Calabria region of Italy, Casalinuovo *et al.* (1996) found animal prevalence in cattle, sheep and goats to be 2.4%, 4.2% and 12.9%, respectively.
- In Egypt, Atallah and El-Kak (1998) state that brucellosis prevalence was 1.17% in cattle and 0.79% in buffaloes and losses due to condemnation of animals due to brucellosis were 1529 Egyptian pounds sterling.
- In Bihar, India, brucellosis prevalence in pigs varied between 10.5% and 4% (Choudhary *et al.*, 1983).
- Nordesjo (1999) found low prevalence levels in dairy cows (5%) in the peri-urban areas of Hanoi, Vietnam.
- Priadi *et al.* (1985) found that in Indonesia the brucellosis prevalence in pigs was 15%, in cattle 2% and sheep and goats were not reported with the disease.
- Adesiyun and Cazabon (1996) report that no animals slaughtered at the Trinidad slaughterhouse were positive for brucellosis.
- A study in the Mexicali valley, Mexico, found that in cattle there was an animal and herd prevalence for brucellosis of 2.54% and 26% (Salman *et al.*, 1984). The authors state the disease was not a problem in sheep or goats.
- Navarrete (1979) reported a prevalence of 10% in pigs found in the Cordoba region of Colombia.

Production losses

The following information was found on production losses due to brucellosis:

- Ajogi *et al.* (1998) estimated brucellosis losses of 12.6 million naira in the grazing reserves of Wase and Wawa-Zange of Nigeria. The prevalence of brucellosis was between 12% and 7% in a cattle population of 18,222.
- In Kirghizia, Zhunushov and Kim (1991) state that a brucellosis vaccination campaign had reduced losses due to this disease considerably.
- Camus and Landais (1981) estimated that herds of cattle in the Ivory Coast with brucellosis and trypanosomiasis incurred a 6% reduction in profits.

General studies that cover the epidemiology and economics of brucellosis

Pfeiffer (1986) carried out a study of brucellosis in Cordoba province of Colombia. He reports low individual prevalence levels of brucellosis (3.3%) in cattle and that the impact of this disease on fertility was minimal, but caused lactations of infected animals to be shorter. His research suggests that the climate and extensive management systems found in Cordoba limit the spread of brucellosis, and he concludes that this disease is not economically important in this region of Colombia and the possibilities of eradicating it are small.

Public health impact

The following information was found on the public health impact of brucellosis:

- Vito *et al.* (1997) report that a human outbreak in 1995 of brucellosis created high levels of costs in terms of treatment and stress for the families concerned.
- Martinez *et al.* (1977) report that pig farmers are more at risk of contracting brucellosis than cattle farmers and that slaughterhouse workers involved with pigs had higher brucellosis prevalence than the general population.

Cost–benefit analysis studies

A number of studies on the cost and benefits of the control of brucellosis were carried out at the time of large eradication campaigns in Europe, North America and other developed countries. In addition, some studies have been done on control at more local levels. The following information was found on this subject:

- One of the most thorough studies of brucellosis control was done by Hugh-Jones *et al.* (1975) on the eradication of bovine brucellosis in England and Wales. This study identifies the main production losses due to brucellosis and also examines the impact of the control campaign in terms of markets for replacements, meat and milk. Finally, it examines through a process of sensitivity analysis the farm-level incentives for becoming brucellosis-free in different sizes of dairy and beef herds at different prevalence levels.
- Caporale *et al.* (1980) report that the prevalence of bovine brucellosis in Italy fell from 1.9% in 1965 to 0.2% in the 2.8 million cattle tested in 1978. The estimated gross benefits were 21,400 million Italian lire. These authors also found that the prevalence of ovine and caprine brucellosis fell from 5.5% in 1968 to 3.7% in 1978 with estimated gross benefits of 2600 million Italian lire. In a later study, the same authors (Ghilardi *et al.*, 1981) estimated that the costs of the brucellosis control campaigns was 3550 million Italian lire for bovine brucellosis and 724 million Italian lire for brucellosis in sheep and goats.
- Bernues *et al.* (1997) found that the bovine brucellosis campaign in the Spanish Central Pyrenees between 1981 and 1993 has been economically efficient.
- Aller (1975) estimated that the annual costs of brucellosis in Spain were US$150 million.
- Amosson (1984) analysed the brucellosis programmes in the USA. The author reports that in 1976 losses due to brucellosis were estimated to be 65 million lb of beef and 35 million lb of milk. Amosson also states that US$75 million

was spent on the control of the disease. Modelling work showed that all strategies for control were profitable (Amosson et al., 1981) and that the most cost-effective programmes were the adjacent herd testing programmes followed by eradication and vaccination programmes.

- Amosson et al. (1983) report positive returns to further reductions in the prevalence of brucellosis in cattle even though the levels at that time were low. The winners of the reduction were consumers.
- Wyble and Huffman (1987) in a study of brucellosis economics of Louisiana beef cattle herds reached the following conclusions: (i) brucellosis infection causes substantial losses in income to the individual cattleman, to the beef industry and to the state; (ii) in the representative herd situations, losses due to brucellosis generally exceed costs of an intensive eradication programme, making the control programme an economically sound option; (iii) the average Louisiana beef herd would benefit from an effective brucellosis prevention programme; (iv) official certification of a herd as 'brucellosis-free' can, and often does, add value to that herd; (v) complete herd depopulation may be the most economic solution to eradicating brucellosis in small, heavily infected herds.
- O'Riordan (1980) analysed the Canadian brucellosis eradication programme and alternative strategies of control. The author found that all strategies gave positive returns.
- In New Zealand, Shepherd et al. (1980) found that because of the need to protect the export market brucellosis eradication campaign gave a positive return even without considering the losses in production caused by the disease.
- In Chad and Cameroon, Domenech et al. (1982) analysed the losses due to brucellosis in cattle herds and also the benefits of control. Their results indicate that control with vaccination was potentially profitable.

Summary for brucellosis

Brucellosis is a disease that was of great economic importance in the cattle systems of the developed countries. This importance attracted eradication programmes that involved huge public and private investments, which were justified in terms of production losses and public health costs caused by this disease. It is argued that the importance of this disease with the successful end to a majority of these campaigns has reduced even though the disease is still found in other regions of the world and in other species. However, it remains important in terms of trade.

Trypanosomiasis

In 1974, Finelle (1974) stated that, due to a lack of accurate data on the economic importance of African trypanosomiasis, FAO planned to carry out surveys to provide information that would give government and international agencies guidelines on resource spending on this disease. Since that time, there have been very extensive studies on the economics of trypanosomiasis on this continent.

Trypanosomiasis is a disease that affects a range of species (see Fig. 16.1) and its impact is different in different regions of the world. The main interest in this disease has been Africa, which has all the trypanosome protozoas, including the trypanosomes that cause sleeping sickness. Many projects have been financed to control this disease through the control of the main vector, the tsetse fly. The main issues for trypanosomiasis in Africa are:

- losses due to mortality and morbidity mainly in cattle, but also in other species;
- public health issues as cattle can harbour the trypanosome that causes sleeping sickness and can also move it from one place to another;
- poor land use because of the presence of tsetse fly and trypanosomes;
- costs of control;
- costs of treatment;
- in many areas, limitations on breed adoption because of the presence of trypanosomiasis.

In other regions of the world, the situation is very different, because of the absence of the tsetse fly and because not all the trypanosomes are found in these regions. In Asia, the main trypanosome is *Trypanosoma evansi* which causes problems:

- mainly with working buffalo; and
- has also been identified as a major constraint in the adoption of improved breeds.

In Latin America, the main trypanosome is *T. vivax*, which is spread by cattle movement and biting flies. The form of trypanosomiasis that this trypanosome produces does not appear as acute as that found in Africa, which means that it debilitates the animals but generally does not kill them quickly. This is a convenient method of propagating the disease. The main issues in Latin America are:

- Losses in production particularly in the tropical grasslands where biting flies are found.
- Costs of treatment.
- Again it is a constraint in the adoption of improved breeds.

- Chagas disease in South America can be carried by domestic pets, and poultry also seem to have a role in maintaining the vector for this disease.

The different causal agents of trypanosomiasis are shown in Fig. 16.1.

There is a range of control options for trypanosomiasis which involve either the control of the vector or the disease (Fig. 16.2).

In Africa, Kristjanson *et al.* (1999) estimated that tsetse-free areas produce 83% more milk and 97% more meat than tsetse-infested areas. This implied that losses in animal production were approximately US$338 million/year. Swallow (2000) also estimated that a further US$800–1500 million are lost in agricultural production. Finally, Geerts and Holmes (1998) estimated that 35 million doses of trypanocidal drugs are used each year, with an estimated cost of US$35 million.

These economic impacts can also be seen at field level. Kamara Mwanga (1996) reported that willingness of communities to be involved in tsetse control was high and consequently backed up by financial and labour

Main species	Main vector	Species affected		Impact
AFRICA				Mortality and morbidity
T. congolense		Cattle	Camels	Major constraint on land use
T. vivax	Tsetse	Sheep	Horses	Reservoir of sleeping sickness
T. brucei		Goats		
		Pigs	Human	Major constraint in the adoption of improved breeds
ASIA, LATIN AMERICA and AFRICA				
T. evansi		Cattle	Camels	Mortality and morbidity
	Biting flies	Sheep	Horses	
T. vivax		Goats	Buffalo	Major constraint in the adoption of improved breeds
		Pigs		

Fig. 16.1. Species and geographical areas affected by trypanosomiasis. (From Rushton *et al.*, 2001.)

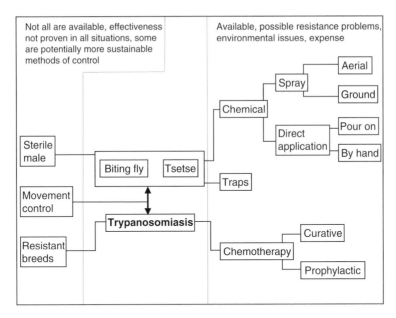

Fig. 16.2. Possible methods of control for tsetse, biting flies and trypanosomiasis. (From Rushton *et al.*, 2001.)

contributions. Barrett (1994), however, comments that this interest is usually strongest in areas with sleeping sickness.

Economic analysis of the control for trypanosomiasis has been presented by various authors for different parts of Africa:

- Putt *et al.* (1980) and Shaw (1986) for Nigeria;
- Barrett (1994, 1997) for Zimbabwe;
- Itty (1992) for eastern and southern Africa.

Budd (1999) has summarized some of this information in an assessment of research carried out on tsetse and trypanosomiasis (see Table 16.2). He states that 260 million people are believed to live in zones with the risk of animal and human trypanosomiasis in Africa. Of that population, 55 million are at risk from sleeping sickness, which kills 55,000 people/year.

Budd (1999) reports that worldwide US$500 million has been spent on trypanosomiasis research and control with an estimated return of US$300 million.

Table 16.2. International research programme for tsetse and trypanosomiasis. (From Budd, 1999.)

Cost/benefit to user	Larger projects 1:1.4 to 1:2.6
	Smaller projects 1:1.7 to 1:2.4
Breadth of benefit	260 million people living in the tropics of Africa
Global net benefit	US$1.5–3.0 billion/year
Cost/benefit of research programme	Net research cost basis – 1:75 to 1:150
	Gross research cost basis – 1:30 to 1:60
Sustainability	Dependent on maintaining tsetse-free status in the long term
Socio-economic factors	Initial beneficiaries are cattle owners
	Subsequent beneficiaries are poorer farmers and all consumers

Information available

The following information was collected and is divided into sections on Africa, Asia, South America and the role of poultry in Chagas disease.

Africa: trypanosomiasis and tsetse

- Kristjanson *et al.* (1999) estimated that trypanosomiasis costs livestock producers and consumers US$1340 million a year; this estimate did not include losses of manure and traction power. The authors estimated that the returns to a trypanosomiasis vaccine had a benefit/cost ratio (BCR) of 34.
- Itty (1992) reports that trypanosomiasis is a major constraint on the development of livestock and mixed farming systems in Africa. The author performed cost–benefit analyses on these diseases in six different countries. The analysis showed that:
  - In Ethiopia and Kenya, susceptible East African zebu cattle are produced, with the help of trypanocidal drugs, but there are major constraints.
  - In Ethiopia, vector control would be more profitable than drugs.
  - In Kenya, the share contract between cattle owner and keeper is a financial constraint to using drugs to control trypanosomiasis in the susceptible East African zebu found in this country.
  - The analysis of keeping trypano-tolerant cattle in Gambia and Côte d'Ivoire, a traditional form of cattle keeping in these countries, is less clear and depends on various social and economic constraints.
  - The introduction of trypano-tolerant cattle in Togo and Zaire showed limited benefits, because fresh milk is not consumed in these countries. However, the social benefits are attractive in both cases.
- A study in Gambia found that in cows infected with *T. congolense* and *T. vivax* the quantity of milk take from the animals was reduced by 25% compared with animals not infected (Agyemang *et al.*, 1990). The authors report that the average quantity of milk per day extracted during a 6-month period was 26% higher in the controls than in infected cows, and that the growth rate of calves suckling infected and control cows was similar.
- A study by Brandl (1988) on the economics of trypanosomiasis control in Africa found that stocking density and maximum carrying capacity were important factors determining the benefits of control. The author states that in areas of 'low challenge', the application of trypanocides is to be given preference over tsetse control and that although the use of sterile males can be organized economically, given certain conditions, it is always less profitable than the aerial application of insecticides with helicopters and, in particular, the use of insecticide-impregnated traps.
- Jordan (1986) identifies three categories of information required to analyse trypanosomiasis control in Africa: (i) livestock losses from mortality and morbidity and potential loss to rural development by preventing the keeping of trypanosomiasis-susceptible breeds of livestock; (ii) the cost of control measures applied; and (iii) quantified benefits that result from the control or eradication of the disease.
- Mortelmans (1984) estimates that without trypanosomiasis in rural Africa, the region would have 3–5 times more livestock.
- A Kenyan study estimated that the loss due to trypanosomiasis was K Sh 8256/ km^2 at a stocking rate of 14.2 tropical livestock units (1 TLSU = 250 kg)/km^2 (Wilson *et al.*, 1983).
- Putt and Shaw (1983) presented an analysis of the control of trypanosomiasis in Nigeria and they report that, in spite of the severity of the assumptions used in their analysis, the high discount rate employed and the limited number of benefits quantified, the results of the economic analysis demonstrate the extreme profitability at both the national and local levels. However, the authors state that the benefits might be less in other countries.

- A study of trypanosomiasis in goats found that the losses in Kenyan shillings per 'tropical livestock unit' over a 6-month study period were 198.07 for the East African goats, 501.95 for the Galla × East African goats and 785.42 for the Toggenburg × East African goats (Kanyari *et al.*, 1983). The authors report that the benefit/cost ratio by using Samorin at the dose rate of 0.5 mg/kg body weight was 1:7.3, 1:18.52 and 1:28.94 for the three goat breeds, respectively.
- Habtemariam *et al.* (1983) developed a model to assess the impact of trypanosomiasis in south-east Ethiopia and the options for control. The control strategies considered were manual vegetation clearing, game elimination, aerial insecticidal spraying coupled with settlement, use of sterile male *Glossina*, avoidance of tsetse-infested areas, increasing the resistance of the cattle population, therapy and combinations of the above methods. The authors assumed that the endemic prevalence of trypanosomiasis was 27.3% and estimated the impact over a 10-year period. The combined use of vegetation clearing, insecticides, therapy and settlement (or resettlement) was the most effective and feasible method of trypanosomiasis control for the simulated situation. A cost–benefit analysis of trypanosomiasis control programmes for an area of 1500 km^2 in south-west Ethiopia, for a project span of 15 years at a discount rate of 10%, was conducted to determine cost-effective and benefit-maximizing alternatives. The trypanosomiasis control methods considered were: (i) reduction of tsetse flies by use of insecticides sprayed from knapsacks; (ii) game reduction; and (iii) no control programme. The cost–benefit analysis using net present values (NPV) and BCR as decision criteria of project feasibility and efficiency indicated that insecticide application was preferable to game reduction. Estimates of present value costs were E$630.17/km^2/year while the present value benefits were E$720.24/km^2/year. The BCR was 1.14 and NPV of the project was E$2.03 million.

- Shaw and Kamate (1982) estimated that the losses due to trypanosomiasis in an area of south-west Mali would be between MF 392,933,000 and MF 577,367,000, with an average loss per infected animal of about MF 19,500 (MF = Mali francs). The authors use these projected losses to carry out a cost–benefit analysis of various control strategies. Only one strategy, systematic treatment plus diagnostic support, had a positive net value at both high and low benefit levels. They also found that prophylaxis treatment of work oxen and treatment of other cattle, which was the policy at the time, were economically feasible if fully implemented. However, no other strategies proved profitable.

Asia (T. evansi)

- In Indonesia, Prastywati Sukanto (1998) reports that trypanosomiasis caused by *T. evansi* is the most important disease in the country and the major limiting factor in the adoption of higher-yielding exotic breeds.

South America (T. vivax)

- Otte *et al.* (1994) studied *T. vivax* in Colombia. They report that clinical trypanosomiasis is rare in the low-lying swampy areas of the country, but that herds with *T. vivax* infections had calves with subclinical symptoms. These animals had a temporary depression of packed cell volume as well as a reduction in growth rate, and there was no evidence of compensatory growth at a later stage.

Role of poultry in Chagas disease (T. cruzi)

Poultry are reported to be important in the maintenance of the insect *Triatoma infestans* (Gurtler *et al.*, 1998, 1999a,b; Cecere *et al.*, 1999; Pires *et al.*, 1999) in Latin America, which transmits *T. cruzi*, which causes Chagas disease in humans. However, *T. cruzi* cannot multiply and maintain itself in poultry (Minter-Goedbloed and Croon, 1981), indicating that its role in the transmission of this important zoonosis is through the maintenance of the vector. Other trypanosomes have been reported from other bird species, but their importance as an economic disease is minimal (Springer, 1997).

Bluetongue

Bluetongue is a disease that can affect large and small ruminants and pigs. In many countries, it is present without clinical outbreaks; however, outbreaks may occur when climate changes encourage insect vectors of the disease. It is endemic in many tropical regions of the world and clinical symptoms are rare in indigenous animals, but are a problem for the introduction of exotic animals. Bluetongue is an important trade disease for fear that countries without the disease may import it and create outbreaks in naive susceptible populations. Australia, which is a country with the disease, has free areas which are protected and monitored to ensure that it can export live animals and semen. Therefore, this disease has a considerable economic impact in terms of:

- restricting trade of live animals; and
- adoption of exotic animals in countries which have endemic bluetongue.

It causes minor losses in endemic areas due to:

- reproductive problems;
- mortality in situations where clinical symptoms occur.

Information available

This section is divided into general information, Europe, North America, Africa, Central America and the Caribbean and Australia.

General information

- Alexander et al. (1996) report that much research has provided strong and growing support for the concept that bluetongue disease is an endemic disease of the tropical regions where it is sustained by an active population of Culicoides vectors and suitable mammalian hosts. There are periodic outbreaks of bluetongue adja-

cent to the tropics. Countries with large populations of Merino sheep and seasonal incursions of competent Culicoides vectors appear to be most at risk, although other breeds can become seriously affected on occasion without any apparent reason. The authors conclude that recent advances in the knowledge of bluetongue have provided a sound basis for a reassessment of the protocols applied by many countries against bluetongue. It now seems that the use of restrictive protocols has disadvantaged access to improved ruminant genetic material.

Europe

- Taylor (1987) reports that bluetongue disease is uncommon in Europe, but the sheep industries of the European Economic Community contain many susceptible breeds and much damage might result from the entry of this disease.
- Ertan and Nazlioglu (1981) estimate that the losses due to bluetongue between 1977 and 1979 were 10.5 million Turkish lire.

North America

- Osburn et al. (1986) estimated that the annual cost of bluetongue infection in the San Joaquin Valley of California was US$5.75 million/year. The cattle population in this area was 350,000.
- A study in the state of Mississippi, USA, estimated that the losses due to bluetongue were US$6 million/year (Metcalf et al., 1980).

Africa

- Barnard et al. (1998) report outbreaks of an unusual disease in December 1995 to March 1996 and the early summer of 1997 in South Africa. Cattle were affected and the pattern of morbidity followed that of a previous outbreak of the disease in 1932–1933. Clinical signs were similar to those of infection with bluetongue virus and epizootic haemorrhagic disease of deer. One dairy herd showed a 42% drop in milk production. Bluetongue virus was isolated.

Central America and the Caribbean

- In Central America and the Caribbean, Oviedo *et al.* (1992) report that although bluetongue (BLU) viruses are enzootic, the direct economic losses are low compared with the losses due to the restrictions imposed on international trade of ruminants in this zone, which depends heavily on livestock production.

Australia

- Geering (1985) states that bluetongue virus has been isolated but appears to cause no clinical disease in Australia.

Echinococcosis/hydatidosis

Hydatidosis is a disease that affects large and small ruminants, pigs and humans. The disease is of importance because infections in humans cause cancer-like symptoms mainly in the liver and lungs. The losses due to hydatidosis are:

- processing losses:
  - condemnations of carcasses.
- public health concerns:
  - costs of treatment;
  - losses in human productivity;
  - mortality.

There exists much information on the prevalence of this disease in different parts of the world. It is generally a major problem in extensive sheep systems that are managed with the use of dogs. Readers interested in the economics of this disease are recommended to read the economic assessment of echinococcosis in Tunisia by Majorowski *et al.* (2001). These authors present a methodology for estimating losses due to this disease and calculate that in Tunisia hydatidosis causes losses of between US$10 and US$19 million each year.

Rabies

Rabies can affect large and small ruminants, pigs and humans. It is of great importance in urban areas of many cities where dogs maintain the disease and occasionally transmit it to humans. In terms of livestock disease, rabies is an economically important issue in South and Central America where the vampire bat transmits the disease mainly to cattle. The distribution of rabies in this region therefore is related to the distribution of the vampire bat. The losses can be very dramatic as rabies kills animals. For this reason, the cattle systems in this region of the world vaccinate their cattle annually and some governments have vampire bat control programmes.

Paratuberculosis

Paratuberculosis affects large and small ruminants. It is a more important problem in dairy cattle systems as the disease causes lower milk yields and higher culling rates. This is reflected in the number of studies that have been carried out from the important dairy producing regions of the world. In sheep and goats there appears to be some impact in terms of increased mortality.

Information available

Europe

- Bennett *et al.* (1999) estimated that the losses due to Johne's disease (JD) in the British dairy and beef suckler herds were between £843,000 and £4.29 million per year and that total costs were between £858,000 and £4.31 million.

North America

- Ott *et al.* (1999) analysed data from the USDA National Animal Health Monitoring System to estimate the losses due to JD. Their analysis showed that Johne's-positive herds experience an economic loss of almost US$100 per cow when compared to Johne's-negative herds. The losses are due to reduced milk production and increased cow-replacement costs. The positive herds reported that at least 10% of their cull cows had clinical symptoms consistent with JD and economic losses were estimated to be over US$200 per cow. High-prevalence herds experienced reduced milk production of over 700 kg per cow, culled more cows but had lower cull-cow revenues and had greater cow mortality than Johne's-negative herds. The authors estimated that JD costs the US dairy industry, in reduced productivity, US$22–27 per cow or US$200–250 million annually.

- Johnson-Ifearulundu *et al.* (1999) reported on a study of JD in Michigan, USA. They found that, for a herd of average size and cull rate, the reduction in mean weight of culled cows attributable to paratuberculosis represented a loss of approximately US$1150 annually for each 10% increase in herd prevalence of paratuberculosis. They also found that the increased mortality rate attributable to paratuberculosis represented a loss of between US$1607 and US$4400 on the basis of lost slaughter value and cost of replacement heifers.

- Stabel (1998) states that, although cattle in the USA with clinical JD are often culled, cows with subclinical paratuberculosis may cause economic losses because of reduced milk yields and poor reproductive performance.

- A study in Holland found that vaccination against JD was highly profitable (van Schaik *et al.*, 1996). The authors report that the costs of the vaccination were US$15 per cow and the benefits (total returns minus costs) were US$142 per cow.

- Thurtell *et al.* (1994) analysed the control of JD in New South Wales. Their report includes:
  - the present situation in terms of the nature, incidence and testing procedures for bovine JD, and the current New South Wales government's measures to deal with JD (notification, quarantine and control, and compensation);
  - the nature of losses attributable to JD in terms of production losses, loss of exports and sales, and increased costs;
  - market failures (the nature of impact on the industry and individual producers and the problem of information in sales involving infected herds); and

  - market-based and regulatory options of dealing with JD.
- The authors conclude that government intervention in the control of JD could be justified if there are limited market failures.

- Collins and Morgan (1991) in their analysis of a test and cull paratuberculosis programme conclude that, given the characteristics of most diagnostic tests for paratuberculosis in use at that time and assuming that paratuberculosis causes at least a 6% decrease in milk production of cows, a test and cull programme should be profitable when pre-test paratuberculosis herd prevalence is more than 5%.

- In a study on JD in New Zealand, Lisle and Milestone (1989) estimated losses on the most severely affected properties to be NZ$6651.38 and NZ$3990.72, respectively, for the 1984–1985 and 1985–1986 dairy seasons. The authors calculated that the costs of a test and slaughter and a vaccination programme to control JD on a 100-cow dairy farm were NZ$400 and NZ$100, respectively. They conclude that in New Zealand a test and slaughter programme is unlikely to be economically viable, but the commercial vaccines at that time sensitize animals to bovine tuberculin.

- Gill (1989) studied the economic impact of JD in Australia. The author calculated direct costs of JD to the Australian dairy industry totalled AUS$3,820,000, of which: reduced productivity due to clinical disease was AUS$690,000, subclinical AUS$2,040,000; increased susceptibility to disease and infertility (not estimated); control AUS$1,090,000. Indirect costs were estimated to be AUS$310,000/year, of which: export testing was AUS$200,000; interstate testing was AUS$10,000; and research was AUS$100,000.

- Everett *et al.* (1989) report that the economic losses in clinically affected cattle in the three worst affected dairy herds in New South Wales, Australia, were between AUS$1500–4000, subclinical milk losses AUS$1000/year. The authors state that the most severely affected beef herd loses only one clinical case per year, valued at AUS$800, but its indirect costs total AUS$80,000. Only 16 of the 46,000 sheep flocks (52 million sheep) in New South Wales had been diagnosed with JD since 1980, and the authors estimate in these flock that the disease caused mortality ranging from 0.4% to 4% in adult sheep. JD had been diagnosed in 43 of the 2000 goat herds in the state, the majority of which were in the dairy sector, which was only 0.5% of the total state herd of 413,000 animals.

• Hillion and Argente (1987) report that the strategy of eradication of JD by the culling of all sick and carrier cattle and with vaccination and hygienic measures gave positive returns in herds with high prevalences.

• Chiodini and van Kruiningen (1986) estimate that the losses due to paratuberculosis in New England (USA) cattle were US$15.4 million due to clinical disease and losses in productivity.

• Benedictus et al. (1985) estimated that the economic losses due to the disposal of a cow with clinical paratuberculosis was on average 2250 guilders, and the loss of disposing of a cow without clinical disease but positive to diagnostic tests averaged 1800 guilders.

• Juste and Casal (1993) analysed the returns to control strategies for ovine paratuberculosis in the Basque country.

Other Diseases that Affect a Range of Species

In addition to the major diseases, a range of minor diseases exist that also affect a range of livestock species. Again information on the economic impact of these diseases is provided with comments on the validity of this information.

Yersinia

Yersinia in animals appears to have two important species Yersinia enterocolitica and Y. pseudotuberculosis. They are common in all types of species (Adesiyun et al., 1986; Staroniewicz, 1986; Gad El-Said et al., 1996) and cause diarrhoea in animals (Adesiyun and Kaminjolo, 1994). Hodges et al. (1984) found a number of different serotypes of Y. pseudotuberculosis in cattle, sheep, goats, pigs and birds that had died or were ill with symptoms of diarrhoea. However, they provide no indication of the prevalence of sick animals, making it difficult to determine how important this disease was. Slee and Skilbeck (1992) found that infection with Y. pseudotuberculosis does not provide protection from infection with Y. enterocolitica. The same study found that older sheep are less likely to have infections from these two forms of Yersinia spp.

The two Yersinia spp. can also cause infections in humans and one of the problems with Y. enterocolitica is that it can grow at refrigeration temperatures (Roberts, 1990). Jensen and Hughes (1980) report the presence of Y. enterocolitica in raw goat's milk, which is a concern in countries where this product is being consumed increasingly in order to combat allergy problems from drinking cow's milk. Lautner and Friendship (1992) list Yersinia as an important zoonosis in their list of pig diseases and a study by Shiozawa et al. (1988) indicates that a high percentage of slaughtered pigs have Y. pseudotuberculosis infections in the throat and respiratory tract. The authors suggest that pig products are a potential source of human infection with this bacterium. Schiemann and Fleming (1981) found a similar level of infection with Y. enterocolitica in the respiratory organs of pigs in Canada. In China, the Y. enterocolitica serotype that affects humans is very close to the pig serotype, indicating that there are public health risks (Hu, 1988). Low levels of contamination with Y. enterocolitica have been reported in poultry meat (Czernomysy-Furowicz et al., 1999).

In a slightly different line of thinking, Yersinia spp. can create costs in brucellosis eradication campaigns because certain serotypes of Yersinia can cause cross-reactions with Brucella abortus tests (Akkermans, 1975; Nattermann et al., 1980).

In summary Y. enterocolitica and Y. pseudotuberculosis are commonly found in livestock around the world. Their impact economically seems to be very limited but these bacteria are known to:

- cause diarrhoea particularly in young animals;
- be a source of food contamination particularly in soft cheeses, raw milk, pig and poultry products; and
- cause cross-reactions in *Brucella abortus* tests.

The overall impact of the disease caused by these two bacteria is probably small and this is reflected in the literature available concerning the prevalence in animals and the losses that result from infections.

Bovine diarrhoea virus and border disease virus

Bovine diarrhoea virus causes problems with fertility mainly in dairy cattle (see Chapter 17, this volume, for more details) and in sheep (Sweasey *et al.*, 1979; Sharp and Rawson, 1986; Burgu *et al.*, 1987). The disease can also infect pigs, but its impact is not that clear and it appears not to be a serious problem.

Rotavirus

Rotavirus infections occur in large and small ruminants, pigs and poultry. The impact of this virus in these groups is summarized as follows:

- The virus affects cattle and buffalo in large ruminants and causes diarrhoea mainly in calves. Losses due to this virus vary, but rotavirus appears to be the second or third most important cause of diarrhoea and subsequent problems with calf mortality. Its impact has been such that research has been carried out to produce rotavirus vaccines.
- In small ruminants the impact of the disease is similar to that seen in large ruminants.
- In pigs, again the impact is similar to large ruminants.
- In poultry, younger birds do not seem to be that badly affected, whereas older birds are affected, causing diarrhoea and

increase in mortality. In the case of layers, it causes a drop in egg production. The outbreaks of rotavirus can cause dramatic losses.

Campylobacter

Campylobacter has importance in fertility in cattle, sheep, goats and pigs. It is reported to be associated with abortions in cattle, sheep and pigs. It is an infection that can be found in the digestive and reproductive tracts and is common throughout the world. However, the major significance of this disease is in terms of public health. Campylobacteriosis in humans is important and the main source of infection appears to come from contaminated food. Anderson *et al.* (2001) estimated that approximately 16,000 individuals in the USA might be infected by *Campylobacter jejuni* derived from both ground beef and fresh beef sources. Campylobacteriosis is estimated to have caused between US$0.7 and 1.4 million of loss in terms of treatment, diagnosis, lost days in work and deaths. The major threat is from contaminated poultry products, but there is also a risk from pork, beef and milk (Shane, 1997).

In summary, campylobacter can be said to have minor impacts in terms of:

- fertility in cattle, sheep, goats and pigs;
- diarrhoea in pigs and poultry;

It can have major impact in terms of public health:

- in countries with intensive pig and poultry systems and intensive processing units with high wages;
- potentially in countries with the consumption of raw milk.

Chlamydia/chlamydophila

Chlamydia affects large and small ruminants, pigs, poultry and humans. The effects of chlamydia in the different groups are summarized as follows:

- In cattle, *Chlamydia* can cause fertility problems.
- In small ruminants, a number of sero-surveys would seem to indicate that this *Chlamydia* is at low prevalences. However, there are exceptions which seem to be in countries with more temperate climates. The data available on the causes of abortion indicate that *Chlamydia* is one of the most important infectious causes of abortion, but this needs to be interpreted in light of the fact that the majority of abortions do not seem to have an infectious cause. Also the data on abortions give no indication of the percentage of animals aborting in general, which makes it impossible to estimate the economic impact of this disease in small ruminants.
- In pigs, *Chlamydia* causes fertility and respiratory problems. The latter appear to be associated with secondary infections.
- In poultry, it seems to be able to cause damage in the respiratory tract and also in the reproductive tract. It has an impact in terms of human health in that severe outbreaks can lead to human infections, probably respiratory also.

The absolute impact of *Chlamydia* is difficult to assess; it seems to be present everywhere, but in some situation it can cause clinical symptoms. Ansell and Done (1988) calculated that in the UK there were 91,000 abortions in sheep due to enzootic abortion in ewes caused by *Chlamydia*. They estimated that it causes losses of £1,274,000 and that the returns from vaccinating against this disease were positive. However, their calculations are not clear on how they have estimated the benefits from the changes and it is suggested that they have not taken into account the need for extra feed resources required for the extra lambs produced or the impact of a greater number of lambs for sale.

Neospora caninum

Neospora caninum affects cattle, sheep, goats and pigs and is a cause of reproductive problems. According to Otter (1996), neosporosis is an emerging problem in cattle and it is in this species where the greatest numbers of articles are published on the epidemiology (French *et al.*, 1998; Bartels *et al.*, 1999) and economics of the disease. Agerholm *et al.* (1997) report that *Neospora caninum* caused abortions in study herds in Denmark, but provide no figures for the prevalence of this disease. Otter (1997) also details a study in the UK which looked specifically at infected herds. This study stated that abortions were sporadic, affecting less than 5% of the cows, but provides no details of herd prevalence in the UK. Thurmond and Hietala (1996), in a study of dairy cows in California, found that cows that are seropositive to *N. caninum* have a shorter life than seronegative cows (6.3 months less) and also have a greater risk of being culled (1.6 times greater risk). Given the costs associated with cow replacement, the authors state that the costs of this disease are greater than just the abortion costs involved.

Kasari *et al.* (1999) studied the economic losses caused by *N. caninum* in beef herds found in Texas. Their analysis found that a herd with a 20% prevalence of infection experienced an estimated 2.4% lower calving percentage, an overall estimated 2.3% lower weaned calf crop and lower calf weight at birth from infected cows (5.6 kg). They predicted that the economic loss was US$13.75/head (US$577.50 herd loss) with a range of between US$23.29/head (US$978.18 herd loss) and US$35.21/head (US$1478.82 herd loss) depending on the impact at individual animal level. At state level, they estimated that the total economic loss to the Texas beef industry was US$7.6 million, but this may range between US$15 million and US$24 million. It is noted that these estimates were derived using deterministic and stochastic models. The former produces a single answer, the latter a range. What is difficult to understand is how the stochastic model has produced solutions that do not include the estimate from the deterministic model in its range. These estimates indicate disease losses, which appear large, but no information is required on how disease status can be changed or how much it might cost.

Yamane *et al.* (2000) estimated the losses in milk production in Japan from cows infected with *N. caninum* and also cows that had aborted due to this disease on the basis of a serological survey that showed an individual animal prevalence of 3.24% and that 2030 aborted fetuses were diagnosed positive to this disease. Their estimates provide information about disease losses.

French *et al.* (1999) used mathematical models to examine the importance of different methods of transmission of *N. caninum*. They used this information to determine the most effective means of reducing infection in dairy cattle. They found that annual culling of infected cattle rapidly reduced the prevalence of infection and was the most effective method of control in the short term. In addition culling calves from infected cows was also effective in the short term. Their analysis did not indicate costs of the control and Antony and Williamson (2001) would argue that insufficient information is available on *N. caninum* to draw definite conclusions on the returns to the control of this disease.

Cryptosporidiosis

De Graaf *et al.* (1999) review information available on cryptosporidial infections in livestock and poultry. They conclude that cryptosporidiosis:

- Is a problem mainly in neonatal ruminants. *C. parvum* is considered to be an important agent in the aetiology of the neonatal diarrhoea syndrome of calves, lambs and goat kids, causing considerable direct and indirect economic losses.
- Avian cryptosporidiosis is an emerging health problem in poultry, associated with respiratory disease in chickens and other Galliformes, and with intestinal disease in turkeys and quails.
- Because of limited availability of effective drugs, the control of cryptosporidiosis relies mainly on hygienic measures and good management.

Summary

The chapter has provided information on the economic impact of livestock diseases that affect a range of species. The review is by no means complete as some diseases that cause important losses such as cysticercosis in cattle and pigs are not included. However, the majority of the most important studies on the economic impact of general livestock diseases are included in this chapter and subsequent chapters will cover the diseases of large ruminants, small ruminants, pigs and poultry.

17 Diseases of Large Ruminants

Importance of Large Ruminants in the World Livestock Economy

The principal products of large ruminants are:

- meat;
- hides;
- milk and milk products;
- manure;
- draught power;
- transport.

Large ruminants are generally regarded as the most important domestic livestock species in the world. Their importance is demonstrated by the list of products they provide. In developed countries, their contributions are mainly restricted to commercial products such as meat, hides and milk. However, in countries such as India, where 15% of the world's cattle population and more that 50% of the world's buffalo population are found, the main purpose of these animals is to provide draught power and manure for crop systems and also transport people and products in rural areas. Milk production is important and increasingly so, but there remains a taboo on eating beef in the largely Hindu population of this country. Cattle are also important as draught animals in Africa and research has shown that the low offtake rates in some smallholder farmer areas are related to the high value placed on draught power

and manure. In South-east Asia, buffalo is the important source of draught power.

Figure 17.1 shows the distribution of the cattle and buffalo population in the world. The largest populations are found in Asia and Central and South America.

Large ruminants supply nearly a third of the world's meat production (30.68%). The pattern of meat production for large ruminants is very different, with the OECD countries being the largest producers followed by Central and South America (see Fig. 17.2). Note that there appears to be an error in the data on buffalo meat production for Central and South America.

Figure 17.3 shows the distribution of the world's dairy cattle. Eastern Europe and CIS have the largest population followed by Asia and OECD.

Again the pattern of production is different for the distribution of production, with OECD dominating the world production. It is also noted that over half the milk produced in Asia comes from other species apart from cattle. This relates to the large buffalo population found in this region. The large ruminants supply nearly all the world's milk production (see Fig. 17.4).

Summary

Large ruminants play an important role in the world livestock economy both in terms of commercial products and intermediate

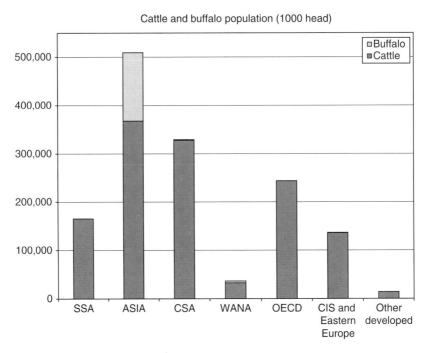

Fig. 17.1. Cattle and buffalo population in the different regions of the world. (From Seré and Steinfeld, 1995.)

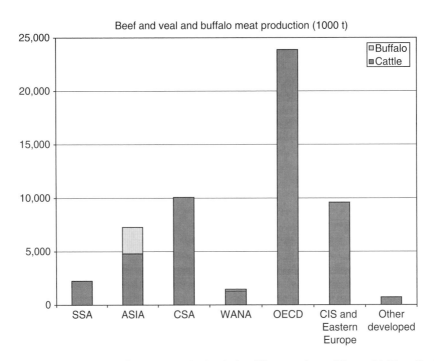

Fig. 17.2. Beef and veal and buffalo meat production in the different regions of the world. (From Seré and Steinfeld, 1995.)

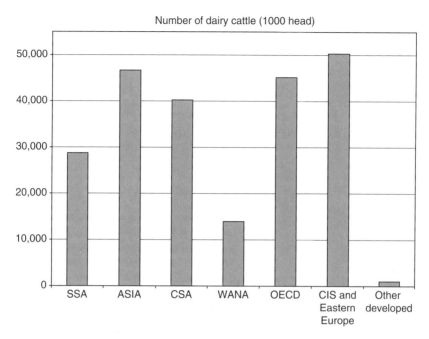

Fig. 17.3. Dairy cattle population in the different regions of the world. (From Seré and Steinfeld, 1995.)

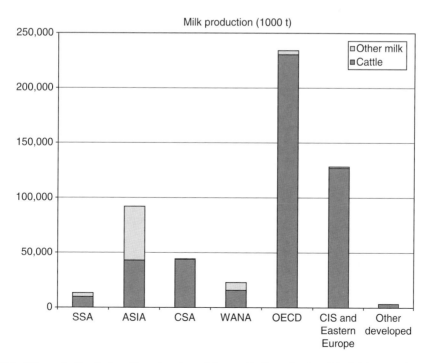

Fig. 17.4. Milk production in the different regions of the world. (From Seré and Steinfeld, 1995.)

products for farm-level production. However, the levels of production from these species do not relate to the populations found in the different regions of the world. The reasons for this relate to the type of management and feeding systems employed in the different parts of the world. In the OECD region, large ruminants are normally found in intensive systems that have high levels of concentrate feeding and investments in machinery and housing. These systems are capable of producing greater quantities of product per animal, but require much high levels of input. In contrast, where the majority of the large ruminant population is found, there are low levels of feed and capital inputs. These are important issues when analysing the economic impact of large ruminant diseases and normally the literature is generally dominated with information from the high-input high-output systems of the OECD countries.

Overview of Large Ruminant Diseases

Some of the most important large ruminant diseases are as follows:

1. Foot-and-mouth disease (FMD; reviewed in Chapter 16, this volume).
2. Rinderpest.
3. Vesicular stomatitis.
4. Contagious bovine pleuropneumonia.
5. Lumpy skin disease.
6. Rift Valley fever.
7. Bluetongue (reviewed in Chapter 16, this volume).
8. Anthrax (reviewed in Chapter 16, this volume).
9. Leptospirosis.
10. Rabies (reviewed in Chapter 16, this volume).
11. Paratuberculosis (reviewed in Chapter 16, this volume).
12. Bovine anaplasmosis.
13. Bovine babesiosis.
14. Bovine brucellosis (reviewed in Chapter 16, this volume).
15. Bovine genital campylobacteriosis (reviewed in Chapter 16, this volume).
16. Bovine tuberculosis (reviewed in Chapter 16, this volume).

17. Bovine cysticercosis (reviewed in Chapter 16, this volume).
18. Dermatophilosis.
19. Enzootic bovine leucosis.
20. Haemorrhagic septicaemia.
21. Infectious bovine rhinotracheitis (IBR)/ infectious pustular vulvovaginitis.
22. Theileriosis.
23. Trichomonosis.
24. Trypanosomiasis (tsetse-transmitted; reviewed in Chapter 16, this volume).
25. Malignant catarrhal fever.
26. Bovine spongiform encephalopathy.

These diseases were on Lists A and B of the OIE. Such diseases are normally contagious and have a high economic impact. However, there are other diseases which are normally named production disease such as lameness or mastitis that are also important and cause high losses particularly in intensive dairy systems. The following section will provide information on a number of diseases listed above.

Information Available

This part of the chapter is divided into:

- General studies of large ruminant diseases.
- Rinderpest.
- Contagious bovine pleuropneumonia.
- Ticks and tick-borne diseases.
- Haemorrhagic septicaemia.
- Bovine leucosis.
- Bovine viral diarrhoea.
- IBR.

General large ruminant disease studies

- Fourichon et al. (1999) reviewed papers that reported losses on production diseases such as dystocia, stillbirth, milk fever, retained placenta, metritis, cystic ovaries, ketosis, displaced abomasum and locomotor disorders in the production levels of dairy cattle. Their data were dominated by North American and European studies and they report that losses were not associated with milk fever or cystic ovaries, but the other problems did cause milk production losses to varying degrees.

- Wells *et al.* (1998) reviewed the available information on diseases that affect dairy production. Their analysis showed that traditional production costs ranked mastitis, reproductive problems and lameness as the most important dairy cattle diseases. However, using a qualitative ranking system, the most important diseases included *Salmonella*, Johne's disease (*Mycobacterium paratuberculosis*), bovine diarrhoea virus-associated disease and mastitis. The authors suggest that ranking systems in the dairy industry should consider zoonotic risks, international trade implications and animal welfare concerns as well as production losses.

Europe

- Rajala-Schultz and Grohn (1999) studied the impact on milk production in Finnish Ayrshire cows by the production diseases: dystocia, retained placenta, metritis, milk fever, ketosis, lameness and mastitis. They found that, except for late metritis, they caused reductions in milk yields. Mastitis had the largest impact.
- Seegers *et al.* (1998) studied the reasons for culling in French Holstein cows. In order of frequency, their research found that reasons were infertility or reproductive disorders, udder disorders, low milk yield, sales for dairy purposes, and others including lameness and emergency culling. The authors report that culling due to fertility problems was the most expensive culling problem as it usually occurred in younger animals.
- Esslemont and Peeler (1993) state that the main losses in British dairy systems occurred in animals with endometritis, lameness, mastitis, extended calving intervals and excessive involuntary culling. They estimated that the cost in a 100-cow herd was approximately £10,000/year.
- A study in Switzerland of dairy herds in 1993/1994 (Stark *et al.*, 1997) estimated that disease-related annual costs per cow were FS 139.44 and per calf FS 4.18. In addition, the annual disease prevention cost per cow was FS 10.18. Antibodies against *Leptospira hardjo*, *Coxiella burnetti*, *Mycobacterium paratuberculosis* and bovine diarrhoea virus were detected in 68.1%, 61.9%, 8.0% and 99.1% of the farms. Nearly two-thirds of the farms (63.7%) had gastrointestinal strongylid infections. Veterinary assistance was required on average 1.96 times per cow and the main treatments were for reproductive and puerperal diseases. The dairy farmers treated most animals with lameness.
- Vagsholm *et al.* (1991) estimated the costs of disease in Norwegian dairy farms using a dual-estimation approach to produce shadow prices. They found that reproductive diseases, ketosis, udder diseases and other diseases had shadow costs per case of 1751, 1268, 295 and 617 Nkr, respectively (US$1 = 7 Nkr).
- Mouchet *et al.* (1986) surveyed 476 dairy farms in Ille-et-Vilaine, France, and they report that veterinary costs in order of expenditure were mastitis (22%), infertility and endometritis (12.6%), prophylactic measures (10.9%), calf diarrhoea (7.9%), obstetrics (6.7%), antiparasitic and antimycotic treatments (6.2%), lameness (6%), vitamin, mineral and amino acid therapy (5.5%), dystocia (4.6%), milk fever (4.4%), digestive disorders (3.8%), foreign bodies (1.7%) and respiratory diseases (1.6%).
- Fisher (1980) examines the economic impact of cattle diseases in Britain between 1850 and 1900. The author describes the Diseases of Animals Act of 1884, which was drafted and implemented in response to the heavy losses in the country due to rinderpest, bovine contagious pleuropneumonia and FMD.

Asia

- Kim JongShu *et al.* (1999) report on the National Animal Health Monitoring Systems in Gyeongnam, Korea. They estimated that:
  - In cows, the most costly seven diseases were clinical mastitis, reproductive disorder, gastrointestinal problems,

multiple system disorders, parturition complications, metabolic/nutritional disease and lameness.

- In young stock, the most costly diseases were the multiple system disorders, reproductive disorders, respiratory disease, gastrointestinal disease and lameness.
- In calves, the most costly diseases were gastrointestinal disorders, respiratory diseases, skin diseases, multiple system disorders and metabolic/nutritional disorders.

- In Pakistan, Khan *et al.* (1994) surveyed livestock producers in villages in the district of Lahore, Pakistan. They found that common diseases in cattle and buffalo were haemorrhagic septicaemia in buffalo calves, diarrhoea in adult buffaloes and FMD in young and adult cattle. They estimated that, in the 5400 cattle and buffaloes in the survey, there were annual financial losses due to disease of Rs 19 million and that Rs 6.8 million were due to haemorrhagic septicaemia.

- Paramatma *et al.* (1987) studied the cattle diseases in an Indian village and found that the most prevalent and economically important diseases were FMD, haemorrhagic septicaemia and gastrointestinal diseases.

- Ronohardjo *et al.* (1986) estimated that losses attributable to fascioliasis, trypanosomiasis, mastitis and FMD among cattle and buffaloes amounted to US$115 million. The authors believed that *Fasciola gigantica* was responsible for losses of US$32 million and trypanosomiasis US$22 million. They report that other major diseases were haemorrhagic septicaemia, *Haemonchus contortus* infestation, ascariasis, brucellosis and anthrax.

- Partoutomo *et al.* (1985) assessed the diseases of major importance in Indonesia. In order of economic importance, they listed fascioliasis, trypanosomiasis, FMD, haemorrhagic septicaemia, gastrointestinal nematodiasis, ascariasis, brucellosis, stephanofilariasis, anthrax, mastitis, lantana poisoning, copper deficiency and scabies in cattle and buffaloes as the major diseases for large ruminants.

Africa

- Otesile *et al.* (1983) studied losses in calves in Nigeria of different breeds. The abortion rate and stillbirth varied between 2% and 45% and the calf mortality rate between 15% and 44.6%. The exotic breeds had higher mortality and abortion rates. The most common causes of post-natal death were neonatal weakness (14.8%), FMD (12.7%), septicaemia (9.2%), parasitic gastro-enteritis (7.0%) and pneumonia (6.3%).

North America

- Hird *et al.* (1991) analysed the data from the National Animal Health Monitoring System for Californian beef herds in 1988–1989. They report that the highest costs for veterinary services were for dystocia, lameness and ocular carcinoma and that mean expenditures for preventive veterinary services were US$1.67/cow-year, which was mainly spent on reproductive problems such as female infertility, vaccination against brucellosis and male infertility, which cost US$0.72, US$0.39 and US$0.22/cow-year, respectively.

- Miller and Dorn (1990) report on the data from the Ohio National Animal Health Monitoring System for dairy cattle. Their analysis found that costs of disease prevention and treatment averaged US$172.40/cow-year, with mastitis accounting for 26%, followed by infertility not otherwise specified 13%, pneumonia 5%, lameness 5%, dystocia 5%, milk fever 4%, left displaced abomasum 4% and death 3%. Mastitis had the highest annual estimated prevalence (37 cases per 100 cow-years), followed by metritis (32 cases per 100 cow-years), infertility (25 cases per 100 cow-years), pneumonia (19 cases per 100 cow-years), cystic ovaries (eight cases per 100 cow-years) and retained placenta (eight cases per 100 cow-years).

- Kaneene and Hurd (1990a,b) describe the design of a National Animal Health Monitoring System for Michigan. They report that, of the three age groups studied, cows had the greatest number of disease problems. Table 17.1 provides details of the importance of different diseases in terms of reporting and cost of treatment or prevention.

- House (1978) analysed data on calf mortality in the USA and for that *Escherichia coli* was responsible for the most devastating economic losses (50.9% and 74.6%). Coronaviral (17.5% and 29.7% loss) and rotaviral (3.2% and 9.1% loss) infections ranked second and third, respectively. In one study, cryptosporidial infections (6.5% loss) were estimated to be similar in economic impact to rotaviral infection. Salmonellosis, mycotic gastro-enteritis, IBR and bovine viral diarrhoea infections accounted for minor losses. The estimated average annual loss from *E. coli* was US$48.6 and US$71.2 million; from coronaviral infection, US$16.7 and US$28.4 million; from rotaviral infection, US$3.1 and US$8.7 million; and from cryptosporidial infection from one study US$6.2 million.

Rinderpest

Rinderpest is a contagious viral disease affecting ruminants and pigs. The disease is characterized by high fever, gastro-enteritis, erosive stomatitis, fetid odour, dehydration and death (Scott, 1990). In the past, the disease was prevalent in many parts of sub-Saharan Africa, South and South-east Asia (OIE, 2001) and it was also present in Europe but eradicated in that region without vaccine. It is a disease that has caused enormous losses and its entry into Africa is sometimes cited as the reason for the slow development of this continent. The reality is that it is a disease that can devastate cattle herds and the efforts that have been put into its control and eradication demonstrate its economic importance. However, with luck this may become the first cattle disease to be eradicated from the world and this section concentrates on the control programmes to give an idea of the investments in the eradication of rinderpest.

Strenuous control programmes have eradicated the disease from much of the world. In Africa, two foci of disease are identified,

Table 17.1. Importance of different large ruminant diseases in terms of reporting and costs of treatment. (From Kaneene and Hurd, 1990a,b.)

Age group	Cows	Young stock	Calves
Most frequently reported	Breeding problems Clinical mastitis Parturition problems Metabolic Gastrointestinal disorders Lameness	Respiratory Multiple system Breeding Gastrointestinal Lameness Birth problems	Gastrointestinal Respiratory Multiple system Lameness Metabolic/nutritional Urogenital diseases
Most expensive diseases	Clinical mastitis Breeding problems Gastrointestinal problems Parturition problems Multiple system problems Lameness Metabolic/nutritional diseases	Multiple system problems Breeding problems Respiratory disease Birth problems Gastrointestinal disease Lameness	Gastrointestinal problems Respiratory diseases Multiple system problems Birth problems Metabolic diseases Lameness
Highest annual preventive cost	Mastitis Breeding problems Lameness Parturition problems Multiple system problems Gastrointestinal disease Metabolic/nutritional problems		

southern Somalia and north-east Kenya, and southern Sudan and contiguous areas of Ethiopia, Kenya and Uganda (Roeder, 2000a). In Asia, Pakistan and Yemen are the areas causing concern (Roeder, 2000b).

Geographical distribution, past and present control campaigns

The Global Rinderpest Eradication Programme (GREP) has set a target of the global eradication of rinderpest by 2010 (GREP, undated). Diagnostic tests and an excellent vaccine are available and there is economic incentive to cooperate in control measures.

Africa

- A new campaign known as the Pan African Rinderpest Campaign (PARC) was established to combat the latest resurgence of the disease, with the ultimate aim of the eradication of the disease. The campaign began in 1987 in Burkina Faso, Ethiopia, Mali, Nigeria and Sudan (Walsh, 1987).
- PARC adopted a country-by-country approach, and the campaign was executed by national teams. Vaccine banks and an emergency fund were established to intervene quickly in threatened countries (Cheneau, 1993).
- Screening of sera from 18 wildlife species in Kenya during the period 1970–1981 found that 8.5% of samples tested positive for neutralizing antibodies to rinderpest (Rossiter et al., 1983).
- Wild animals including buffalo (Syncerus caffer), warthog (Phacochoerus aethiopicus) and giraffe (Giraffa camelopardus) were affected by outbreaks in Tanzania in the early 1980s (Rossiter et al., 1983; Wafula and Kariuki, 1987).
- The milder endemic form of the disease, which is more difficult to detect, is considered to be a particular problem. This form of the disease can persist among small populations and the percentage of animals affected may be very low, meaning that a relatively large sample of cattle may need to be tested in order to detect the presence of the disease (Rossiter and James, 1989).

- The campaign has had considerable success, the disease is limited to two foci, and many African countries have been able to declare provisional freedom from the disease over recent years. Tambi et al. (1999) found positive returns to PARC in ten countries that they analysed.
- Outbreaks such as those which occurred in Kenya between 1994 and 1996 were contained by two rounds of mass vaccination and surveillance with the assistance of the FAO and the European Union, and a zone of the country was declared provisionally free of the disease (Empres, 1999a).
- The collapse of the government in Somalia in the early 1990s has made it difficult to gain access to cattle in the south of the country, but it is suspected that rinderpest continued to circulate in the region (Empres, 1999b).
- Conditions in southern Sudan also make data on the disease difficult to obtain, but the northern part of the country has been declared provisionally free (Roeder, 2000a).
- It is argued that mass vaccination should be stopped in favour of intensive surveillance and emergency preparedness to safeguard against outbreaks of rinderpest, as suboptimal vaccination campaigns resulting in immunity rates of below 70% will not result in the eradication of the disease (Roeder, 2000a).

South Asia

South Asia has also seen extensive efforts to control the disease in recent years:

- Prior to the mid-1950s, 400,000 bovids were affected each year in India and around half of them died in 8000 outbreaks (Adlakha, 1985). A national rinderpest eradication campaign was launched in 1956 and the disease incidence was much reduced.
- Rinderpest is reported to have entered Pakistan from India in 1956. The disease was brought under control in the 1960s and the country appeared to be free of the disease by 1977, although it remained seriously threatened (Raja, 1985).

- Durrani *et al.* (1988) report that a rinderpest-like disease had threatened the buffalo and cattle in the Landhi dairy colony for the previous 18 years, and that the presence of the disease had now been confirmed.
- Outbreaks of rinderpest have continued in Pakistan during the period from 1994 to 2000 (Roeder, 2000b).
- One factor limiting the effectiveness of the control campaign was reported to be the poor quality of the vaccine available in the country, prior to 1995. Quality-assured vaccine enabled the eradication of the disease from northern areas. Elsewhere in the country strategic vaccination was continued primarily in the buffalo tract of Sindh province (Roeder, 2000b).
- In 2000, rinderpest was reported from three dairy farms near Karachi. Further investigations revealed that other outbreaks had occurred in northern Sindh during the 1998–2000 period (GREP, 2001).
- Bangladesh experienced a severe rinderpest epidemic in 1958, which is estimated to have killed 3 million cattle and buffaloes (Siddique, 1985). The country was considered to be at considerable risk from the disease as the climate was favourable to the spread of the virus and animals are vulnerable due to their poor nutritional status. The congregation and dispersal of animals during the monsoon period would also facilitate the spread of the disease. A control campaign was instigated and vaccination was carried out both in border areas and in the interior of the country.
- However, a serological survey reported by Debnath *et al.* (1994) revealed that only 8.5% of animals in border areas tested positive for rinderpest antibodies, revealing that the country was vulnerable to another epidemic and that vaccination procedures needed to be reviewed.
- Nepal saw systematic control of the disease in the period between 1965 and 1969. An outbreak in the vicinity of the India border was controlled in 1978 (Lamichang, 1985). The last reported incidence of the disease in Nepal was in 1990, in Bhutan in 1969 and in Sri Lanka in 1994 (OIE, 2001).

South-east Asia

- South-east Asia has also seen the disease controlled by vaccination and movement controls. The disease has never been reported in Malaysia, and the last reported incidences of the disease occurred in Indonesia in 1907, Singapore in 1930, the Philippines in 1955, Burma in 1957, Thailand in 1959, Cambodia in 1965, Laos in 1966 and Vietnam in 1977 (OIE, 2001).

Ticks and tick-borne diseases (TBDs)

Ticks and tick-borne diseases are widely distributed throughout the world, particularly in tropical and subtropical countries. It has been estimated that 80% of the world cattle population is at risk from ticks and tick-borne diseases and that they cause US$7 billion worth of losses (McCosker, 1979). Perry and Young (1995) state that tick-borne infections are a greater constraint to livestock development in Africa than in other geographical zones. This is supported by the fact that Africa has all the most important ticks and TBDs, and is the only region affected by East Coast fever.

The tick species that cause the most serious problems for all livestock producers may be divided into four groups:

1. The *Boophilus* spp. that transmit the protozoan *Babesia* spp. and the rickettsia *Anaplasma* spp. The species are widely distributed and their most significant impact is on imported and exotic breeds of cattle.
2. The *Hyalomma* spp. that transmit the protozoan *Theileria annulata*. Tropical theileriosis caused by the organism is a particular problem for cross-bred dairy cattle in India, and worldwide it is estimated that 250 million cattle are at risk of this disease.
3. The *Amblyomma* spp. that transmit the rickettsia *Cowdria rumintium* that causes heartwater, a disease of small ruminants and exotic cattle in sub-Saharan Africa. *Amblyomma* spp. also transmit the protozoan *T. mutans* and have

been identified as a cause of dermatophilosis, which is a significant problem in West Africa. These tick species are also associated with tick worry or damage.

There exists a range of options for the control of ticks and tick-borne diseases (Fig. 17.5). The choice of which option to use is generally site-specific and requires knowledge of the technology available, its cost and its impact.

Getting the choice of options wrong can lead to problems of tick-borne disease instability (Fig. 17.6) and possibly problems of resistance to drugs:

- Minjauw *et al.* (1999) analysed a trial with different strategies of tick and East Coast fever control. They estimated that the strategically sprayed and immunized cattle in a traditional extensive system of management had the highest NPV, and the non-immunized group with no tick control the lowest. A break-even analysis showed that the immunization costs could rise to US$25.9 before profitability was affected. For herds under intensive

tick control, immunization was shown to be of no economic value. The results demonstrated the value of immunization, and indicated that this strategy is best used in combination with tick control measures.

- Where an outbreak of a tick-borne disease occurs, the re-establishment of endemic stability will take time and losses may be quite severe, and it is poor families who are likely to be affected most severely (Minjauw and McLeod, 2001).

- Within the smallholder dairy sector in East Africa, where herd size would typically be around three cows, loss of a single animal would have a serious effect on household income. Milk sales make a particularly important contribution to household income at certain times of the year when other sources of income are lacking (Heffernan and Misturelli, 2000) and incidence of tick-borne disease at this time could be particularly serious for household income.

- Loss of a single high-quality young female animal can have serious long-term

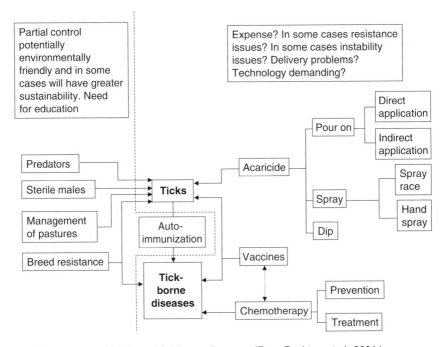

Fig. 17.5. Options to control ticks and tick-borne diseases. (From Rushton *et al.*, 2001.)

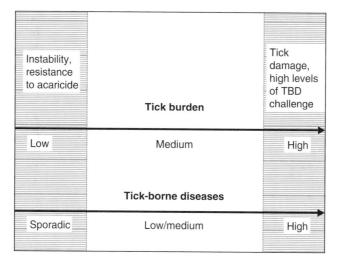

Fig. 17.6. The balance in the control of ticks and tick-borne diseases. (From Rushton *et al.*, 2001.)

consequences for the herd and given the shortage of good-quality genetic stock in Kenya available to smallholders, it is likely to be difficult to replace (Minjauw and McLeod, 2001).

East Coast fever

East Coast fever regularly kills animals and causes morbidity. The option of relying on enzootic stability does not appear a possibility for this disease and the need for appropriate farm-level solutions is high.

- Mukhebi *et al.* (1992) estimated that the losses due to *T. parva* in the area of Burundi, Kenya, Malawi, Mozambique, Rwanda, Sudan, Tanzania, Uganda, Zaire, Zambia and Zimbabwe were US$168 million and that 1.1 million cattle die due to the disease.

- In a more recent study, Minjauw and McLeod (2001) estimate much higher losses of US$233.81 million for Kenya, Malawi, Tanzania and Zambia. The area affected by the disease has approximately 24 million head of cattle and is one of the poorest regions of the world. The poorest people in this region are from rural areas and reliant on livestock and agriculture for their living.

Amblyomma variegatum

The tick *A. variegatum* is involved in the spread of heartwater and associated with dermatophilis, but is also responsible for serious damage to animals, often causing secondary infections, and is also associated with dermatophilosis. This tick is widespread in Africa and is also present in the Caribbean, where it is considered a risk to the livestock industry in the USA.

Contagious bovine pleuropneumonia

Contagious bovine pleuropneumonia (CBPP) is a bacterial disease affecting cattle and water buffaloes. The disease can occur in acute, subacute or chronic forms and is characterized by pneumonia, serofibrinous pleurisy and oedema of the interlobular septa of the lungs (Edelsten *et al.*, 1990). Recent years have seen the appearance of the disease in several countries in Central, Eastern and Southern Africa, which has necessitated strenuous efforts for containment. Between 1989 and 1998, the Democratic Republic of Congo, Rwanda, Burundi, Tanzania and Zambia all became infected with the disease (Empres, 1998b):

- Botswana saw the first outbreak for over 50 years, although it was later provisionally able to declare itself free of the disease (Empres, 1998a).
- The disease was reported to be endemic in Angola, while Malawi and Mozambique were under threat from the disease spreading across the border from Tanzania (Empres, 1997).
- The disease is also considered endemic in northern Namibia, but a control programme initiated in 1997 is stated to be reducing the incidence of the disease (Empres, 2000).
- Outbreaks of the disease have been reported in recent years in Kenya, Uganda, Ethiopia and in many West African countries (OIE, 2001).
- South and South-east Asia are largely free of the disease, but outbreaks have been reported from Bangladesh and Pakistan (OIE, 2001).

Control strategies

Control of CBPP is based on a combination of vaccination movement restrictions and slaughter programmes. Treatment of the disease is rarely justified as there is the risk of converting actively infected animals into carriers (Edelsten *et al.*, 1990).

- War and instability are thought to have led to the reappearance of the disease in Burundi in the mid-1990s (Empres, 1998c).
- Cross-border movements are reported to have been responsible for the first outbreaks of the disease in Tanzania since the 1960s (Bölske *et al.*, 1995). Cattle were moved into southern Kenya due to poor water and grazing conditions as well as cattle thefts. When CPBB was suspected, many herders recrossed the border in an attempt to avoid the disease. In this manner, a more serious outbreak was prevented by movement restrictions imposed by the herders themselves (Bölske *et al.*, 1995).
- Mass slaughter may be the only effective option in the infected area, combined with strict movement controls and intensive surveillance. Test and slaughter policies are considered ineffective and can lead to the spread of the disease (Empres, 1997).
- The 1995 outbreak in Botswana was only controlled by complete depopulation of the infected area and strict surveillance (Empres, 1998b).
- In Zambia, the disease is prevented from spreading beyond the area close to the Angola border, where outbreaks have occurred, by vaccination, test and slaughter policies, and movement controls, combined with an extensive publicity campaign (Empres, 1997).
- In southern Sudan, the disease is reported to be endemic, but severe clinical disease is rare (Empres, 1997). It is suggested that in areas such as this, surveillance, and vaccination only of those animals that are identified as being at particular risk, may be more appropriate than mass vaccination (Empres, 1997).
- A cost–benefit analysis, which compared mass vaccination against CBPP with 50% coverage; a 5% selective vaccination and treatment scheme against CBPP, anthrax, blackleg and haemorrhagic septicaemia, and selective treatment against trypanosomiasis, was performed by Zessin and Carpenter (1985). The analysis demonstrated that surveillance and selective treatment strategy appeared to be the most beneficial, and would help establish improved links between herders and the veterinary service.

Haemorrhagic septicaemia

Haemorrhagic septicaemia (HS) is a form of acute pasteurellosis affecting cattle and water buffalo (Edelsten *et al.*, 1990). It is endemic in South and South-east Asia and sporadic outbreaks occur in sub-Saharan Africa (Edelsten *et al.*, 1990; OIE, 2001). This geographical distribution is reflected by the available literature on this disease, which is dominated by work from Asia. Water buffaloes are particularly susceptible to the disease and economic losses result from decreased milk production and the loss of draught power (De Alwis,

1993a). While sporadic disease outbreaks attract the attention of the authorities, the low levels of the disease in endemic areas among young animals may be more economically significant (De Alwis, 1993a).

- Major outbreaks of haemorrhagic septicaemia occur in India during the monsoon season (Kundu, 1993). During the 1940s and 1950s, about 60,000 cattle and buffalo died annually, but the incidence and mortality rate have been reduced considerably by the use of vaccines and drugs (Kundu, 1993).
- Sri Lanka saw an outbreak in 1955–1956, which killed nearly 10,000 livestock (De Alwis, 1993b). Since that time, the disease has become endemic in the dry zone of the country, an area where indigenous animals are kept under extensive management conditions, contact between animals is unrestricted.
- In Sri Lanka, haemorrhagic septicaemia occurs in areas where early detection is difficult, case fatality is near 100%, but the morbidity rate is highly variable, ranging from 5% to nearly 90% (De Alwis, 1993b).
- Hiramune and De Alwis (1982) reported that, among cattle and buffalo examined in the endemic area of Sri Lanka, the carrier rate was 22.7% in herds where disease had occurred in the previous week, declining to 1.9% in herds which had the disease 6 weeks previously. In this area, outbreaks are more frequent, but the morbidity levels tend to be lower than in non-endemic areas.
- The disease is also confined to young animals in the endemic areas, while elsewhere animals of all ages may be affected (De Alwis, 1993b).
- Sabah, Malaysia, saw an outbreak in 1973 in which 1200 buffaloes died; since the outbreak, approximately 100–150 cases have been recorded annually. Case fatality is close to 100%. However, no cases have been recorded among cattle, which are not usually kept in close proximity to buffaloes (Yeo and Mokhtar, 1993).
- In other regions of Malaysia, the disease is enzootic and of major economic importance (Jamaludin, 1993).

- Haemorrhagic septicaemia also causes heavy losses among cattle and particularly buffalo in Vietnam (Phoung, 1993).
- Cattle and buffalo in Cambodia are also affected (Kral et al., 1993).
- In Burma, haemorrhagic septicaemia is reported to be the most important bacterial disease of livestock (Van Khar and Myint, 1993).
- Cattle and buffalo, as well as sheep and goats, have been reported as infected in the Philippines (Interior, 1993).
- In Indonesia, haemorrhagic septicaemia is reportedly one of the most important diseases affecting buffalo (Putra, 1993).
- Mustafa et al. (1978) report continual outbreaks of the disease in all parts of Sudan.
- In Namibia, Voigts et al. (1997) reported outbreaks during 1994 and 1995 and it was suggested that the oryx antelope was a possible source of infection during one outbreak.

Control strategies

Vaccination is the main control method employed against haemorrhagic septicaemia. The oil adjuvant vaccine, used in many countries, provides protection for a 1-year period, but vaccination rates are generally low (20–50%; De Alwis, 1993a). Ideally the vaccine should be given to cattle and buffalo at 4–6 months of age and a booster given 3–6 months later.

- A study of 13 districts in Malaysia revealed that the vaccination coverage rate ranged from 12 to 65%, and the vaccination coverage appeared to be lower in areas that had experienced outbreaks (Yeo and Mokhtar, 1993).
- Putra (1993) notes that, due to the economic importance of the disease, the control programme in Indonesia is directed by the central government, which aims to vaccinate 60% of susceptible animals.
- Neramitmansook (1993) notes that sporadic outbreaks continued to occur among animals in Thailand despite the strong recommendation by the Department of

Livestock Development that at least 70% of village cattle and buffalo be vaccinated.

- There is some debate over the efficacy of the vaccine in endemic areas. De Alwis (1982) reports that, in the endemic area of Sri Lanka, no difference in mortality was found between vaccinated and unvaccinated herds.
- Treatment of infected animals with antibiotics is possible if treatment is given early. However, knowledge of the antibiotic sensitivity of the strain of infection is important as antibiotic resistance is reported to be an increasing problem (De Alwis, 1993a).

Bovine leucosis

Bovine leucosis is a strange disease in that it appears to cause little or no loss at farm level, but it has a number of analyses concerning its control. Its importance relates to trade issues where some countries place bans on animals with this disease or coming from countries with the disease. The following information is available:

- A study in Costa Rica on bovine leucosis infection in bovines concluded that bovine leucosis virus did not have any adverse effects on production, reproduction or the incidence of mastitis (Schramm and Aragon, 1994).
- Thompson et al. (1993) report an outbreak of bovine leucosis in New Zealand. They state that although clinical enzootic bovine leucosis is rare in New Zealand bovine leucosis infection is more widespread with a prevalence level of at least 5–10% in dairy herds. However, the authors felt that the economic impact of enzootic bovine leucosis on the productivity in New Zealand's dairy cattle is small. Their concern was that the introduction of control or eradication schemes in Europe and North America would lead to restrictions on the export of live cattle and genetic material from New Zealand.
- Da et al. (1993) estimated that the losses due to bovine leucosis virus infection were US$42 million in the USA dairy industry.

- Johnson and Kaneene (1991) report that most of the economic losses associated with bovine leucosis related to trade restrictions on the importation of cattle to the EEC countries.
- Muller and Wittmann (1990) estimated that losses due to bovine leucosis in the Osterburg region of East Germany were 3.2 million East German marks a year. They estimated that the savings from disease control were 1.7 million marks or 69 marks per cow.
- Kautzsch and Schluter (1990) state that, between 1975 and 1987, 508 million marks were spent in the German Democratic Republic on the control of bovine leucosis.
- Reinhardt et al. (1988) state that bovine leucosis has no influence on abortion, mastitis or fertility. However, they found that positive animals had an average milk loss of 156 kg, which in a herd of 137 cows with 30% prevalence was equivalent to US$74,880/year.
- In Poland, Meszaros et al. (1986) report that one of the problems of the bovine leucosis eradication campaign was the high cost of the test to identify positive animals.
- Hugoson and Wold-Troell (1983) analysed the returns to different strategies of controlling bovine leucosis virus in Sweden. They found that a strategy of organized control was the worst option and that options of no control and private initiatives gave similar returns at low exports. However, the private control strategy was favourable where exports become more important.
- Kellar (1981) studied the economic impact of bovine leucosis virus in Canada. The author's analysis showed that annual beef sector losses from clinical disease were US$49,000 and dairy losses were US$529,000. The trade impact was minimal and Kellar states that it could be absorbed by the domestic sector. The author concluded that, in the absence of any shift in export requirements, the economic impact of this disease had reached a point of equilibrium.
- Davies et al. (1980) examined the returns to two eradication strategies for bovine leucosis virus: slaughter of all herds contain-

ing reactors or slaughter of seropositive cattle with herds containing reactors not being declared free of enzootic bovine leucosis (EBL) until they returned two clear tests 6 months apart. The costs of these strategies were £37 million and £29 million, respectively, over a period of 25 years. Both strategies had benefits of £4.8 million.

- Langston *et al.* (1978) report that cows with bovine leucosis virus antibodies tended to produce more milk and to produce at a higher rate for the first two lactations; for subsequent lactations the negative cows had higher production and higher production rates, though differences were not significant. The authors conclude that bovine leucosis virus-infected cows had no greater mean age, no lower milk production and no lower reproductive efficiency than did non-infected cows.

Bovine diarrhoea virus

Bovine diarrhoea virus has been studied in depth in the dairy systems in Europe, indicating its importance in this region. The following information is available:

- Bennett *et al.* (1999) estimated that the losses due to bovine viral diarrhoea in British dairy and beef systems were between £5.19 million and £30.94 million.
- Dufour *et al.*'s (1999) analysis of the eradication of bovine virus diarrhoea in France indicates that such a programme would only be cost-effective (which probably means the benefits are greater than the costs) after 15 years of operation.
- Sorensen *et al.* (1995) describe a stochastic model to simulate the economic consequences of bovine diarrhoea virus infection in a dairy herd.
- Pasman *et al.* (1994) describe a model to simulate the economics of bovine diarrhoea virus control.
- Houe *et al.* (1993) estimated that the total losses due to bovine diarrhoea virus infection in the Danish dairy herd were 13 million Danish kroner per year.

- Wentink and Dijkhuizen (1990) estimated that losses due to bovine diarrhoea virus infections averaged 136 Dutch florins per cow with a range of 42–285.
- Wittkowski and Orban (1984) investigated problems of abortions, premature birth and neonatal losses in a herd with a high prevalence of antibodies to bovine viral diarrhoea (92%).

Infectious bovine rhinotracheitis (IBR)

IBR is a disease that causes much debate concerning its economic importance. It is widespread in many countries, but details of its real impact are generally not available. The following information was collected:

- Bennett *et al.* (1999) estimated that the losses due to IBR in British dairy and beef systems were between £1.14 million and £4.23 million/year and that total costs of this disease including control costs were between £5.73 million and £9.79 million.
- Noordegraaf *et al.* (1998) developed a simulation model for IBR to test five control strategies, including both a voluntary vaccination programme and a compulsory vaccination programme for all dairy herds. The voluntary vaccination programme with 50% participation was predicted not to be able to eradicate IBR. The authors suggested that a compulsory vaccination programme would be necessary to eradicate IBR in The Netherlands.

Ephemeral disease

Ephemeral disease appears to be of importance in Asia and Australia; the following information was collected on the disease and its economic impact:

- Davis *et al.* (1984) describe an outbreak of ephemeral fever in a herd of 250 Friesian and Australian Friesian Sahiwal cattle in northern Queensland in 1983. They report that the morbidity rate was 15% and the mortality rate 2% and calculated that the cost of the outbreak included the loss of milk production of 1192 kg of milk for 3 weeks of the outbreak (AUS$277), loss of milk production over the rest of lactation of 2043 kg (AUS$506) and the replacement values of two cows that died (AUS$1600), a total loss of approximately AUS$2400.

- In East Java, Indonesia, Ronohardjo and Rastiko (1982) report an outbreak of ephemeral fever between 1978 and 1982 that affected 1089 animals, killing 264 adult and 65 young cattle. The authors attempted to estimate the losses taking into account value of animals and losses in traction power.

- Theodoridis et al. (1973) experimentally infected 19 dairy cattle with ephemeral fever. The disease reduced milk yield by between 44.5% and 73.0% depending on the stage of lactation. Ephemeral fever lowered the resistance of the udder to bacterial mastitis, and the infected cows also showed delayed oestrous activity, abortion and delivery of weak calves.

Summary

The amount of information available on costs of outbreaks, analysis of disease losses and cost–benefit analyses of control strategies provides a good idea of the economic importance of large ruminants in the world livestock sector and also the importance of disease within the large ruminant sector. However, within the large ruminant systems many of the major contagious diseases are now under control and in some countries eradicated. One disease, rinderpest, will probably be the first cattle disease of importance to be eradicated worldwide. These efforts have involved much investment in terms of money and human capital. The new issues in large ruminant diseases appear to be:

- the more minor diseases and production problems in the dairy sector;
- final stages of control and eradication of diseases such as FMD;
- surveillance of diseases that are under control but unlikely to be eradicated such as tuberculosis; and
- public health issues concerning diseases such as BSE and E. coli H157, which are new or emerging disease problems.

18 Diseases of Small Ruminants

Importance of Small Ruminants in the World Livestock Economy

Principal products from small ruminants are:

- meat;
- wool and hair;
- milk and milk products;
- manure.

Despite this wide range of products, small ruminants are a minority group in the world livestock economy. They provide approximately 5% of the world supply of meat, but are more important in the African region, where their contribution reaches 30% in parts of North Africa. In terms of milk production, their contribution is small in relation to cattle and buffalo, but significant in the poorer societies of the world. Wool production is important as one of the main natural fibre supplies in the world. However, the importance of wool reduced with the widespread use of cotton in the late 19th and early 20th centuries and more recently with the use of synthetic fibres. Finally, manure is a key part of many small ruminant production systems in the world, e.g. the sheep and wheat systems of Australia and the smallholder farmer systems in Latin America.

Figures 18.1 and 18.2 show the world goat and sheep population and the estimated meat production, respectively.

Therefore, sheep and goats are found throughout the world, but their importance economically is small in comparison to cattle, pigs and poultry. This importance is reflected in the resources that have been dedicated to research into diseases that are important to these species.

Overview of Small Ruminant Diseases

Main diseases of great economic importance, which are included in Lists A and B of OIE diseases, are as follows:

1. Peste des petits ruminants (PPR).
2. Ovine epididymitis (*Brucella ovis*).
3. Caprine and ovine brucellosis (excluding *B. ovis*).
4. Caprine arthritis/encephalitis.
5. Contagious agalactia.
6. Contagious caprine pleuropneumonia.
7. Enzootic abortion of ewes (ovine chlamydiosis).
8. Ovine pulmonary adenomatosis.
9. Nairobi sheep disease.
10. Salmonellosis (*Salmonella abortus ovis*).
11. Scrapie.
12. Maedi-visna.

Nearly all these diseases have been covered in the review of general diseases in Chapter 16

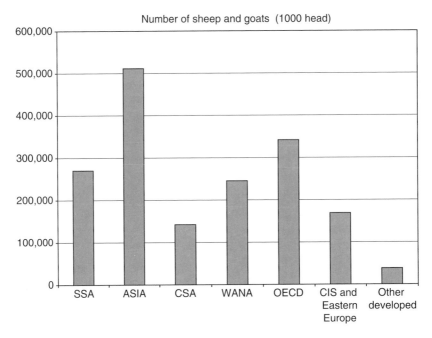

Fig. 18.1. Number of sheep and goats in the different regions of the world. (From Seré and Steinfeld, 1995.)

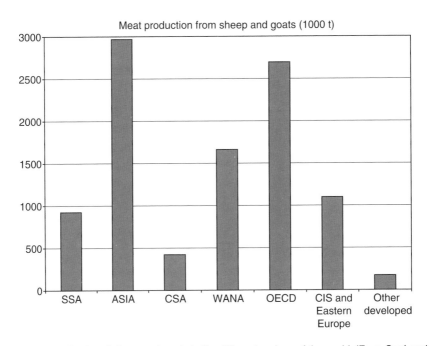

Fig. 18.2. Meat production of sheep and goats in the different regions of the world. (From Seré and Steinfeld, 1995.)

(this volume). The exceptions are PPR, Nairobi sheep disease and scrapie. No information was found on the economic importance of the latter two diseases. The importance of scrapie has increased with the concerns relating to BSE in cattle. Its impact on production appears small. Nairobi sheep disease is a viral disease transmitted by ticks. In endemic areas, it causes no serious problems and control measures are not required. However, exotic animals need to be vaccinated if they are taken to such areas. Specific information about PPR is presented below.

In addition to the list of diseases presented above, a number of other important diseases affect small ruminants. Internal parasites are probably the area most studied and further information can be found in the CABI *Animal Health and Production Compendium*. External parasites are also important and some information is provided in this chapter on their economic impact. Blood parasites such as trypanosomiasis also affect small ruminant production and again some information is provided in this section.

The following references were found on general reviews on the importance of diseases that affect small ruminants:

- Akerejola *et al.* (1979) reviewed the economically important diseases of small ruminants in Nigeria. They found that internal parasite problems and nutrition were the most important. With respect to contagious diseases, PPR was reported to cause between 10 and 20% mortality in goats. Blood parasites are common, but only affect exotic breeds. The same pattern is also seen for bluetongue and Rift Valley fever with only exotic animals affected. *Pasteurella* infections are important in certain areas.
- Mukasa-Mugerwa *et al.* (2000) report that between 28% and 59% of lambs in a Research Institute in Ethiopia die before they are 1 year old. The major cause of death is pneumonia followed by digestive problems, endoparasite problems and starvation. A very small percentage of deaths are related to septicaemia. It was found that there were significant breed differences and that low birth weights increased the risk of death.

Peste des petits ruminants

PPR is a viral disease in goats, and less common in sheep. Historically, the disease was primarily associated with West Africa, but now occurs in a belt across Africa immediately south of the Sahara, extending into the Arabian Peninsula (Taylor, 1984). OIE (2001) report the disease in India, Pakistan, Nepal, Benin, Cameroon, Côte d'Ivoire, Eritrea, Ethiopia, Ghana, Guinea, Mali, Mauritania, Niger, Nigeria and Senegal.

The economic impact of PPR in small ruminants is as follows:

- production losses:
  - mortality;
- control costs:
  - vaccination;
- trade.

More specific information on the impact of the disease and the potential for its control is as follows:

- A high seroprevalence of PPR antibodies was found in central Niger, suggesting frequent exposure to the disease (Stem, 1993). As such, the disease appears to be a major constraint to small ruminant production in Niger. Rumours of an outbreak are sufficient to deter the movement of flocks into an area. Outbreaks in the country are reported to occur approximately every 5 years (Stem, 1993).
- Martrenchar *et al.* (1997) conclude that mixed PPR and capripox infections, along with stongyles and external parasites, are limiting factors in small ruminant production in northern Cameroon. Serological studies, however, could find no relationship between seroconversion for PPR and the appearance of any clinical symptoms. Most animals also survived for more than 2 months following seroconversion.
- Nawathe (1984) report that over 100 outbreaks were reported annually in Nigeria, and that many more go unreported. Epidemics tend to occur during the rainy season when goats are herded together, and around Christmas when movement towards markets increases.

- Roeder *et al.* (1994) describe an outbreak among a large herd of goats in the Addis Ababa area, where the morbidity rate was nearly 100% and the mortality rate up to day 20 of the outbreak was approximately 60%. The source of the infection appeared to be from the south-west of Ethiopia, where it was suggested that the disease persists in endemic forms. The disease is also reported to have entered the country in 1989 via the Omo river valley in the south and to have spread by 1996 to the Ogaden and central Afar region.
- A serosurvey at Debre Zeit abattoir, Ethiopia, in 1997 showed high prevalence rates of 86% among nomadic animals, 43% among those from sedentary systems and 33% among animals from mixed farms (Empres, 1998).
- Rinderpest was reported for the first time in Eritrea in 1993 and a nationwide epidemic followed in 1994 with mortalities of 90% among sheep and goats in some outbreaks; efforts to control the disease by vaccination had limited success and outbreaks re-emerged in 1996 (Empres, 1998).
- South Asia has increasingly become a focus of the disease, which is causing serious losses in Pakistan, Afghanistan, Nepal, Bhutan, Bangladesh and India (New Agriculturalist, 2000).

Control strategies

- Where the disease is endemic and small ruminants are kept in large numbers, quarantine and segregation are not realistic means of controlling the disease. As such, vaccination is the preferred method of control (Nawathe, 1984) using tissue culture rinderpest vaccine (TCRV). The vaccine provides protection for over 1 year and is tolerated by healthy goats of all breeds, but side effects have been noted such as abortions and mild signs of PPR. In addition, the delivery of the vaccine has been problematic with a failure to maintain a cold chain leading to some non-viable doses being administered (Nawathe, 1984). In areas where the disease is endemic and animals harbour subclinical infections, subse-

quent vaccination with TCRV can trigger off the disease. Use of PPR hyperimmune serum produced in cattle is an alternative. Goats given hyperimmune serum along with a virulent PPR virus developed durable immunity. The cost of this treatment may, however, be prohibitive for most farmers (Adu and Joannis, 1984).
- Economic modelling suggests that the introduction of a vaccination campaign in Niger in the 1980s was a sound decision in terms of animal health and potential economic returns (Stem, 1993). Furthermore, herders appeared to be willing to pay for the vaccine. The use of a thermostable vaccine would further reduce costs.
- Awa *et al.* (2000) found that the control of PPR and gastrointestinal parasites gave a positive return in Cameroon with a benefit/cost ratio (BCR) of between 2.26 and 4.23.
- In northern Cameroon, field evaluation of a homologous vaccine against PPR significantly reduced mortality in vaccinated flocks. An economic analysis, which evaluated the cost of the vaccine, the potential for increased production and the current market prices for livestock suggest that vaccination may accrue considerable economic benefit to herders (Martrenchar *et al.*, 1999).
- Vaccination programmes do not always produce the desired benefits, at least in the short term. The introduction of a vaccination against PPR along with dipping against sarcoptic mange, among goatherds in south-west Nigeria, failed to clearly demonstrate reductions in mortality rates (Reynolds and Francis, 1988).
- In a semi-arid area of Mali, the introduction of deworming along with vaccination against PPR, pasteurellosis and anthrax failed to produce significant changes to mortality or weight gain (Ba *et al.*, 1996), although it was acknowledged in this case that the vaccination regime may be at fault. Vaccinations were only performed once or twice a year; as such, kids were often not vaccinated until they were 4 or 5 months old. Malnutrition, injuries and loss are reported to account for 40% of kid deaths, indicating that management improvements remain a priority.

Given the unpredictable nature of outbreaks of PPR, anthrax and pasteurellosis, it is suggested that vaccination may be desirable to reduce risk, but may discourage farmers and government from investing in other improvements.

Summary

PPR is a disease that appears to be becoming increasingly important. It is one of the few contagious diseases that is spreading rather than being controlled, and effective vaccine to control this spread is at this moment not readily available. The reasons for this appear to be that it mainly affects goats, a species of little importance in relative terms with other species.

Other diseases

Information on the impact of trypanosomiasis, border disease and orf were collected:

- Kanyari et al. (1983) report that returns from trypanosomiasis control in goats using samorin varied depending on the breed of goat. The BCR for this control was 7.3, 18.5 and 28.9 for East African, Galla × East African and Toggenburg × East Africa breeds, respectively.
- In a trial on the impact of border disease on sheep in the UK, Sweasey et al. (1979) found that lambs from infected ewes had lower growth rates than other lambs and poorer carcass conformation.
- Bennett et al. (1999) report on the economic impact of contagious pustular dermatitis (orf), which is a contagious skin disease caused by a parapoxvirus. This disease is probably most important for the damage it does to the skin and the secondary infections it produces. Vaccines exist for its control and farmers with this problem have to pay attention to careful treatment of the damaged areas. The disease can also present itself in humans. The authors estimate that the losses in Britain are £1.8 million and that the costs including control costs are £3.6 million.

However, they state that these estimates are inadequate due to a lack of data.

External parasites

External parasites are very important, particularly in sheep systems, where disease such as sheep scab cause heavy losses in wool production. The following information was collected:

- Cole and Heath (1999) estimated that ectoparasites cost the New Zealand sheep industry US$60 million a year, a figure which includes treatment costs and production losses. The authors present data which suggests that costs can be reduced by integrated pest management and the control of nematodes to reduce dags on the sheep. The data presented indicate that these savings are between a quarter and a half of the present costs of controlling fly strike and lice.
- Bennett et al. (1999) describe the economics of blowfly strike in Great Britain. They report that between 60% and 90% of flocks in Britain will have at least one animal attacked each year; they predict that between 1% and 5% of the animals affected will die and that other losses will be related to fleece damage and decrease in growth rate. There are costs in terms of management to control this problem by dipping or spraying.

Summary

Sheep and goats are not in economic terms very important in the world livestock economy. In the tropical areas, they are normally found with poorer sections of society and in the industrialized countries their importance is in the production of wool, meat from young animals and in niche markets for milk and milk products. The most important diseases appear to be parasitic, either internal or external, and much research has been done on their impact and control in particular in Australia and New Zealand. However, PPR appears to be a disease that is of increasing importance and one of the few contagious diseases with little or no control programme.

19 Diseases of Pigs

Pigs in the World Livestock Economy

The main products from pigs are:

- meat and meat products;
- pig fat for cooking;
- manure.

According to FAO statistics, pigs are the most important species in the world for the supply of meat, supplying 40% of the world's meat supply (Seré and Steinfeld, 1995). Their importance is also growing as countries become richer and search for cheaper forms of meat and developed countries continue to prefer to eat white meat because of health concerns. However, the pattern of demand for pigmeat is not even throughout the world, in part because of religion, with pigmeat not being consumed by Muslims or Jews. Also in some parts of the world, pigmeat has a much greater importance. For example, in the region described as Asia, 60% of meat production comes from pigs, whereas in the North Africa region less than 1% of meat production comes from pigs. However, it should be noted that the analysis of meat production takes no account of milk and eggs, which are two other important sources of global animal protein.

Figure 19.1 shows the production of meat for the different regions of the world (see Sere and Steinfeld, 1996, for the countries in these regions).

Therefore, pigs are the most important species in the world in terms of meat production, but this production is concentrated in Asia, particularly South-east Asia and the Organization for Economic Cooperation and Development (OECD) countries. The reasons for the popularity of pigmeat are that it is relatively easy and cheap to produce as these animals are capable of surviving on a range of diets. This economic importance has led to considerable research on pig nutrition and health and the effective control and eradication of some contagious diseases.

Overview of Pig Diseases

The main pig diseases in the world are the following:

1. Swine vesicular disease.
2. Classical swine fever (CSF).
3. African swine fever (ASF).
4. Aujeszky's disease.
5. Atrophic rhinitis of swine.
6. Porcine cysticercosis (reviewed in Chapter 16, this volume).
7. Porcine brucellosis.
8. Transmissible gastro-enteritis.
9. Enterovirus encephalomyelitis.
10. Porcine reproductive and respiratory syndrome.

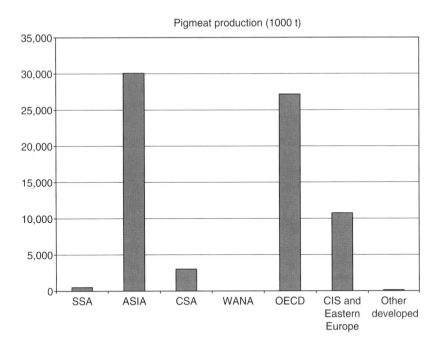

Fig. 19.1. Pigmeat production in the different regions of the world. (From Seré and Steinfeld, 1996.)

These diseases were on the OIE Lists A and B for livestock diseases. Other important diseases affect pigs such as FMD but these have been covered in the review of general diseases in Chapter 16 (this volume).

Information Available

Information is presented below on:

- general information on the importance of pig diseases;
- African swine fever (ASF);
- classical swine fever;
- Aujeszky's disease;
- PRRS; and
- multiple infections and other disease.

Readers interested in the impact of digestive, respiratory and reproductive diseases of pigs are referred to CABI's *Animal Health and Production Compendium*.

General information

The following information was collected on the general importance of pig diseases:

- Smits and Merks (2001) identified the most important pig diseases in Holland, classifying the diseases into three categories. They identify *Salmonella* (only specific strains), *Pasteurella multocida* DNT + PAR, *Actinobacillus pleuropneumoniae*, *Haematopinus suis* (lice) and *Sarcoptes scabiei* (var. suis; mange) as diseases that can be eradicated and recommend thatthe Dutch pig industry does not adopt the OIE list of diseases to direct pig veterinary services.

- Christensen *et al.* (1994) describe the Danish Health and Production Surveillance System and present results on the disease frequency measured on a daily basis. The most frequent diseases were: among sows, reproductive problems at farrowing (incidence 1.5 per 1000 sow-days); among non-weaned piglets, gastrointestinal diseases (incidence 0.8 per 100 piglet-days) and mortality (incidence 0.3 per 100 piglet-days); among fatteners, respiratory diseases (incidence four per 1000 fattener-days).

- Hall (1984) analysed data from a survey of veterinarians in north central USA. The author found that the main disease problems were: diarrhoea before weaning; non-specific piglet mortality; pneumonia; agalactia syndrome; and transmissible gastro-enteritis. The order of economic importance (losses due to the problems) of the conditions was: pneumonia; reproductive disorders; atrophic rhinitis; piglet diarrhoea; and 'housing/environment'.

- Penny and Penny (1978) surveyed the opinions of the members of the Pig Veterinary Society about priorities for pig research. The problems of the highest priority were reproduction/infertility, preventive medicine and economics of disease, atrophic rhinitis and neonatal enteritis. The authors added swine dysentery in a medium-priority group and Aujeszky's disease in a lower-priority group.
- Farez and Morley (1997) describe the risks of pork and pork products in the spread of foot-and-mouth disease (FMD), CSF (hog cholera), ASF and swine vesicular disease, emphasizing the importance of trade control on pig products. The authors suggest that risk analysis is required when importing pork and pork products from countries endemic with these diseases.
- Awa et al. (1999) provide a health status of pigs in north Cameroon. The most prevalent problem was ectoparasites, Haematopinus suis, with over half the pigs affected. Seroprevalence of ASF was only 2% and gastroenteritis prevalence was only 4%, but a major cause of piglet mortality. However, tuberculosis and cysticercosis prevalence were 33.2% and 12.3%, respectively.
- A study of diseases identified in the slaughterhouse in Turin, Italy, found that pneumonia had the highest prevalence (17.6%), followed by pleuritis (10.2%) and pleuropericarditis (6.5%; Griglio et al., 1992).
- Texdorf (1981) reported that 1.13% of pigs slaughtered in the Marburg slaughterhouse in Germany were condemned. The most important condemnation was tuberculosis and pale, soft, exudative (PSE) meat (25%), followed by cryptorchidism (17.7%), multiple abscesses

(15.14%) and influenza (10%). In addition, 18.1% of livers and 4.9% of hearts were condemned due to ascarid infections and swine influenza, respectively. The overall cost of condemnations was estimated to be 550,000 DM.

Classical swine fever

CSF is probably the most important livestock disease in terms of economic impact and trade after FMD. It is found in Europe, Asia and the Americas (OIE, 2001). The disease causes dramatic losses in both intensive and backyard systems and there are wildlife reservoirs of CSF, making it difficult to control and eradicate. The disease symptoms are indistinguishable from ASF, and in countries with both diseases there is a need for laboratory analysis to confirm an outbreak. There have been a number of studies on CSF concerned with its control and eradication in Europe.

An effective vaccine for classical swine fever exists, but once an outbreak occurs it is important to combine vaccination campaigns with strict movement controls. Vaccination of commercial herds is relatively straightforward, but is very difficult in backyard systems which have multi-age herds and regular introduction of young animals that are susceptible. The latter systems, which are associated with poor farmers, therefore need to vaccinate at least once every 6 months to achieve vaccination coverage that would protect the herd.

The following information on the disease was collected:

- Ellis (1972) made a retrospective study of the successful CSF eradication programme in Great Britain. He reports that the benefit/cost ratio for this programme was between 4.03 and 2.62.
- Ellis et al. (1977) analysed the eradication of CSF in the European Union (EU) and concluded that this programme would not exceed existing programmes and in some cases would be much lower.
- Mangen et al. (2001) assessed two different emergency vaccination strategies for the control and eradication of CSF

outbreaks in Holland using data from the outbreak in this country in 1997/1998. The two strategies were vaccination of contact herds because of a lack of capacity to destroy animals and vaccination by permission in order to move vaccinated animals and meat. Neither strategy proved to be advantageous over the slaughter policy adopted during the outbreak.

- Nielen *et al.* (1999) used a simulation model to assess the control policy adopted for the 1997/1998 CSF epidemic in Holland. Their analysis showed that pre-emptive slaughter was not as expensive as expected. They conclude that losses and the size of the epidemic could be reduced by improving farm-level biosecurity.

- Lai Thi Kim Lan (2000) estimated that losses per pig due to CSF ranged between US$23 and US$28 in Vietnam. At household level, this was between US$53 and US$295. The highest losses were recorded in systems that both raised pigs and fattened them.

- Saatkamp *et al.* (1997) analysed the use of an identification and recording system to control CSF in Belgium. Their analysis showed that such a system was only justified with a high frequency of CSF outbreaks.

- Lai Thi Kim Lan (2000) found that such an intensive vaccination strategy in the backyard systems of Vietnam could give positive results.

- In countries with disease-free status for CSF, there is a ban on imported pigs and pig products. Where outbreaks occur in such countries, a slaughter and destruction policy is usually adopted (Scott, 1990).

African swine fever

ASF is a peracute haemorrhagic disease with extremely high mortality rates (Wilkinson, 1993). The disease is found mainly in Africa, but there have been outbreaks in Europe. Less virulent forms of ASF exist where mortality is lower and chronic infections cause no clinical symptoms. Pigs that recover from ASF infection with less virulent strains may not show clinical symptoms if reinfected, but may replicate and shed the virus. As such, the carrier state may be significant for the epidemiology of the disease. The following sections are divided into the geographical spread of the disease, its impact on production and methods of control.

The disease and its geographical spread

- Transmission can occur directly from pig to pig, by infected meat or via soft ticks (Sumption, 1992). In much of Africa south of the Sahara, the disease is maintained among wild populations of warthogs and the soft tick *Ornithodoros moubata*.

- The disease is able to persist in the absence of this wildlife reservoir. In parts of Central and West Africa, ticks and warthogs are not present, yet the disease spreads easily among domestic pigs (FAO, 1998). The elimination of the disease from this ecological situation is extremely unlikely (Wilkinson, 1993).

- The scavenging habits of village pigs are considered to be a major route of infection. Pigs that are continuously confined are at much lower risk of the disease than those that are free range (Empres, 2000).

- Serious outbreaks of ASF continue to occur in parts of sub-Saharan Africa (Empres, 2000). The disease was first reported in West Africa in Senegal in 1978. The presence of the disease was confirmed in Cape Verde in 1980. Large-scale outbreaks occurred in Côte d'Ivoire in 1996 and in Benin, Togo and Nigeria in 1997. The countries involved lost a third or more of their pig populations. Despite stringent measures to prevent the entry of the disease Ghana was struck in September 1999.

- Senegal continues to suffer repeated small outbreaks each year, and a larger outbreak occurred in Gambia in April 2000 (New Agriculturalist, 2000).

- Since the 1980s, in Cape Verde outbreaks tend to occur twice a year, in spring and winter (FAO, 1998).

- The disease has been endemic in Cameroon since 1982 (Empres, 1998).
- ASF also occurs in Southern and East Africa. The disease has been reported in recent years in Malawi, Zambia, Angola and Mozambique (OIE, 2001). Outbreaks are reported to have occurred in Namibia and South Africa in 1998, in Kenya in 1994 and in Zimbabwe in 1992.
- An enzootic region is reported in the central region of Malawi, which extends into the Eastern Province of Zambia and south into the Tete Province of Mozambique (Haresnape *et al.*, 1987). An outbreak in the Ntchisi district of Malawi in 1981 killed 86% of the pigs in the infected area of 120 km² (Haresnape, 1984).
- An outbreak occurred in Botswana in June 1999 (Empres, 1999).
- Recent information indicates that ASF outbreaks have occurred in Nigeria, Kenya and Zambia.

Impact of the disease

- Indigenous pigs may be more resistant than exotic. However, the perception that indigenous pigs can 'fend for themselves' is reported to have contributed to the high mortality among this class of animals during the outbreak in Ghana in 1999 (Empres, 2000).
- Wilkinson *et al.* (1981) report that pigs experimentally infected with ASF virus showed 94% mortality rate and most died within the first 10 days of infection.
- Braco-Forte Junior (1970) reports that the 1957 outbreak of ASF in Portugal resulted in 471 properties being infected with 16,989 pigs affected. Of these pigs, 6352 died and the contact pigs were destroyed. The outbreak lasted 13 months.
- Disease outbreaks are reported to be a major factor limiting swine production in the Eastern Province of Zambia (Wilkinson *et al.*, 1988).

Control

At present, a vaccine is not available and control is based upon the slaughter of infected animals, movement restrictions and on the strict regulation of the importation of pigs and pig products. The following information was found on this aspect of the disease:

- The cooperation of the public, particularly pig keepers, is essential. It is reported that, during the 1982 outbreak in Cameroon, the initial good cooperation of farmers in the proper burial of infected pigs broke down as the outbreak continued and frustration mounted (Nana-Nukechap and Gibbs, 1985).
- Pigs suffering from ASF will often be slaughtered before they are investigated by the veterinary authorities or may be sold on to other villages, facilitating the spread of the disease (Haresnape, 1984).
- The ability to compensate farmers for the slaughter of their animals is important in ensuring an effective control programme. Compensation at market prices paid to pig farmers by the World Bank is considered to have been vital in bringing an outbreak in Nigeria in October 1999 under control (New Agriculturalist, 2000).
- Where ticks are involved in the spread of the disease, the use of acaricides may be able to reduce the incidence of the disease, but complete elimination of ticks from pigsties is difficult, as they are able to hide in cracks in mud and wood (Haresnape, 1988). As the ticks also infest human habitations and can be transferred from houses to pigsties, the burning of infested pigsties is also unlikely to be effective. Equally, the local practice of putting blankets over the roofs of pigsties may facilitate the transfer of ticks.

Summary

ASF is one of the most important pig diseases in the extensive pig systems found in Africa. It is also an important trade barrier disease. It is one of the few contagious diseases that is yet to have a vaccine and its control is difficult as wild pigs are reservoirs and the disease can also be spread by ticks.

Porcine reproductive and respiratory syndrome (PRRS)

PRRS is a relatively new disease, but one that has caused sufficient economic impact to be researched. The EU held a meeting to discuss this impact in 1991 (Dijkhuizen *et al.*, 1991). In the acute form this disease can be devastating but it appears that in the endemic form it does not cause serious losses. Losses include:

- fertility problems;
- increased mortality of young pigs;
- increased abortions or early farrowing;
- lung infection reducing feed conversion and daily weight gain; also leading to secondary infections.

Control measures include:

- vaccination;
- test and slaughter;
- restocking of herd.

The following information on the disease was collected:

- Dee *et al.* (2001) carried out an analysis of a test and removal policy to eradicate PRRS at farm level, which showed that it could be used to eradicate the disease. The diagnostic protocol cost US$10.66 and the authors suggest that more research is needed to see if the test and removal strategy is justified.
- Regula *et al.* (2000) found that subclinical PRRS caused a reduction in average daily growth rate of 40 g/day.
- Pejsak *et al.* (2000) report an outbreak of PRRS in Poland that caused recently infected gilts to give birth to dead or mummified piglets. The average number of piglets born alive to the infected gilts was 6.8, the number of pigs weaned was 6.2 and the number sold as fatteners 5.7.
- Nodelijk *et al.* (2000) found that although PRRS in its acute form caused economic impact the same disease caused little impact when it was endemically present.
- Pejsak *et al.* (1997) report that a clinical outbreak of PRRS caused sows to farrow

prematurely and that 1562 of 2067 piglets were born dead or died before weaning.

- Dee *et al.* (1997) found no differences in gross margins for pig herds seropositive and seronegative to PRRS.
- Teuffert *et al.* (1993) describe an outbreak of PRRS in a sow-breeding herd in Germany. The outbreak reduced the litter size and the percentage of unweaned and weaned pigs reared. There was also a decrease in the duration of pregnancy, the proportion of pregnant sows, the number of live piglets per sow and the conception rate in the presence of infection. Acute infections were associated with anoestrus and an increased culling rate due to infertility. The acute phase of the disease lasted 10–12 weeks and was followed by a chronic phase. Sows that recovered from PRRS virus infection produced litters of normal size. The estimated financial losses within the breeding herd without the 50,000 DM veterinary costs (treatments, examinations and parvovirus vaccinations) were estimated to be 442,831 DM, equivalent to 492 DM per sow in production (in 1991).
- Blanquefort (1995) evaluated a voluntary programme of control of PRRS in the Loire region of France.
- Brouwer *et al.* (1994) reported that Dutch pig farms affected with PRRS had severe problems for 4–6 months with losses of 215 guilders per sow. The losses related to smaller litter sizes, longer farrowing periods and higher replacement rates.

Aujeszky's disease

Aujeszky's disease affects pigs, cattle, rodents and other animals. It causes severe itching in the animal affected and in severe cases can kill animals. A majority of pigs survive after an outbreak and remain carriers of the disease. In young pigs, this disease can cause sudden deaths. The disease can be controlled by vaccination and there has been some interest in the assessment of control programmes in Europe and the USA, where decisions on vaccination or test and removal have required more complex epidemiological and economic analysis. The following information was found on this disease:

- Done and Ellis (1988) requested an economic analysis of Aujeszky's disease.
- Rodrigues *et al.* (1990) analysed the control and eradication of pseudorabies in pigs. They report that the expected monetary values for the vaccination and test and removal alternatives were similar. When the prevalence rate of pseudorabies virus was less than or equal to 57%, test and removal were optimum; otherwise, vaccination of sows only was recommended. However, sensitivity analysis showed that, when higher gross margins for the producer were assumed, test and removal were preferred at all prevalence rates. Vaccination was preferred with lower gross margins, lower vaccination costs or with better protective effect of pseudorabies virus vaccines.
- An economic analysis of the Aujeszky's disease control campaign in northern Germany concluded that mass vaccination of all pigs in regions with endemically infected herds followed by test and removal of seropositive animals is the most cost-effective way to control the spread of Aleutian disease virus (ADV) within pig populations (Willeberg *et al.*, 1996).
- Buijtels *et al.* (1997) examined the Dutch policy on Aujeszky's disease using a simulation model. Their analysis found that the disease could not be eliminated without vaccination and that to eradicate the disease sows needed to be vaccinated three times a year and fatteners twice per cycle. This policy was predicted to be sufficient to eradicate the disease in 2–3 years and the strategy became compulsory in Holland in October 1995.

Multiple infections and other diseases

The following information was found on other diseases and multiple infections:

- Madec *et al.* (2000) describe post-weaning multisystemic wasting syndrome (PMWS) in France which led to respiratory and digestive infections and increased mortality.
- Coronavirus infections, either transmissible or porcine respiratory coronavirus, are common in different regions of the world, Chae ChanHee *et al.* (2000) reporting animal prevalence of 53% and herd prevalence of 61% in Korea and Wesley *et al.* (1997) reporting that 91% of pigs tested in Iowa were seropositive to coronavirus.
- Bennett *et al.* (1999) report that the losses caused by *Streptococcus suis* type II meningitis in Great Britain were up to £940,000 and that the total cost including treatment was between £18,000 and £2.3 million. The authors note that there is severe lack of data on disease incidence, effects on production, treatment and control.

Summary

Pigs are a dominant species in world meat production, and their importance is greatest in South-east Asia and China. The importance of pig production is likely to grow as industrial systems of production have good feed conversion efficiency. With increased production from such systems, there are likely to be changes in the importance of pig disease, with greater needs to control the main infectious diseases covered in this chapter.

20 Diseases of Poultry

Importance of Poultry in the World Livestock Economy

Principal poultry products are:

- meat;
- eggs;
- manure;
- feathers.

Poultry provide a quarter of the world's meat supply and the most important areas of consumption and production are the OECD countries followed by Asia and the Central and South American countries (Fig. 20.1).

The order of production is similar for eggs, but the level of production in Asia is similar to that in the OECD countries (see Fig. 20.2). The combined production of eggs and poultry meat provides nearly 40% of the world's supply of meat and eggs.

In addition to these enormous contributions to the world's supply of protein, it is noted that ownership of poultry is much more widespread than other species. In rural areas of developing countries, it is common that 80–90% of families own poultry. The systems in which they are kept have low levels of production, but require little or no input. The numbers and production from this extensive poultry sector are small in comparison to the intensive poultry sector found throughout the world.

Poultry is one of the most important sources of animal protein in the world and this importance is growing, with people in developed countries looking to buy white meat and the developing countries investing in intensive poultry systems to reduce the costs of meat. The majority of the birds and production are concentrated in intensive poultry systems, which require high levels of disease control. The rest of the poultry population is found in low output–low input systems providing important sources of protein for rural people throughout the world.

Overview of Poultry Diseases

The main diseases of great economic importance are:

1. Newcastle disease.
2. Highly pathogenic avian influenza.
3. Avian infectious bronchitis.
4. Avian infectious laryngotracheitis.
5. Avian tuberculosis (reviewed under tuberculosis in the main diseases section).
6. Duck virus hepatitis.
7. Duck virus enteritis.
8. Fowl cholera.
9. Fowl pox.
10. Fowl typhoid (reviewed in Chapter 16, this volume, under Salmonella).

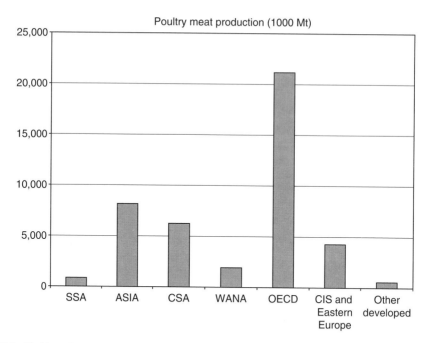

Fig. 20.1. World production of poultry meat in 1000 Mt. (From Seré and Steinfeld, 1995.)

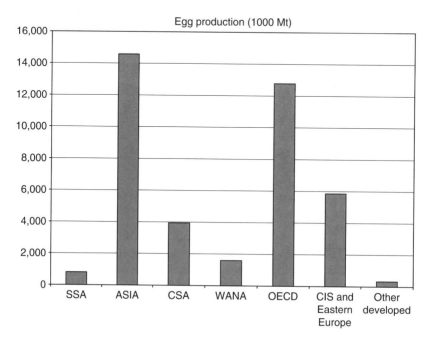

Fig. 20.2. World production of eggs in 1000 Mt. (From Seré and Steinfeld, 1995.)

11. Infectious bursal disease (Gumboro disease).
12. Marek's disease.
13. Avian mycoplasmosis (*Mycoplasma galli-septicum*).
14. Avian chlamydiosis.
15. Pullorum disease (reviewed under Salmonella in Chapter 16, this volume).

These poultry diseases were found in Lists A and B of OIE. Other important poultry diseases are not on this list, such as, for example, *Salmonella*, which due to its ability to cause infections in humans causes huge losses each year, and is reviewed in Chapter 16 (this volume). Below, information will be provided on diseases that cut across the disease classification and also information on the general incidence of disease in different geographical areas.

Information Available

This section is divided into:

- general information about poultry disease occurrence;
- Newcastle disease;
- Marek's disease;
- infectious bursal disease (IBD);
- *Mycoplasma meleagridis;*
- multiple infections and other diseases.

General information about poultry disease occurrence

The following information was gathered on the general occurrence of poultry diseases in the world:

- McIlroy (1994) identifies infectious bronchitis, Newcastle disease, avian influenza, Marek's disease, salmonellosis and the chicken anaemia virus as economically important diseases in broiler and broiler breed production.
- Christiansen *et al.* (1996) studied the diseases in turkey meat flocks as part of the National Animal Health Monitoring system in California. The data are from 1988–1989. They report that enteritis occurred in over one-third of the flocks,

and colibacillosis in nearly one-quarter of flocks. These were the most common diseases reported. *M. synoviae* was reported in two flocks and *M. gallisepticum* and *M. meleagridis* each were reported in one flock. Total mortality rate in the sample flocks was 9.0% (95% confidence interval (CI) 8.2–9.8%). The tom-specific mortality rate was 10.9% (95% CI 9.8–12.1%) and the hen-specific mortality rate was 6.6% (95% CI 5.7–7.4%).

- Aichberger (1986) reports on diseases encountered in broilers in Austria over the period of 1983–1985. The author found that just over half the slaughtered birds were seropositive to IBD, between 10% and 1% were positive to aviadenovirus and less than 1% were positive to infectious bronchitis virus and *M. synoviae*.
- Goren (1979) investigated virus infections in broiler flocks in Holland. The author found that 28 of 160 flocks had *M. synoviae* infections, but it had no impact on growth rates. However, the occurrence of colibacillosis and a high percentage of rejections due to polyserositis were associated with a higher occurrence of *M. synoviae* and infectious bronchitis virus than in flocks where these conditions did not occur. Infectious bursitis, infectious bronchitis and CELO (avian adenovirus) infections were prevalent in the south of The Netherlands, and they had an adverse effect on growth rates. Vaccination against infectious bursitis and infectious bronchitis did not seem to be very effective in flocks where the risk of infection was high.
- Palic *et al.* (1998) analysed the poultry diseases in Serbia between 1989 and 1998. They report that commonly recorded diseases with various degrees of severity were:
  - viral (Newcastle disease, infectious bronchitis, Marek's disease, avian infectious bursitis, infectious laryngotracheitis);
  - bacterial (salmonellosis, pasteurellosis, tuberculosis, mycoplasmosis, clostridial infections);
  - parasitic (ascaridiosis, histomoniasis);
  - protozoal (coccidiosis);

- mycotic diseases (aspergillosis, myco-toxicoses); and
- that deficiency diseases were also a serious problem.

- Kapetanov *et al.* (1998) analysed records from broiler flocks in Yugoslavia between 1988 and 1995, a total of 11.37 million birds. The mean mortality was 11.20% (range 6.50–14.89%). Technological faults were the commonest cause of mortality (24.61%) followed by mortality due to mycotoxicoses (14.45%) and *Escherichia coli* infections (13.06%). Other causes of mortality included omphalitis, salmonellosis, coccidiosis and aspergillosis. Mycotoxicoses accounted for 19.35% of financial losses, technological faults for 17.26% and *E. coli* infections for 15.93%.
- Nawathe and Lamorde (1982) reported that, in poultry in Nigeria, Newcastle disease is still responsible for heavy losses, followed by Gumboro disease and Marek's disease. Outbreaks of avian leucosis were common in heavy layers and egg drop syndrome has been identified on some commercial farms.
- Permin (1997) investigated diseases that affect poultry in the rural systems of the Morogoro Region of Tanzania. He found that 100% of the animals had endoparasites, of which the most common nematodes were *Tetrameres americana* (57%), *Heterakis gallinarum* (76%) and *Ascaridia galli* (30%) and the most common cestode was *Raillietina echinobothrida*. Nearly a third (28.5%) of the birds had antibodies against *S. gallinarum/pullorum* and 4.2% had antibodies against Newcastle disease virus.

Newcastle disease

Newcastle disease is probably one of the most important diseases in poultry in both commercial and rural backyard systems. Like many other diseases, there are many forms of Newcastle disease virus. Some are non-pathogenic, others mildly pathogenic and finally a group that causes serious losses in terms of lower egg production and high mortality.

This section is divided into work that has been carried out for the commercial sector and the work in the rural poultry sectors. The latter is dominated by the pioneering work of Peter Spradbrow supported by ACIAR in South-east Asia; the economics for this project was done by Joe Johnston. The Australians have also contributed one of the most thorough studies (Hafi *et al.*, 1997) on risks of introduction of Newcastle disease to a country free from the pathogenic forms of this disease and readers are recommended to refer to this publication for similar studies.

Commercial sector

FLOCK-LEVEL IMPACT
- Ring *et al.* (1988) analysed Newcastle vaccination of different poultry systems in Germany using cost–benefit analysis techniques. They found that, in all systems, the cost–benefit analysis was positive if they assumed that without vaccination there would be a Newcastle disease outbreak every 2 years.
- Kvarnfors *et al.* (1997) state that outbreaks in Sweden had occurred in 1956, 1981 and 1995. The last outbreak caused a dramatic drop in egg production in one of the country's biggest egg producers. In one house, production fell from 3000 to 70 eggs per day. Mortality was low and post-mortem of birds revealed no typical findings. High antibody titres for Newcastle disease initiated the destruction of 100,000 birds, 1.3 million brood eggs and day-old chicks and 350,000 hatchery eggs.
- Ganesan *et al.* (1993) describe a subclinical outbreak of Newcastle disease which had a serious impact on egg production. The outbreak was controlled with the revaccination of the flock with mesogenic Newcastle vaccine and egg production returned to normal.

SECTOR-LEVEL IMPACT
- Leslie (2000) presents an analysis of the costs of the 1973 Newcastle disease outbreak in Northern Ireland and compares how these costs would translate if a similar outbreak took place in 1997. She found

that the full cost of an outbreak had increased, although in real terms the costs of its control have fallen.

- Hafi *et al.* (1997) produced a document on the economic impact of Newcastle disease in Australia due to demands from the USA, Denmark, Thailand and New Zealand for a relaxation of Australian quarantine laws. Australia is free of pathogenic forms of Newcastle disease. The authors simulated an outbreak of Newcastle disease in the state of New South Wales to determine the economic impact of the introduction of this disease to Australia. They provide information on the Australia poultry industry stating that in 1992–1993 its gross value was AUS$1059 million, which represented 10% of the gross value from the Australian livestock sector. Their analysis looks at the advantages of importing meat from the countries mentioned, which would mean that poultry meat would be imported more cheaply than meat produced in the country. It also looked at the risks of Newcastle disease outbreaks with this importation of meat and the costs of the simulated outbreak. The results of this analysis are not straightforward and depend on the volume of imports. At low levels of imports, the predicted producer losses are high (AUS$152 million) and the benefits of imports are low (AUS$0.13 million). Even at high levels of importation, the benefits of imports (100,000 t/year) do not equal the predicted losses. The authors combine these results with risk analysis, which suggests that at low levels of imports the risk of disease entry would need to be very low (less than one chance in 1852). This is a very thorough analysis of the entry of an exotic disease to a free country and is recommended reading for people interested in such analysis.
- Omohundro and Walker (1973) report on the Newcastle disease epidemic in Southern California and Arizona in the USA. It took 20 months to eradicate the viscerotropic velogenic form of the disease and involved the slaughter of 11.58 million birds from 1321 flocks. The cost of this eradication was US$48 million.

Rural production systems

- Copland *et al.* (1988) describe a model to evaluate the economic impact of V4 vaccine of rural poultry in South-east Asia.
- Spradbrow (1990) describes the importance of Newcastle disease in rural poultry systems and the possibilities of control using heat-stable oral vaccines.
- Johnson (1990) made an economic analysis of the ACIAR programme of research into Newcastle disease and how it might best be controlled. The research involved the development of a heat-stable vaccine that could be delivered on food. The majority of the initial research was carried out in Malaysia, which adopted a widespread programme of vaccine delivery. In addition, work was carried out in Thailand, the Philippines, Indonesia and Sri Lanka. Johnston estimates that the flow of net benefits from the research in the five countries concerned was in the region of AUS$389 million.
- Johnston *et al.* (1992) describe the economic analysis of oral vaccination of the 43 million birds in Philippine villages. They estimated that the returns to this programme would be 13.8 times greater than the costs.
- Johnston (1993) describes a model to assess the benefits from campaigns to vaccinate rural poultry against Newcastle disease in Asia.
- Spradbrow (1993) details the information on the economic impact of Newcastle disease in backyard poultry systems. He mentions that it is one of the most important reasons for mortality in these systems and quotes that this disease annually kills 70–80% of unvaccinated village chickens. The author also states that the fact that most local languages have a name for Newcastle disease is a good indication of its prevalence and importance.
- Awan *et al.* (1994) in their review of Newcastle disease in rural poultry comment that although this disease is an important constraint in these systems it is not the only one. It is likely that effective control of Newcastle disease will not increase bird numbers dramatically as other constraints such as feed supply will then have an impact.

Marek's disease

Marek's disease is worldwide and caused important economic losses in the 1960s that led to research into a vaccine to control the disease. Ansell (1988) identifies the following losses due to this disease:

- broilers:
  - carcass condemnations;
  - mortality;
  - lower feed conversion.
- broiler breeders:
  - carcass condemnation;
  - mortality.
- layers:
  - carcass condemnation;
  - mortality;
  - lower egg production.

The following information on the economic impact of Marek's disease has been collected:

- Ansell (1988) used the analysis structure above and information on the costs of research into vaccination against Marek's disease between 1960 and 1983 to calculate the returns on the research. He states that the returns were very high with a benefit/cost ratio (BCR) of 30.
- Bennett et al. (1999) estimated that the losses due to Marek's disease in Great Britain are between £0.5 and £3.2 million and that total costs including control are between £1.2 and £4.5 million.
- Calnek and Witter (1997) provide information on the percentage of condemnations due to Marek's disease which shows a peak in the late 1960s and early 1970s followed by a steady decline presumably due to vaccination through to 1995.
- Voigtlander et al. (1991) reported that vaccination against Marek's disease in broilers after an outbreak of this disease reduced mortality by 30%, carcass rejection by 7% and increased profit per bird by 2.5%.
- Tadic and Bidin (1988) studied Marek's disease in poultry farms in Croatia. The disease caused 2.18% mortality of the parent hybrids and was found to have affected carcass quality in 7% of the birds produced. The total loss due to Marek's disease per layer was estimated to be

US$14.85 and the total losses due to parent birds dying in Yugoslavia in 1986 were estimated to be US$712,206.

- A study in the German Democratic Republic in 1972 found that vaccination against Marek's disease in broiler chicks was justified economically when they were kept at high concentrations under unfavourable conditions, and for a fattening period exceeding 40–50 days (Werner et al., 1987).
- Powell (1986) reports that Marek's disease is still a disease of major economic importance in the world even though vaccination had avoided the outbreaks that were seen in the 1960s. The author's concern is the appearance of more virulent strains of the virus.
- Ring et al. (1985) analysed data from the German Federal Republic and The Netherlands for 1982, and found that Marek's disease vaccination produced a saving of at least ten times the cost of administering the live vaccine. Heinze (1984) reports that costs of vaccine were on average DM 0.034 per chick and the application DM 0.019 per chick.
- Lee (1980) in a trial with white Leghorn chicks found that vaccination against Marek's disease did not affect growth or mortality in young birds, but vaccinated birds went on to produce more and heavier eggs. These vaccinated laying birds also had lower mortality rates.
- Purchase and Schultz (1978) state that between 1965 and 1974 research expenditure on avian leucosis was US$32 million. Their economic analysis of this work on the control of Marek's disease indicates a BCR of 22 if only the costs from 1965 are taken into account and a BCR of 4 if costs going back to 1939 are included.
- Lee and Reid (1977) found that there were no differences in growth, mortality or egg production between a group of vaccinated and non-vaccinated Single Comb White Leghorn pullets.

Infectious bursal disease

IBD is extremely difficult to assess in terms of its economic impact in that it has a number of different serotypes with different levels of pathogenicity. Obviously designing tests that can distinguish between serotypes is also difficult. The disease is also associated with other infections as one of its impacts is immunosuppression. The following information from the literature was collected:

- Binta *et al.* (1995) describe an outbreak of IBD in the towns of Gaborone, Francistown and Mochudi in Zimbabwe. The outbreak occurred between 1989 and 1993 with an average of 11 outbreaks per year mainly in commercial flocks. The outbreaks were associated with infections of Newcastle disease, colisepticaemia, salmonellosis, *Staphylococcus aureus* and mycoplasmosis. Post-mortem revealed ecchymotic haemorrhages in the thigh muscles and the subcutaneous tissue around the thigh either unilaterally or bilaterally. There was also dwarfism or stunting of the broilers as a result of poor feed conversion and concurrent diseases were a sequel to infection.
- Bennett *et al.* (1999) report that it was not possible to estimate the losses due to IBD in the UK because of a lack of data on the disease incidence. They did, however, estimate that the control costs through vaccination were £3.8 million/year.
- McIlroy *et al.* (1993) found that there was a positive impact of increasing vitamin E in the diets of birds with subclinical IBD. Their analysis showed that the performance of flocks with subclinical IBD was consistently worse in terms of net income, feed conversion ratio and average weight per bird than flocks without subclinical disease (McIlroy *et al.*, 1989). In their trial the average net income of flocks with subclinical IBD and fed a high vitamin E-containing diet was 10% better than that from flocks with subclinical IBD and fed a normal vitamin E-containing diet. The difference between the average net income achieved by flocks without subclinical IBD and being fed on either a high or a normal vitamin E-containing diet was only 2% and not significantly different.

Mycoplasma meleagridis

Mycoplasma meleagridis has a series of papers on its economic impact in the USA which have been authored or co-authored by Carpenter:

- Carpenter and Riemann (1980) report that a programme of eradication of *M. meleagridis* by dipping hatching eggs was economically justified.
- Carpenter (1980) estimated that the impact of *M. meleagridis* infection on hatchability was 5%. He calculated that the impact occurred between the 25th and 28th days of infection and would account for losses of up to US$7.5 million/year in the USA. The cost of the control of egg-transmission was estimated to be US$1.4 million, giving a total annual cost of this infection as approximately US$9 million.
- Carpenter *et al.* (1981a) examined two different control programmes for *M. meleagridis*. One included egg dipping, which was predicted to give a return of US$1.58 per hen, and the other option where egg dipping was not necessary would give a return of US$2.06.
- Carpenter *et al.* (1981b) report that turkey eggs experimentally infected with *M. meleagridis* showed a decrease in production of first-quality poults of approximately 20% when compared with uninoculated controls. They estimated that the total economic losses associated with decreased hatchability caused by *M. meleagridis* and the cost of a control programme were estimated to be US$9.4 million/year in the USA.
- Carpenter (1983) reports a difference in weight between turkeys with and without *M. meleagridis* infection. This weight difference translated into a profit of US$ 0.06 per bird.

Multiple infections and other diseases

The following information is available on multiple infections and other diseases:

Mycoplasmas

- In an experiment with the dual infection with *M. gallisepticum* and *M. synoviae* Branton *et al.* (1997) found that no significant difference was found between control and infected birds for hen-day egg production, egg weight or eggshell strength.
- Mohammed *et al.* (1987) investigated the losses in commercial layer flocks in California, USA, due to *M. gallisepticum* and *M. synoviae*. They found that a *M. gallisepticum* infected flock produced between 12 and five fewer eggs per hen than an uninfected flock, but that *M. synoviae* had no impact on egg production. They estimated that commercial layer producers in southern California lost an estimated 127 million eggs because of *M. gallisepticum* in 1984. This lost egg production and associated control programme costs amounted to an estimated financial loss of approximately US$7 million. This represented a loss of approximately US$6 million in consumer surplus.
- Harada *et al.* (1986) reported that oxytetracycline and doxycycline treatment of layer and broiler birds to control *M. gallisepticum* and *M. synoviae* infections improved growth rates and egg production. No costs and benefits are presented.
- Landgraf and Vielitz (1983) report on the experimental infection of laying hens with *M. gallisepticum* and *M. synoviae*. They found that hens infected had higher monthly mortality rates (0.5–0.7%) and lower monthly egg production (infection caused it to fall from 87% to 69%).

Multiple infections

- Jorgensen *et al.* (1995) studied subclinical infections of IBD virus, adenoviruses, reoviruses and chicken anaemia virus in broiler birds. They found that there was no significant effect on flock performance for any of the viral infections either alone or in combination.

Skeletal diseases

- Bennett *et al.* (1999) estimated that skeletal problems in the broiler, breeder and commercial layer parts of the poultry industry in the UK caused between £11.8 and £24.1 million worth of losses.
- Bisgaard *et al.* (1981) examine the condemnations due to arthritis in ducks in Denmark. Between 1959 and 1968 the condemnations due to this problem were 0.4% of the ducks slaughtered. However, the introduction of compulsory measures to control salmonella reduced this to 0.12% between 1969 and 1978. They estimated that the national annual cost of arthritis from 1959 to 1968 was 207,579 Danish crowns and that during the next 10 years the cost was only one-third of this sum.

Summary

The world poultry sector supplies 40% of the world's meat and egg protein in terms of weight. This supply is largely from intensive or industrial production systems, which have huge investments in breeding programmes, housing, feeding and processing. The industrial systems also invest considerable amounts of money in research on poultry diseases. The result of this investment is obvious to see, in that a number of important contagious disease such as Newcastle disease, avian influenza and Marek's disease have been brought under control and in some areas eradicated. In contrast, the other components of the poultry sector are the rural scavenge-based systems found in nearly all countries that are low input–low output systems. These systems also suffer disease problems, but investments in research are very small and the investments at farm level in terms of control almost non-existent. However, the impact of diseases at this level can be devastating, causing hardship to poor families and also risks of infection to the intensive sector.

Part III

Economic Analysis and Policy Making: Examples from Around the World

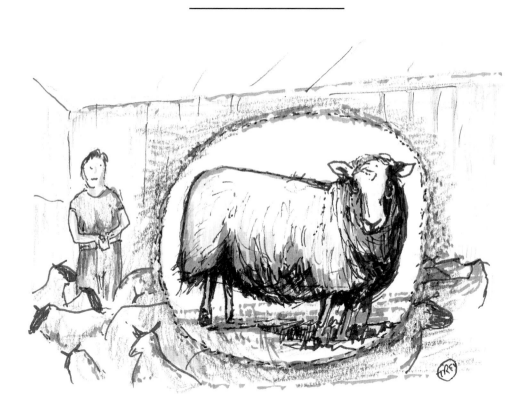

Introduction

The challenges that face livestock sectors around the world are different and dependent on many factors from agroecological to socio-political. Rushton (2006) classifies countries into three groups, which are specified below.

The developed world has eradicated most of the important contagious diseases from their domestic livestock. They are faced with challenges with regard to preventing the entry of contagious diseases from outside (FMD), from wildlife populations (CSF, tuberculosis) or through vector-borne spread (bluetongue). These countries face challenges in terms of maintaining adequate veterinary services for farm livestock systems where, although livestock numbers are the same, the number of producers is becoming smaller. There are also problems with endemic diseases and questions about who should pay for their prevention and control.

In the developing world, there is a divide between countries actively involved in the livestock product trade, who since the late 1980s have aggressively controlled and in some cases eradicated contagious diseases in order to have access to the most important and rich markets for their products. The examples of FMD and CSF control and eradication in the Americas are probably the most obvious, but we should not forget the efforts of the Thais to control highly pathogenic avian influenza (HPAI) and modify their poultry sector in order to maintain their exports. These changes are dramatic and deserve further work on how these countries have achieved such rapid advances, often in the face of socioeconomic and political difficulties.

There is a final category of countries identified that have weak governments, weak livestock sectors and no strong ability to participate in international trade. These countries' efforts on livestock development and animal health control have largely been driven by aid agendas that have often been inconsistent in their advice. There are examples of drives to control diseases such as ECF, CBPP and some zoonoses, but these efforts are patchy. The most successful campaign is the eradication of rinderpest across the world, a disease that had favourable technical factors for its eradication such as a relatively thermostable vaccine that confers life-long immunity.

The following contributions have been selected from different regions and countries with an intention to provide a snapshot of the main challenges being faced in very different environments.

- Joachim Otte and Ugo Pica-Ciamarra provide an overview of the livestock policies required to help poor livestock producers around the world.
- Liz Redmond and Harvey Beck detail the difficulties of planning an animal health service in a country where the budget is dominated by controlling tuberculosis.
- Hernán Rojas discusses animal health disease status and trade from his experience in South America and more specifically Chile.
- Pascal Bonnet and Matthieu Lesnoff discuss how to define a strategy for CBPP in an environment where much external assistance is still required.
- Vinod Ahuja describes the challenges of veterinary service delivery in an environment where most livestock keepers are smallholders.
- Devendra discusses the challenges of increasing livestock product supply in environments not traditionally associated with livestock production.

For readers interested in further analysis of animal diseases in different regions, they are referred to the following documents:

- Developed countries – with a focus on the control of contagious disease in naive populations:
  - FMD in the UK is well documented by Power and Harris (1973) for the 1967–1968 outbreak, Thompson *et al.* (2002) for the 2001 outbreak and the House of Commons (2008) for the 2007 outbreak.
  - Classical swine fever control in Europe has been well covered by work done at Wageningen University (Mangen *et al.*, 2001; Mangen, 2002).
  - Avian influenza control in The Netherlands (Stegeman *et al.*, 2004).
- Developed countries – with a focus on the control of endemic diseases:
  - UK-based work on endemic disease control by Alistair Stott (Stott, 2005) and Richard Bennett (Bennett, 1992; Bennett, 2003).
  - Tim Carpenter's work on *Mycoplasma meleagridis* in the USA (Carpenter *et al.*, 1979; Carpenter, 1980).
- Developing country challenges:
  - FMD studies carried out by Brian Perry and colleagues for South-east Asia (Perry *et al.*, 1999) and Southern Africa (Perry *et al.*, 2003).

- Newcastle disease control in backyard production systems (Spradbrow, 1993) and avian influenza in a region (Rushton *et al.*, 2005).
- General challenges for developing livestock and animal health policy in Africa (Perry *et al.*, 2002, 2005; Scoones and Wolmer, 2006; Rushton *et al.*, 2006a).

- The need to combine different skills in mapping, economics and disease risk (Wint and Robinson, 2007; Shaw *et al.*, 2006).
- Service delivery in developing countries well documented for Africa in a book by David Leonard (2000) and Vinod Ahuja's study in India (Ahuja *et al.*, 2000).

21 Livestock Policy and Poverty Reduction: Experiences from the Developing World

Joachim Otte and Ugo Pica-Ciamarra

Introduction

Increasing population, income growth and urbanization in developing countries are boosting the demand for food of animal origin. This trend provides significant opportunities for poverty reduction, as an estimated 42% of the poor worldwide are dependent on livestock as part of their livelihood.

However, imperfect or missing markets often trap poor livestock keepers in low-income equilibria, preventing them from deriving major benefits from the increased demand for animal protein. Thus, if poverty alleviation is a policy goal, policy makers should identify, design and implement public actions that allow poor livestock producers to take advantage of the increasing demand for meat and milk. This is, however, not a simple task: livestock sector development is shaped by an intertwined mixture of macroeconomic and agricultural sector policies, with livestock sector-specific interventions playing a subordinate role, while policy makers in the livestock departments tend to design livestock sector policies in isolation with minimal consultation with other ministries or representatives of the livestock sector.

A Framework for Pro-poor Livestock Policies

In the last decades, most developing countries have gone through orthodox macroeconomic and institutional reforms. These have promoted economic growth but largely failed to significantly benefit poor livestock keepers. The policy challenge, therefore, is not only to create a conducive macroeconomic and institutional environment, but also to make the growth process pro-poor.

To ensure that poor livestock keepers are included in, and contribute to, economic growth, governments should design and implement policies targeted at achieving three major objectives:

1. *Establishing the basics for livestock production*, i.e. providing poor livestock holders with adequate and secure access to basic production inputs. This objective contains two subsidiary policy objectives, which are:
  (a) securing access to land, water and feed; and
  (b) providing risk-coping mechanisms for natural disasters and price shocks.

Insecure access to basic inputs and variability of returns prevent livestock keepers from making efficient use of their scarce resources and from effectively responding to market signals. For instance, high variability of returns may induce pastoralists to overstock and to use livestock as a form of insurance rather than as a means of production.

2. *Kick-starting domestic markets for livestock and derived products.* This objective has three subsidiary policy objectives, namely to provide secure access to:

(a) livestock services;
(b) credit and secondary inputs, such as compound feeds; and
(c) domestic output markets.

Poor livestock producers, in fact, even when 'having access to the basics', may be locked into low-income equilibria as missing or imperfect markets prevent them from availing themselves of the production-increasing inputs necessary to escape poverty. For instance, high fixed transaction costs and lack of information hinder price transmission, potentially preventing smallholders from fully benefiting from a prospective increase in meat/milk price.

3. *Sustaining and expanding livestock production.* Three sub-objectives are subsumed under this overall objective:

(a) securing food safety and quality of livestock products according to national, regional and international standards;
(b) promoting research activities in animal feeding and breeding to support the production of high-quality commodities; and
(c) ensuring the environmental sustainability of livestock production.

These are mostly public goods and necessary elements for countries to be competitive in international markets as well as to avoid smallholders being crowded out from their domestic markets by foreign competitors. For instance, livestock research activities driven by the profit-seeking efforts of private institutions rarely serve the poor, who are thought unwilling or unable to pay for research outcomes.

Unfortunately, evidence from Asia, Africa and Latin America has shown that livestock sector policies are not explicitly designed to be pro-poor. In many poor countries, national policy documents emphasize the importance of interventions to 'kick-start domestic markets', with a focus on input over output markets. Reforms are undertaken in credit markets and in animal health and extension service delivery, while marketing and market information are only marginally addressed. Some attention has also been paid to policies for expanding and supporting long-run livestock production, such as the reform of research institutes, and the opening of markets supported by measures to satisfy international sanitary standards.

Conclusions and Recommendations

With a view to rural poverty reduction, the current policy framework of many countries appears unbalanced. It implicitly focuses on livestock production and productivity, rather than on poor livestock holders and their livelihoods. Current policies, in fact, are biased towards 'kick-starting domestic livestock markets' and 'expanding to international output markets'. Yet, poor livestock holders will only respond to policies designed for 'kick-starting' and 'expanding' markets, and hence escape poverty, when access to basic production inputs is secured and vulnerability to shocks is reduced.

To improve this situation and ensure that livestock policies have a combined growth and poverty reduction impact, governments should be more aware of the 'economic' behaviour of the rural poor and take the poor livestock-producing household rather than a production function as the entry point for policy design. This would imply focusing not only on technical issues and market policies but also on strategies promoting access to basic resources, and reducing vulnerability and transaction costs of small livestock producers. Only then will input and output market policies be effective, sustainable and pro-poor.

22 Economics in Animal Health Policy Making in Northern Ireland

Liz Redmond and Harvey Beck

Introduction

Economics is just one of many but central inputs into the policy-making cycle in Northern Ireland. It is applied at a number of stages in the policy development and review cycle, from the early stages of policy development, the establishment of a need for policy and the appraisal of policy options, through to the monitoring and evaluation of the effectiveness of existing policy and policy review. This policy development framework in Northern Ireland is well documented, with an accompanying practical document. These guides are very clear that economics is central to policy development in that all *proposals should be supported by evidence of suitable appraisal, approval, management and evaluation. There are no exceptions to this general requirement'* regardless of where the financing has come from.

The process in Northern Ireland will be illustrated by a case study involving a review of policy of bovine tuberculosis (TB) control. It is important to remember that the process is iterative, with a monitoring process once a policy has been implemented.

for a large proportion of expenditure by the Northern Ireland state veterinary service. This policy review illustrates the difficulties, limitations and imperfections encountered in applying economics to animal health policy making. The review adopted an interdisciplinary approach with a team led by a policy professional, and including people with skills in veterinary science, economics, finance and laboratories. An external audit firm was also engaged to undertake some of the economic analysis. Economics featured in the terms of reference to the TB review at two main stages in the policy development process:

1. Evaluation of the existing approach is the assessment of costs, benefits and evaluation of value for money (VFM) of the current approach, and identification of VFM indicators.
2. Appraisal of options is the assessment of public expenditure implications of options and identification of recommendations.

The review had various stages, which are detailed in the following sections.

The Review of Tuberculosis in Northern Ireland

In 2002, a major review of TB policy in Northern Ireland was completed, a disease that accounts

Defining the need

In Northern Ireland, there is a 5-year policy review cycle and the TB control policy review should have been carried out in 2000, but was not complete until 2002 due to the FMD crisis in Great Britain. The review found that TB control costs were increasing and, of the £17 million spent in 2001/2002, a third was used in farmer compensation. The hope at the time was that some of this compensation money could be quickly saved in the more innovative way of public–private partnerships.

Having defined a need for change the next step is to establish an evidence base.

Establishing an evidence base

The evidence drawn on included epidemiology, developments in scientific research, field expertise from within the department, and economic evaluation of the existing approach. However, the extent to which the evidence base could be developed was limited by the considerable political and industrial pressure to move quickly to complete the review, in light of rapidly increasing disease levels and expenditure over the preceding few years. In order to meet the tight deadline set for the review, a deliberate decision was taken to complete the review based on indicative costs and qualitative assessment of benefits, with the option of further detailed analysis of accepted recommendations following later.

In particular, one of the main criticisms of this work was the fact that it relied heavily on descriptive epidemiology and expert epidemiological opinion. Had there been more time and resources available, it would have been preferable to develop a more detailed analysis of the disease picture at this stage in the review, in particular a detailed analysis of the factors causing the increasing disease trend. This would have allowed for better estimation of benefits in the economic evaluation and appraisal of options later in the review.

In terms of the economic evaluation (evidence base), two key questions had to be answered:

1. Whether the programme was cost beneficial (i.e. do benefits outweigh costs?); and
2. Whether it represented good VFM (i.e. could costs be lower and/or benefits greater?).

For the first, the conclusion was that the benefits exceeded costs by a reasonable margin simply by preventing adverse production effects. To come to this conclusion, data were drawn from the Republic of Ireland studies into production losses associated with TB. These were estimated to be at least £20 million per annum. Other non-quantifiable benefits could be assumed to add to these saved production losses, including potential trade access with resumption of exports, human health and animal welfare benefits.

This benefit was set against the annual cost to government of the control programme of £17 million, and although somewhat rough and ready this could be used to indicate that the programme was cost beneficial and economically worthwhile.

VFM can be taken as applying at the level of the overall economy or simply to public expenditure. The latter narrower definition was adopted in this review as the approach was simpler and quicker. However, transfer of costs to the private sector would maximize value in public money terms alone even though this may not change the overall VFM to the economy, which raises the issue of distribution.

Three components of VFM as defined in the Treasury Greenbook were: economy, efficiency and effectiveness. Conclusions from looking at these were:

- In terms of **economy** (i.e. achieving lowest possible cost), total annual compensation costs and costs in terms of staff time and fees were identified as the main areas for potential savings. A complex relationship exists between these costs areas, as restricting staff costs, in particular, may have led to increased disease levels and hence compensation costs. Of these, compensation levels therefore offered most scope for reduction.
- In terms of **efficiency** (i.e. ratio of outputs to inputs), it was difficult to find a suitable measure due to lack of management information (e.g. administrative and testing costs per outbreak). Cost per reactor was counter-intuitive, in that it had actually been decreasing as incidence increased (fixed cost spread over more reactors).

- In terms of **effectiveness** (i.e. difference between what is expected from a policy and what it delivers), it was considered that the existing eradication goal of the programme could only be achievable in the very long term, and in face of rising incidence it should be replaced with 3- and 5-year targets of reduced reactor numbers.

Another potentially useful indicator of the VFM from this programme is the ratio of input (disease control programme expenditure) to gross output in terms of the commodity (Northern Ireland beef and milk). The higher the indicator, the lower is the VFM. The VFM had been decreasing by this measure, and this decrease had accelerated in the year preceding the review. In crude terms, the cost of the programme to government had reached 4% of the gross value of the commodity, which certainly must have been an unsustainable situation.

Stakeholder analysis and consultation

At this stage key stakeholders were asked to give their views on the current programme and on what areas they thought the review should consider. Feedback from stakeholders was considered when building up options for appraisal.

Policy linkages

In terms of policy linkages, approaches in Great Britain and the Republic of Ireland were considered and comparisons made. In terms of learning, the approach taken in New Zealand was also examined.

Generate policy options

Policy options, offering the potential to improve performance in terms of economy, efficiency and/or effectiveness, were identified by the review team based on their expert opinion and consideration of the evidence, stakeholder views and policy linkages.

The review team consolidated a list of 12 options into a short list of five, by a two-step process. Step one was weighting and scoring each of the 12 components against four criteria:

- impact on incidence of disease;
- robustness (i.e. how well the information used to produce the recommendation would stand up to scrutiny);
- consensus among scoring team; and
- sustainability of net benefits over time.

High-scoring options were then rated 'A', medium-scoring were rated 'B', and low-scoring were rated 'C'. The following five options were identified:

- Do nothing – status quo.
- Do minimum (European Union (EU) compliance – inconclusive reactor requirement, dealer registration, restrictions on overdue tests).
- Option A (do minimum + boundary fencing, Animal and Plant Health Inspection Service (APHIS) augmentation, pre-movement testing, review testing arrangements, badger research).
- Option B (option A + changes to valuation and compensation).
- Option C (option B + charge for late tests, biometric identification, contract cattle housing).

The 'do nothing' option was the status quo and the baseline case from which costs and benefits were then measured. The 'do minimum' option consisted of changes to current policy needed to bring Northern Ireland fully into compliance with EU statutory requirements.

Economic appraisal of options

The next step was economic appraisal of the options. Both qualitative and quantitative analyses were carried out. The technique of qualitative analysis, applied to assess non-monetary benefits, was fairly simplistic, and the results were of lesser significance in the choice of preferred option. The remainder of the paper will therefore focus on the quantitative analysis of costs and benefits, and the assessment of public expenditure implications of the options.

Ideally both the costs and benefits of all option components should be quantified. Unfortunately in this case, as for the evaluation of the existing programme, only limited benefits calculation was done, due to tight time frames and data limitations (lack of sufficient epidemiological modelling and cost data).

There were only two components for which benefits were quantified (changes to valuation and compensation, and pre-movement testing). For the other components a cost only approach was taken, i.e. calculating the total cost of the option. This was consistent with the Treasury Greenbook total cost approach. A full cost–benefit analysis was not done because benefits could not be quantified in all cases.

The analysis was limited to costs attributable to government, as the review was primarily concerned with development of policy that offers best VFM to the public purse and farmer costs (consequential) were estimated to be *de minimus* compared with the size of compensation payments.

A 5-year appraisal period was chosen. Net present cost (NPC) was calculated (quantifiable costs plus quantifiable savings) and discounted over 5 years at 6% in line with the Treasury Greenbook approach at the time (now revised to 3.5%).

A static baseline was used that reflected a situation in which disease incidence (i.e. total TB reactors as percentage of all animals tested) remained at 2000 levels, whereas the trend baseline represented an increase in disease incidence, which had been the trend since 1995. This forecast was a linear extrapolation derived by simple regression analysis of the past trend. It assumes that under the status quo the disease incidence will continue to rise.

Using the static baseline, all options were more costly in terms of public expenditure than doing nothing, and if this assessment alone was used then there would be no justification for doing anything new or different. Using a trend baseline, which reflected the position more likely to occur if there was no new intervention to turn around the rising incidence at the time, option 'do minimum plus A + B' is equivalent to doing nothing but with the advantage of meeting EU requirements. All other options were more costly than doing nothing.[1]

The 'do minimum' option is so costly because it included a policy on removal of second-time inconclusive reactors, which was estimated to substantially increase the number of animals removed and compensated but with little benefit in terms of reduced TB incidence. Although this measure is included in other options, the savings associated with the other measures reduce the disease incidence and net cost.

Choose preferred option

The review made the recommendation that the 'do minimum plus A and B' option be adopted. This package meets EU requirements and the status quo would not have been a politically acceptable option in light of rising incidence.

Implement: plan and deliver

Approval was obtained from the Department of Finance and the Minister, followed by further consultation with stakeholders. Stakeholder feedback resulted in slight modifications to details within the final package of measures for implementation. Implementation of main measures started in the second half of 2004.

Monitoring and evaluation

Post-review evaluation indicators are framed around the reduction in the number of TB

---

[1] Note that this calculation is based on attributing a monetary cost of £16 million over 5 years to the status quo and 'do minimum' options. The assumption was made that both the status quo and 'do minimum' options would have no impact on existing levels of TB and would be associated with a continued rise in incidence, at an additional cost of £16 million over 5 years. The assumption was made that all other options would maintain disease incidence at 2000 levels.

reactor animals and the reduction in costs to government (programme costs and compensation costs). Reporting against these indicators to the Department of Finance started in January 2005 and is done at 6-monthly intervals. Progress against the targets has been good because of a significant decline in disease incidence during 2005, though attribution to the review measures is difficult. Another major review of the TB programme is expected in 2007/2008.

Immediately after the review was published, the incidence of TB was still increasing and the actual incidence quickly diverged from the static baseline of 2000 levels and exceeded the trend line, with associated increased programme costs (increasing from £16.7 million in 2000/2001 to £24.5 million in 2004/2005). If the cost savings had been measured against this baseline, then the savings would have been even greater than estimated against the trend baseline. In other words, actual savings are likely to have exceeded estimates.

The VFM has increased since the review, though is lagging slightly behind the substantial drop in TB incidence seen in 2005 due to the need to maintain a high input of labour to maintain the effort to reduce disease levels.

What can be learnt from this case study?

The Treasury Greenbook approach is very broad and animal health policy does not fit very easily into the framework (particularly in a cost-constrained environment). The application of this approach to the TB programme presented many challenges, and when the review is assessed strictly against this approach it shows many weaknesses.

In particular, data limitations impacted heavily on the ability to estimate benefits. This is often a problem for animal disease policy analysis, since there are so many uncertainties and much unpredictable background 'noise'. Detailed understanding of disease epidemiology is an important element in improving benefit estimation. In Northern Ireland, the epidemiological capacity has been significantly strengthened and enhanced since this review was done, and data are now greatly improved. These data are currently being used to undertake further work on some of the policy options identified in this study.

Better and cost-effective methods for drawing in non-monetary costs and benefits of animal health programmes would also make a significant contribution to improving the approach.

Despite the weaknesses in the detail of the analysis, adhering to the government guidelines certainly led to acceptance of this review by central government funders, and continued acceptance. In addition most of the features of good policy making were present, such as the need to be *forward* and *outward looking* through a process that is *inclusive* with *effective communication*. This process has to have an *evidence base*, be *joined up*, encourage *innovative* and through *evaluation and review* allow *lessons to be learnt*.

Conclusion

Economic input is an integral part of the policy development process and evidence-based policy decision making, and to government decision makers the concept of economics and VFM are synonymous.

When applying policy development frameworks in real situations, it is important to remember practicality and proportionality. Frameworks are important but their application requires flexibility in light of logistics, human and economic resource constraints. Therefore, there needs to be the application of economic principles in a policy review process, which recognizes that economic studies are the best approximations of reality given the resources available. Improving these approximations cannot be done during the review process, but requires a continual improvement in data collection and analysis that are used in such reviews. The review itself can help highlight where these continual processes need to be strengthened.

23 Animal Diseases Management in a New Livestock Trade Environment: the Case of Chile

Hernán Rojas

The Starting Point

Chile has a very good animal health status, being free of the main transboundary diseases.[1] Newcastle disease (NC), foot-and-mouth disease (FMD) and classic swine fever (CSF) have been eradicated in the country as a result of campaigns that involved public–private partnerships. These campaigns started in the 1960s. In addition, the country has effective control programmes for the main endemic diseases, such as bovine brucellosis and tuberculosis. Disease control efforts, with such positive results, have generated experience, a good reputation, and a great pride in both the public and private organizations of the livestock sector. Such a situation has provided an excellent basis for international trade, and has given a platform for further improvements in the Chilean animal health status.

Chile has a relatively small livestock population compared with other South American countries, but this sector involves an important number of producers, who are distributed throughout the country. The majority of animals belong to, and are managed by, families, which own around half of the livestock population. Around 85% of the livestock properties belong to either small or subsistence farms.

The New Livestock Export Process

The good animal disease status of the Chilean livestock population, as well as a respected animal health system and a strong economy, has created conditions for the development of the livestock industry. This has encouraged investment in the infrastructure and marketing to export livestock products.

The free trade agreements signed by Chile in recent years with the strongest economies in the world, followed by aggressive animal health status negotiations, opened main markets for livestock products. As a consequence, renovated livestock chains, which include producers and the processing industry, have begun a new livestock development era in Chile. The export process has pushed changes in the production, quality assurance, marketing and trading issues. Today, there are high standards in all the components of the livestock chain, a great change from the late 1990s.

A consequence of the globalization of livestock production and processing has been that animal health management has become a key element in livestock development and trade policy. For example, in the early 2000s a number of transboundary disease events showed the need for strong management. There was FMD in Europe and South America, high impacts of bovine spongiform encephalopathy (BSE) in Europe, the USA,

---

[1] All the ex-List A OIE diseases and BSE.

Canada and Japan, and widespread outbreaks of highly pathogenic avian influenza in many countries in Asia and Europe.

In the context of globalization of livestock production and processing, the chapter will examine the role of animal health management in the Chilean livestock trade.

New Demands for Animal Health

To begin, maintain and develop an international livestock trade process, Chile had to adjust its animal health management policy. The key element was to organize everything around the livestock trade. The main changes are presented as follows:

1. *The improvement of the prevention and control strategy* – The strategy and the implementation of main animal health actions were improved in order to avoid production and economic losses. The main aspects of this process were:
- Prevention policy for main exotic diseases was revised and improved.
- For each disease an individual plan for prevention of entry, surveillance, response and control was developed.
- New strategy and support to control programmes for endemic diseases were implemented.
- Diagnostic laboratory and inspection posts at borders were also improved.
- A new traceability and movement control programme was created.
- New rules and procedures for veterinary drugs and vaccines assessment were created.

2. *The demonstration of animal health status* – Based on international standards a system has been developed to provide evidence of Chile's animal disease status and veterinary service quality. This included:
- Detailed files of evidence to demonstrate that the country was free of all exotic diseases were elaborated and are continually in a process of revision.
- OIE standards were used and adjusted for each country that Chile trades with, i.e. responding to the needs of the importing country.

- In the case of FMD and BSE, files have been presented to OIE, with a statute of declared free and temporally free, respectively.

3. *Response to an animal disease or health event* – Rapid and effective response to an exotic disease incursion into the country has become a fundamental aspect of the Chilean animal health system. The preparation and reaction to animal health problems include animal health and trade measures. The following actions have been taken:
- Contingency plans have been revised and updated for all exotic diseases.
- The country used the plan and all the principles of animal health and market management during the avian influenza H7N3 incursion in 2002.
- The same principles were used in the American foul-brood outbreak in 2005.

4. *The incorporation of the private sector into the animal health system* – Animal health management is very complex and therefore the private sector has been involved in different issues. It is recognized that the private sector in the country has a crucial role in prevention and disease control as well as sanitary negotiation. The following actions have so far been carried out:
- The private sector had an important role in the avian influenza (AI) outbreak in 2002.
- Today there are common public and private surveillance programmes for poultry and pig diseases.
- Active participation in the BSE prevention and active surveillance programme.

5. *A recognition of the growing importance of food safety* – Chile's trading partners along with national legislation have increased the need to improve food safety standards of livestock products. This is an issue which has a close link with animal health, both in management and in trade. The following actions have been implemented:
- The development of an official food safety system from the farm to the processing plant was based on international standards but also in line with national legislation.
- The responsibility of slaughterhouse inspections was transferred from the Ministry of Health to the veterinary service.

- Animal welfare management has been incorporated, especially in transport and slaughtering.
- A residue control programme for all species has also been implemented.

6. *An animal disease and health status negotiation team and procedures* – In order to open and maintain markets, using all the animal health and veterinary service background, a specialized team and procedures were created. Some issues covered are:

- better connection with commercial negotiation units;
- improvement of the link and knowledge of international reference institutions, such as OIE, Codex Alimentarius and sanitary and phyto-sanitary (SPS) measures of WTO;
- creation of country managers in the veterinary service to handle sanitary negotiations;
- coordination of other sanitary and food safety units of veterinary service.

Other issues have been recognized and have influenced the changes in the veterinary services. These were: the greatest importance of the *wild animal population* for animal health and trade; the great importance of the *international reference organization (OIE)*; and the inclusion of *family livestock production* in national biosecurity.

Cost–Benefit Analysis: Changes in the Approach

The main motivation to eradicate animal diseases in the past was increases in production and the reduction of production costs. In Chile, the analysis focused mainly on primary production. Traditional cost–benefit analysis, based on Inter American Development Bank recommendations, was used to support governmental decisions and to obtain credits. Trade benefits from animal disease eradication and the positive role of the livestock industry as a whole were not considered.

The cost–benefit analysis approach has changed with Chile being free of main transboundary diseases and the initiation of livestock product exports. Animal health actions have become extremely important to the livestock industry. The livestock product export strategy needs to be supported by high standards of animal health management, resulting in high levels of livestock competitiveness and trade.

The incursion of a transboundary disease and hence a change in animal health status in Chile would have a huge impact on the livestock industry, trade and the general economy and society. Therefore, the government and the private sector have agreed that the prevention of exotic diseases and its control should be given a high priority. A clear justification has been made to react quickly if a transboundary disease is detected in order to return to a disease-free status as quickly as possible. Animal health actions are also supported by trade policies to reassure trading partners. In conclusion, cost–benefit analysis has expanded to include the livestock industry as a whole and all the externalities of livestock trade.

Examples of Specific Disease Management

Prevention of an old disease: FMD

Chile has been FMD-free without vaccination since 1981, after a 20-year eradication programme. Two incursions of the disease occurred in 1984 and 1987, and were both successfully controlled and stamped out (Cancino and Vidal, 1984; Cancino, 1988).

Since the last outbreak, there has been a FMD Prevention Programme, with activities that are implemented with a different level of intensity depending on an ongoing process of risk assessment. This programme was reinforced in 2001, in response to FMD outbreaks in other South American countries. General measures are risk assessment in pre-border, post-border inspection, surveillance and biosecurity at farm levels. An area of exclusion to avoid contact between livestock from Andean neighbouring countries is part of the measures. The size of this area depends on the risk. There are general and specific actions in these areas. Finally, specific media programmes support the prevention measures. The principles and components of the programmes are detailed in Rojas *et al.* (2002) and Espejo (2006).

Measures are mainly financed by the government, although the private sector understands and appreciates the programme and agrees and collaborates with its activities.

Control of a recent outbreak: avian influenza (AI)

An AI outbreak of H7N3 strain occurred in 2002. Two farms were found positive in a period of 15 days. The strategy applied was the immediate elimination of flocks from positive farms, avoiding the dissemination of the disease to the rest of the country. In parallel, a strategy was applied to minimize the trade impact through visits to countries importing poultry products from Chile and also to OIE. These visits shared the results of the disease detection and response and a high level of transparency was maintained.

The culling of the two infected farms to stamp out the disease resulted in the destruction of 560,000 breeding chickens and turkeys. This measure was financed by the Poultry Association. Other animal health measures were implemented to support the control of the initial foci. Outbreak and surveillance teams were manned and the rest of the country was zoned to facilitate the outbreak management and to reopen markets. Strict surveillance and biosecurity measures were put in place in the rest of the country (Rojas and Moreira, 2006).

The impact of the disease was calculated by Verdugo *et al.* (2004), who estimated that the cost of the AI outbreak was US$31,782,475. These costs were largely borne by the private sector (US$31,391,889), reflecting the high value of animals eliminated and the cost of the elimination process.

Control of new disease: foul-brood

Honey producers are mainly focused on export markets, and the majority are family producers. American foul-brood was first detected in Chile in 2003 in three small api-

aries, in a restricted area in the north of the country. The outbreak was totally controlled. In 2005, two outbreaks were found simultaneously in two regions. A restricted area was set in the main outbreak, with movement restriction. An intensive epidemiological trace-back investigation was applied, resulting in the detection of 98 outbreaks in seven regions of the country. All the infected apiaries in the country were eliminated and a 3 km restricted area was set around them. Strict surveillance and biosecurity was applied. No antibiotic use was allowed, either for prevention in disease-free apiaries or in controlling disease in infected apiaries (Cancino and Rivera, 2006).

In order to facilitate the notification of cases, an economic incentive was created to replace positive hives. This measure had never been applied before, with the exception of FMD during the 1987 outbreaks. It significantly helped outbreak control. Bee products for export were not restricted, with the temporary exception of the restricted area. After the emergency and under a strict surveillance programme, 16 new outbreaks were found in 2006. No cases of American foul-brood have been found in 2007 and 2008.

Control of an endemic disease of recent entry: porcine reproductive and respiratory syndrome (PRRS)

PRRS was detected in Chile in 2003. A national investigation determined that the disease had spread throughout the country's commercial herds. A project was approved to eradicate the disease that involved a public/ private partnership. Official legislation was approved that detailed compulsory measures in infected farms.

At the beginning of the project, there were a number of multi- and mono-site producers identified as positive to PRRS. All farms, infected and clean, were included in the eradication programme. A private initiative, guided by the Pork Association (ASPROCER), and supported by the veterinary service, removed positive mono-site herds and replaced them with negative sows. This measure was paid for by ASPROCER and supervised by the veterinary service. Positive multi-sites had an individual eradication plan, which was implemented and paid for by the producer and supervised by the veterinary service.

Strict surveillance in all farms and biosecurity measures were implemented and continue to date. This is part of the public and private surveillance programme for the Chilean pork industry. In 2007, the country was declared officially free of PRRS and this was recognized internationally (Estrada, 2007).

Final Words

In recent years, Chile has demonstrated that public investment in animal disease control and general strengthening of animal health systems during the 1960s have been a very important component of the country becoming a livestock exporting country. The positive changes in animal health management have recognized the need for strong partnerships between public and private sectors in animal disease prevention and control measures.

The change in focus of the Chilean livestock sector has required a modification of cost–benefit analysis that includes trade and general society impacts of a change in animal disease status and management. This information is critical in helping the government take decisions on investment in animal health projects.

24 Decision Making, Scales and Quality of Economic Evaluations for the Control of Contagious Bovine Pleuropneumonia (CBPP): the Use of Economic Analysis Methods in Combination with Epidemiological and Geographical Models to Help Decision Making for CBPP Control in Ethiopia

Pascal Bonnet and Matthieu Lesnoff

Introduction

This chapter describes how economic evaluation methods (cost–benefit and cost-effectiveness analyses) have been used in analysing the economic rationale for the management of contagious bovine pleuropneumonia (CBPP) in mixed crop–livestock farming systems of Ethiopia. The analysis was carried out from the perspective of the government and the farmer. The results were used to develop recommendations on CBPP policies and management through an appropriate decision-making process with a multidisciplinary approach (medical geography, mathematical modelling). It reflects a possible combination of public and private management of the disease and opens a new vision of CBPP management. It also shows how analysis at different geographical, temporal and socio-economic scales may reflect various rationales of actors for managing the disease, and the need for policy makers to consider conflicting interests.

For academic purposes, and in order to emphasize the characteristics of appropriate economic analysis to support decision making, the analysis structure used is that recommended by Drummond *et al.* (1998) for analysing the quality of any economic analysis when evaluating health programmes.

The Research Question

Two different questions were examined through two different studies.

The *first study* was carried out in the context of the privatization of the CBPP management where there was low incidence of disease (apparent endemic status) and no public policy for CBPP eradication. The study compared the efficiency of vaccination and curative treatment to control CBPP and hence mitigate its impact in an average herd of the Western Wellega region of the Ethiopian highlands. The initial herd of the mixed crop–livestock system was composed of 15 animals. A *cost–benefit analysis*[1] was carried out with a comparison of several CBPP management strategies at farm level: a treatment of incident CBPP cases with antibiotics (oxytetracycline) versus various alternatives of vaccination of a herd with T1SR or T144 vaccines. The analysis was carried out from the perspective of the farmer and used a short-term time horizon representing the agricultural cycle of 1 year.

The *second study* was carried out in the context of CBPP public management where the goal is CBPP eradication in a given economic zone. The state veterinary service manages CBPP with the objective of eradication in the zone in order to manage biosecurity and develop and seek recognition of zones and compartments for livestock trade. The study examined which vaccination campaign would achieve a zonal eradication, in order to respond to regulatory requirements with regard to the SPS agreement (OIE-WTO) and to risk regionalization underlying the definition of zoning and compartments in the OIE code. A preliminary *cost-effectiveness analysis*, which was simplified to a cost-minimization analysis, was carried out. A comparison of several vaccination scenarios was made to assess various spatial alternatives for targeting vaccination campaigns. The analysis was carried out from the governmental perspective and with a long-term time horizon.

A Comprehensive and Explicit Description of Control Options

In the first study, private use of antibiotics and vaccines was included. In this scenario, the *farmers* privately manage any clinical CBPP cases with antibiotics (oxytetracycline 20%), or prevent their herd from getting CBPP with vaccination. It was assumed that there was good access to antibiotics and vaccines, which were distributed by the private sector and the state veterinary services, respectively.

A CBPP-free herd in a high-risk environment was considered to be certain of having contact with CBPP, and the farmer was aware of that risk. The herd infection corresponded to the introduction of one clinical case and the CBPP spread was simulated up to 1 year after an introduction. In that risky situation, the farmer was assumed to use four alternative control strategies:

- A curative strategy (ANT) consisting of antibiotic treatments of incidental clinical cases in the infected herd. The treatment administration delay was set to 1 week after the occurrence of the first clinical signs.
- Two purely preventative strategies[2] were also considered:
  - a vaccine strategy (VACC3) based on international recommendations with three successive vaccinations of the herd to reach a 100% protection rate with available vaccines (T144 and T1SR);
  - a vaccine strategy (VACC1) with a single vaccination to achieve a 50% protection rate.
- A mixed strategy (VACC1-ANT) which combined a single vaccination with antibiotic treatments of clinical cases that occurred despite vaccination.

In the second study, only vaccination strategies were simulated for T1SR or T144 vaccines. The vaccine delivery and administration were by the state veterinary services with a frequency based on international recommendations. However, the government did not have the capacity to vaccinate the full territory or the entire animal population. Therefore, it needed to target prevention to protect highly valuable economic territory, with the delineation of OIE-defined free zones or compartments.

The spatial scenarios developed for testing were based on a preliminary hierarchical risk mapping made prior to any knowledge of CBPP distribution in the area. A thematic interpretation of the socio-economic interactions and

---

[1]Referred to as partial budget analysis for short time periods and investment appraisal for long time periods (see Chapter 7, this volume).

[2]The herd infection was assumed to occur in the first month following the last vaccination.

of the agricultural development underlying the spatial organization of the study district helps to prioritize the choice of the prevention strategy to be evaluated out of the various vaccination options available (Bonnet, 2005). Three geographical areas were identified that represented three different livestock management strategies and risk levels. These three zones (A, B and C) were delineated based on a study of cattle movement between farms and cattle density (analysis of homogeneity with local indicators of spatial autocorrelation LISA (Anselin, 1995)). The three zones identified in the study district had the following characteristics:

- A: a homogeneous periurban zone, with intensive and dynamic dairy production systems, and characterized by high levels of animal movement (48%) though low density. Therefore, strong and frequent interactions with a high risk of contagious disease.
- B: a homogeneous zone, with traditional cereal cropping systems, less intensive livestock systems and with low animal movement (20%, therefore less risk for disease) and a medium density of cattle.
- C: a heterogeneous and contrasted zone, with traditional mixed farming systems, characterized by moderate levels of animal movement (32%), high cattle density and large areas under crops. The area was sparsely populated but had dynamic population patterns.

Given the risk model, the study compared the cost and performance of the prevention with various spatial options with a theoretical model as described by Haggett (2000), and applied to risk factors of CBPP. Four scenarios were evaluated:

1. A mass (blanket) vaccination in the whole district.
2. Two defensive vaccination strategies with vaccination in the outskirts of an area assumed to be at high risk. One strategy covered more of the outskirts than the other.
3. An offensive vaccination in the area assumed to be at very high risk.

The options were only varied by the scope of the vaccination area that was being targeted,

both spatial and population coverage in order to determine the vaccination cost. The effectiveness of the vaccination was considered the same in the area whatever the spatial option chosen, and therefore the study was similar to a cost-minimization analysis.

The Efficacy of Programmes, Evidence of Programme Effectiveness

Both studies used the same disease control technologies and efficacy was estimated through a literature review. There were no published data either in experimental or field conditions found on antibiotic effectiveness, i.e. the proportion of clinical cases recovering after treatment. It was assumed that antibiotic treatment was fully effective with all treated clinical cases recovering just after treatment. The problem of chronic carriers after antibiotic treatments was not considered.

Vaccines were assumed to give full protection and the different rates of effectiveness were determined by the vaccination strategy (modus operandi) applied. The vaccine protection was assumed to last 1 year, and any side effects of vaccines not properly administered were not considered. In the second study, targeted vaccinations in restricted areas were considered to be as effective as mass vaccination, by offering optimal immune protection in the targeted regions.

Concerning uncertainty two aspects were envisaged, referring first to the observed variability of some needed parameters (e.g. market price of animal product), and second to the statistical distribution of model outputs. Two models were used and their outputs are sensitive to assumptions underlying the results.

Costs and Benefits from an Intervention

All important and relevant elements with regard to the consequences of an intervention were estimated. The costs and consequences of an intervention need to be valued and where appropriate a financial value applied.

If necessary, other cultural and social values should be included. In both studies, some sensitivity analysis was performed and presented in preliminary reports.

Study one: farm impact

A representative mixed crop–livestock farming system commonly found in the East African highlands was used for the study. These systems have herds which are sedentary and small. Cattle are the cornerstone of the agricultural system: they provide milk, meat and manure production and animal draught power for crop cultivation. All the economic outputs from the herds were included in the analysis. When dealing with direct costs of health interventions, not all the costs were included since the local distribution costs were neglected because of the small area studied. The analysis is carried out within a limited area where it is assumed that medical technologies were available at the various veterinary centres (private and public), and that transport costs were small.

The farmer was assumed to bear the full cost of antibiotics delivery as this was provided by private veterinary services. They also bore partial cost of vaccine delivery provided by the state veterinary service under a cost-recovery system. Antibiotic treatment costs were estimated from field data using local market prices. The vaccine cost for the farmer was set to 2 Ethiopian birr (ETB[3]) per vaccinated animal, and reflected the international price of the vaccine when exported from Ethiopia. This represented a hypothetical situation in which vaccines are produced and delivered by the government with a cost-recovery policy (i.e. without a commercial benefit). The average cost of a complete sequence of antibiotic treatments (following the manufacturer's recommended dosage) was estimated to be 40 ETB per treated animal.

The intervention benefits were calculated by comparing annual herd-level gross margins (see Chapter 7, this volume), and used to assess the acceptability of CBPP-control strategies. Revenues included dairy and draught

power outputs and manure was ignored. Costs included the restocking of animals lost due to CBPP and direct costs of health interventions against CBPP. All production measures were made using local production parameters derived from previous studies of herd dynamics in the area. After herd infection, the annual revenues of clinical cases surviving CBPP were reduced proportionally to the mean duration of the clinical phase and were calculated with epidemiological models. Therefore, a monetary value was placed on the intervention impact.

The time horizon for the farm-level analysis was short and therefore there is no need for time discounting methods. The incremental costs and benefits of the CBPP management strategies were calculated as a difference with a baseline 'do nothing' strategy, which was the current situation without any systematic disease management applied.

Sensitivity analysis

In the first analysis, a SEIR mathematical model of spread of CBPP was used within the herd to simulate the epidemiological impact of a herd infection. It is sensitive to some epidemiological parameters like reproductive ratio Ro[4] (i.e. virulence of the CBPP strain), to herd size and to the transition parameters that were obtained from a literature review and from a longitudinal survey. Before outputs were used in the economic model, the uncertainty of outputs of the epidemiological model was partly reduced by rerunning the model with Monte Carlo simulations, and using various parameter values. To run the model, strong assumptions were made about the likelihood of reinfection of herds. It was assumed that there were no reintroductions of animals during the study period.[5] Average results of model outputs were then used.

---

[3] 1 ETB = 0.1 Euro in 2003.

[4] Ro: expected number of new infectious animals caused by a typical infected individual during its entire infectious period in a completely susceptible herd which is in a demographic steady state at the moment the infection is introduced.
[5] Nevertheless frequent movements of animals were observed between herds.

When running the economic model, average market values of resources were used. They are generally highly fluctuating parameters along time. A sensitivity analysis was performed on these parameters and results indicated that the cost of restocking had a major influence on the herd gross margin variations, indicating the impact of mortality rate on the results and conclusions. Additionally other simulations showed that vaccination ranking is improved when CBPP virulence and the clinical incidence are higher.

Study two: state intervention

For the second study, all costs and consequences were simplified by the use of a unique animal herd variable. Consequences of eradication in terms of market access were included directly in the model. The vaccination costs were assumed to remain the same per animal, and to simplify the analysis no financial conversion was used for the numerator of the cost-effectiveness ratio. Numerator and denominator were therefore kept in physical units with a basic effectiveness criteria of the number of animals vaccinated divided by the number of animals protected. The need to evaluate the real costs of vaccination was not felt to be necessary. Therefore, the technical effectiveness criteria are the ratio: *number of animals vaccinated/number animal protected*.

In a cost–benefit analysis that would follow this step, there would be a need to use relative economic value associated with the underlying production systems and sub-territories (dairy or crop–livestock mixed system), since such information is important to help decision making when economic development is associated with spatial segregation. The long-term benefit of the intervention requires some thought on discounting and should be theoretically used for both numerator and denominator of the ratio used. The choice of various rates should be part of the sensitivity analysis.

An incremental approach was adopted because of the nature of the study, whose objective was to compare various vaccination scenarios with a gradual reduction of animal population being vaccinated, the protection level within the territory remaining the same. The model used was a geographical model of epidemiological risk, based on the analysis and mapping of spatial structures associated with risk factors of the disease (mainly the mobility of animals and the density of cattle population). The model was sensitive to the geographical scale and the type of lattice grid used, due to the well-known 'modifiable areal unit problem' (MAUP). It is sensitive to the methods used for the delineation of borders of the areas at gradual risk (hot spot cluster analysis or categorization of discrete values of LISA parameters was used). Nevertheless, when running the efficiency model, and since monetary values were not used, the economic model was less sensitive to economic parameters. Therefore, outputs of the study were expected to provide good evidence of the technical efficiency of the alternative scenarios evaluated.

Discussion of the Results

The results from the farm-level study demonstrated a relative advantage of the antibiotic treatment. All comparisons with the baseline gross margin analysis indicated that the interventions gave a positive return, i.e. the herd gross margin for the CBPP intervention strategy was on average greater than the herd gross margin strategy of 'do nothing'. When comparing vaccination and treatment strategies, ANT had a mean incremental HGM of 118 ETB versus a mean incremental HGM of 18 ETB and 55 ETB, for VACC3 and VACC1, respectively.

As discussed above the preliminary ranking of zone scenarios was based on a *variant* of the 'cost'-effectiveness ratio (CER) calculated for four vaccination strategies, and did not consider the real monetary cost of the interventions. The four options evaluated were:

- Mass vaccination in all zones of the territory: CER is equal to 1.0.
- Defensive vaccination offering containment at the full periphery of the zone at higher risk (the high movement area shaded in darker grey in the top right part of Fig. 24.1) is 0.67.

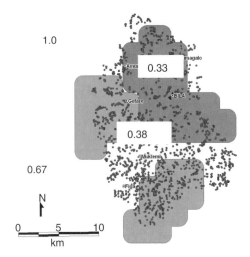

Fig. 24.1. Map showing the targets of the different zone vaccination strategies in Ethiopia.

- A similar defensive scenario when ring vaccination is exclusive of very low-risk zones (the lighter grey shaded areas to the left and bottom in Fig. 24.1): CER is then equal to 0.38.
- Offensive vaccination in the core of the zone at higher risk: CER is equal to 0.33. This last scenario is technically the most efficient one, since it minimizes the cost of the vaccination campaign by the government.

The distribution of endemic CBPP was revealed *ex post* by a sero-prevalence survey. It was mainly concentrating and surviving in a low densely populated rural area (with regard to animal and human population) representing the outskirts of the central town. It is a territory associated with a spatial and social system of dairy development with large use of social capital and high animal movement. Figure 24.2 presents the 'socio-pathogenic complex' of CBPP: the spatial analysis identified a hot spot of cattle move-ment (in dark grey) and a hot spot of cattle density (hatched grey), that are represented here with the CBPP known area (the larger, darker grey dots are infected herds). The small dots represent farms and towns of the district.

The two variables represented two con-trasting risk factors of the disease:

- The endemic nucleus of CBPP is sup-ported by the first hot spot with a high level of animal mobility (within the dairy subsystem of the local town).
- CBPP can be 'exported' from the nucleus to another epidemiological system (e.g. a small village with significant local den-sity at greater geographical scale, a situa-tion that could also sustain the disease locally).

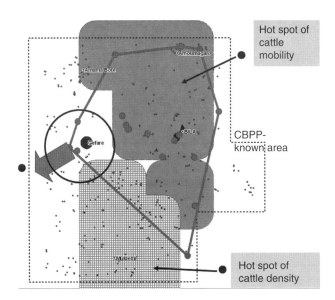

Fig. 24.2. Hot spots of cattle movement and density in a CBPP endemic area of Ethiopia.

- In the study site, the disease transmission rate due to animal density could not sustain the disease alone, whereas animal movements could.

The results provoke the need to reflect on the need to adapt disease management policy in two different ways. First, the study at farm level indicates that the use of antibiotic treatments could be reconsidered in African smallholder contexts. Nevertheless, the lack of scientific knowledge on the long-term biological effects of antibiotics remains a major limitation when envisaging the eradication of the disease in potentially certifiable areas of production, i.e. when zones that have an economic comparative advantage in trading livestock in international markets. As a result of the economic analysis, an experimental trial was designed and launched to assess the effectiveness of some antibiotics against CBPP. The model also did not take into consideration exchange of animals, a common practice of the local farming systems, which would allow frequent reinfection in the long run.

Second, the state intervention study provides evidence for optimizing vaccination campaigns to free a particular zone from the disease and under public budget constraints which are the norm in sub-Saharan Africa. Nevertheless, it should be noted from the study that density of cattle generally used in targeting strategies did not represent the most appropriate risk factor at the scale chosen in the geographical model, as compared to animal movements. The movements must be interpreted here as important components of the farming systems and social solidarity. They represent a major way of optimizing use of the animal resources in the territory therefore cannot be stopped.

Finally, results from economic evaluations of specific intervention cannot be interpreted without a holistic view of the animal health system (Leonard, 1993; Bonnet, 2003). For instance, for strategies using antibiotic treatments administration delays and under-dosages, which are frequently observed in the field, were important parameters since they affect the utilization effectiveness. This directly challenges the real impact of health education and promotion programmes. In addition, the pricing of health technologies (antibiotics and vaccines), which depends on national animal health policy (e.g. on the delivery channels and the governmental incentives), also determines the economic efficiencies of the different strategies. Models can help to better design such pricing policy when technologies are subsidized.

Only the repetition of various economic evaluations of CBPP management programmes, carried out from various perspectives and time horizons, can provide complete evidence for a comprehensive analysis of the CBPP management in a diversity of farming systems. Approaches and results are therefore complementary to each other and decision makers may then use them to better envisage a mixed policy to address CBPP in the African context.

25 Animal Health Policy in South Asia: What Can Economic Analysis Contribute?

Vinod Ahuja

Introduction

Animal health policy in the South Asia region has been characterized predominantly by direct government action either in providing services to livestock farmers or in undertaking livestock productivity-enhancing measures. It is a widely held view among policy makers that, given the poverty status of South Asian livestock farmers, the potential of livestock in contributing to poverty reduction, and poverty reduction being a public good, there is a strong rationale for direct action by the government as opposed to a regulatory, monitoring and market-enhancing role. Accordingly, most governments in South Asia have developed large networks of publicly supported service providers backed by free or heavily subsidized input supply.

Any casual observer of livestock farmers in South Asia would perhaps sympathize and support the above policy stance. Given the role of public policy in the creation and fair distribution of the economic pie, such a policy would make eminent sense on the grounds of fairness and social justice. A more careful analysis of the distributional outcomes, however, raises questions about the desirability of this policy, and the need to fine-tune service delivery systems that include creating space for other non-government service providers. A study in four states of India, representing different economic, social, market and production contexts, analysed distributional outcomes of this policy. This chapter summarizes the results of those studies to illustrate the contribution economic analysis can make to animal health policy.

The Context

The studies were conducted in four states of India representing a wide range of livestock production, marketing and socio-cultural contexts as shown below:

1. Gujarat – front runner in the dairy cooperative movement, relatively commercialized production system, experience with different systems of service delivery including cost recovery by cooperative service providers.
2. Rajasthan – although located adjacent to Gujarat, the state represents an arid production zone with annual rainfall approximately 800 mm and a vast geographical area under desert conditions.
3. Kerala – a small state in South India with a long history of cross-breeding and the highest proportion of cross-breds in the livestock population. A state known for its achievements in male and female literacy and high outmigration. Highest density of veterinary institutions (dispensaries, hospitals and polyclinics).

4. Orissa – a mid-size state on the eastern coast. Highest rural and urban poverty incidence among all states of India, highly subsistent production system, high tribal population, and poor social and physical infrastructure.

Further comparative statistics across these states are given in Table 25.1.

Study Design

Household surveys of livestock farmers were conducted to understand the differential access by various categories of service users and the potential impacts of alternative policy choices. The first of the two surveys covered service provider units operated by various agencies – government, cooperative unions, private entrepreneurs and non-government organizations (NGOs). The second survey covered livestock-

owning households and collected information on livestock assets and services, household characteristics and agriculture activities of selected households. The basic questions that the surveys sought to address were:

1. Who are the primary service providers? What kinds of services are available from which providers?
2. What is the level of access to these services for the beneficiaries?
3. How is the use pattern for these services different for different groups of farmers?
4. At what price are these services available? Do the poor receive services at a different price?
5. How do various service providers fare with respect to price and non-price factors? How do the users perceive the price and quality of these services?

The findings from the household surveys have been published in Ahuja *et al.* (2003a,b).

Table 25.1. Comparative profile of the study states in India.

Indicator	Gujarat	Rajasthan	Kerala	Orissa	All India
Geographical area ('000 km²)	196.0	342.2	38.9	155.7	3,287.3
Poverty incidence (%)					
Rural	22.18	26.46	25.76	49.72	37.27
Urban	27.89	30.49	24.55	41.64	32.36
Literacy (%)					
Male	81	68	95	67	73
Female	87	33	89	45	51
Number of livestock (millions)	21.2	49.1	3.6	23.4	464.5
Proportion of cross-breds in total cattle (%)	8.66	4.28	81.01	7.65	12.34
Proportion of buffaloes among total livestock animals (%)	33.1	21.2	1.8	6.0	20.1
Average milk yield (kg/animal in milk /day)					
Buffaloes	4.2	4.4	6.2	2.5	4.3
Cross-bred cows	8.2	6.1	7.0	4.9	6.4
Indigenous cows	3.3	2.9	2.6	0.8	1.9
Average rainfall (mm)	1,004.2	817.8	2,911.3	1,337.6	47,647
Road density (per 100 km²)	47.6	41.2	381.7	168.6	76.8
Road length (per 100,000 of population; km)	195.3	266.3	462.1	737.4	256.1
Number of veterinary institutions[a]					
Veterinary hospitals/polyclinics	14	1,437	260	13	8,720
Veterinary dispensaries	478	285	833	527	17,820
Veterinary first aid centres	589	1,727	26	2,939	25,433

[a]Veterinary polyclinics are the veterinary hospitals with multiple specialities and specialists such as surgery, gynaecology, radiology, etc. These employ several postgraduate veterinarians and are located mostly in state headquarters and at times in some important district headquarters. Veterinary hospitals are institutions with in-patient facilities and with usually one or two qualified veterinarians. These are located mostly in district headquarters. Veterinary dispensaries are the same as hospitals but without in-patient facilities and with only one qualified veterinarian. First aid centres are minor dispensaries in villages manned by para-professionals.

In this chapter, the main findings are summa-rized and conclusions developed.

Survey Results

Primary providers and access to services

In all the study states, the veterinarians employed by the State Animal Husbandry Departments (SAHDs) are the primary service providers. In Gujarat, Kerala and Orissa, there was good access to government services with more than 95% sample respondents in these states stating they would be able to obtain government vet-erinary services when needed. In Rajasthan, the comparable figure was 63%. The state veterinary service provides services through the network of veterinary dispensaries, veterinary hospitals and polyclinics and veterinary first aid centres. Except in the case of emergencies, all govern-ment services are supposed to be delivered at the centres. In the case of emergencies, the government veterinarians are allowed to make home visits and charge a nominal fee to cover their transportation cost. After office hours,

however, the veterinary doctors were allowed to engage in private practice. But, in reality, pri-vate practice by government veterinarians was widespread even during office hours.

Alternative sources of livestock services include cooperative unions, private veterinari-ans and some NGOs. Among the four states included in this study, cooperatives offer a sig-nificant alternative only in some districts of Gujarat. The cooperative service is mostly deliv-ered at home. The proportion of those having access to cooperative veterinary services was 47% in Gujarat and about 14–17% in Rajasthan and Kerala. The extent of private veterinary practices for farm animals is extremely limited and they generally operate in areas where other service providers – government, cooperative, NGOs, etc. – are not able to meet the demand.

An important question in this context per-tains to differential access to these services by poor and non-poor. More specifically, do the poor households have similar access to these services to the rich? Table 25.2 compares the proportion of those in the bottom, middle and top 20% of households, as ranked by a wealth index based on ownership of household assets,

Table 25.2. Access to veterinary services disaggregated by wealth categories in Gujarat, Rajasthan and Kerala as a percentage.

Do you have access to	Bottom 20%	Middle 20%	Top 20%
Gujarat			
Ethnic/traditional healer	71	58.0	52.4
Private veterinarian	6	11.1	7.3
Cooperative veterinarian	52	55.5	40.2
Government veterinarian	–	–	–
At the centre	90.5	91.4	93.9
At home	90.5	93.9	93.5
Rajasthan			
Ethnic/traditional healer	75.6	86.1	91.5
Private veterinarian	2.7	12.5	26.8
Cooperative veterinarian	2.7	11.1	23.9
Government veterinarian	–	–	–
At the centre	63.5	62.5	93.9
At home	58.1	56.9	92.7
Kerala			
Ethnic/traditional healer	8.2	4.8	2.4
Private veterinarian	22.4	19.0	26.5
Cooperative veterinarian	12.9	17.9	19.3
Government veterinarian	–	–	–
At the centre	100	99.0	100
At home	100	98.8	99.0

who responded 'yes' to the access question. It is clear that in Gujarat and Kerala, all households had good access, while in Rajasthan the poor felt more constrained with respect to receiving veterinary services. For example, in Rajasthan 64% of the households in the bottom group reported having access to government veterinary services at the centre against 94% in the top group. Comparable figures for home service were 58% and 93%.

Use pattern

Analysis of data on the number of veterinary visits made by different providers indicated that a larger number of these cases were attended at home. It was quite common for the government veterinarians to attend even ordinary animal health problems at farmers' homes, and the majority of such visits were undertaken in a private capacity. In fact, farmers in all income groups revealed a clear preference towards home service, and the government veterinarians catered to that preference mainly in a private capacity. Analysis also indicated that, on a per adult bovine basis, the number of visits in Rajasthan and Kerala increased with income, whereas this trend was less sharp in Gujarat. Further, in Gujarat, there was no significant difference in the proportion of home versus in-centre services across income groups. Both these trends were, at least partly, explained by the availability of relatively inexpensive home service from the cooperative unions. In all the three states, the proportion of those opting for the services of private veterinarians increased with income. This was especially evident in Rajasthan and Kerala, where private usage of the top 20% was more than double the rate of lowest 20%. At least part of this tendency could be explained by the fact that private veterinarians established themselves in relatively higher-income areas.

Price structure

Generally all three types of providers – government, private and cooperative – were providing the full range of curative veterinary services, i.e. general sickness, gynaeco-logical problems, injuries and minor surgery. Farmers were required to go to veterinary hospitals and polyclinics only in the case of major surgery. Such cases were, however, few in number, and farmers generally did not seek major surgery for their animals.

The prescribed costs at the service centres were either zero or very nominal (in the range of Rs 2–5 per visit, including medicines, depending on the type of animal). In reality, however, the service users incurred expenditures that were significantly higher than the officially prescribed price. As per the data collected in the survey, the average visit price to a service centre was Rs 40, Rs 18 and Rs 5 in Rajasthan, Kerala and Orissa, respectively. Total cost, including the cost of drugs and medicines purchased from the market, turned out to be approximately Rs 125, Rs 50 and Rs 70 in Rajasthan, Kerala and Orissa, respectively.

The story for home service is similar. Even though the government veterinarians were allowed to charge a nominal amount for a home visit to cover transportation cost, in reality the charges were significantly higher than what could be justified as the transportation cost. The estimated average cost of a home visit (including the cost of medicines purchased at the stores) by a government veterinarian was Rs 178 in Kerala, Rs 160 in Gujarat and Orissa, and over Rs 300 in Rajasthan (Table 25.3). As a share of total cases (in-centre and home), only about 15% were treated for free in Rajasthan and 25% in Kerala.

Two further questions deserve more analysis: (i) were the majority of those receiving services at official prices poor? and (ii) were the prices paid by the poor significantly lower, if not zero, than those paid by the rich?

With respect to the first question, analysis indicated that, of those receiving service for free, only about 10% in Rajasthan and about 30% in Kerala belonged to the bottom quintile. Coming to the second question – whether the average price paid increased with economic status – it appears that average expenditure per animal per veterinary visit was indeed lower in the case of poor households. At the same time, however, to be able to conclude that the poor received services at the discounted price, one will need to control for variation in the service quality. This question is further explored below.

Table 25.3. Total charges per home visit (Rs).

Disease	Gujarat			Rajasthan		Kerala		Orissa
	Govt	Coop	Private	Govt	Private	Govt	Private	
General sickness	153	49	173	275	214	175	140	–
Gynaecological problems	248	59	284	306	316	180	–	233
FMD	–	–	–	292	–	134	–	71
Mastitis	–	–	–	–	–	235	–	190
Injury	117	–	–	–	–	150	–	121
Pneumonia	–	–	–	258	–	–	–	–
HS	–	–	–	302	–	–	–	204
Other	146	50	157	314	–	120	–	–
Overall average	161	51.5	202.2	333	286	178	204	–

Note: '–' indicates not calculated due to insufficient observations.

User perceptions

The data presented above clearly indicate that the users paid significantly more than was officially prescribed. However, it provides no information on the users' perceptions of the prices and service quality. To get a sense of these aspects, the survey asked the users if they considered the quality to be 'satisfactory' and the cost to be 'reasonable'.

In general, there was widespread satisfaction with the service quality. In Gujarat, over 80% of the cases attended by cooperative veterinarians received a 'satisfactory' quality as well as a 'reasonable' cost rating from the users. Comparable figures for private and government veterinarians were 76% and 68%. Kerala and Orissa did even better on the quality rating and there were no appreciable differences across private and government veterinarians. A large number of users in Gujarat, Kerala and Orissa considered the price of the services to be reasonable. In Rajasthan on the other hand, however, a significantly larger proportion of respondents considered the price to be unreasonably high. Given that average charges per visit in Rajasthan were substantially higher than in other states, this result makes intuitive sense.

Finally, a comparison of perceptions across income groups reveals an interesting pattern. In both Gujarat and Rajasthan, the proportion of those who responded that quality is satisfactory and cost is reasonable increased with the income, but the association was much less pronounced in the case of quality than in the cost.

Price and Demand Structure

The descriptive analysis in the preceding sections provides a reasonably good idea of the structure of the market in terms of overall availability, prices and the perceptions of users. However, this analysis is not sufficient to evaluate the potential distributional impact of any change in service delivery policy, especially with respect to subsidies. That question requires an understanding of the factors influencing the demand for these services, especially the magnitude of price elasticities (net of other factors influencing demand) and how these vary with income. We therefore now turn to analysing: (i) the price differences across government, private veterinarians and cooperative unions; and (ii) price elasticities of demand for veterinary services for different income groups.

Price differences across provider types

Regression results with price as dependent variable are presented in Table 25.4. Looking first at the coefficients on the variables

Table 25.4. Explaining the variation in price per visit.[a] (From Ahuja et al., 2003a,b.)

Explanatory variables	Gujarat	Rajasthan	Kerala	Orissa
Intercept	82.38	−65.89	14.83	−
	(2.81)	(−1.10)	(1.24)	
Service time	0.68	0.34	1.00	−
	(2.72)	(1.32)	(5.34)	
Travel and waiting time	−0.03	0.03	−0.20	−
	(−0.70)	(0.72)	(−4.50)	
SUPMED (1 if supplied medicines during	−1.29	70.20[b]	13.70	−70.5
the visit, 0 otherwise)	(−0.12)	(2.40)	(3.18)	(−4.4)
VETVIS (number of visits to cure)	−9.86	79.00[b]	−5.73	−
	−1.17)	(3.20)	(−2.09)	−
GOV (1 if government veterinarian,	−44.85	42.80	−4.31	−
0 otherwise)	−4.07)	(1.23)	(−0.42)	
COOP (1 if cooperative veterinarian, 0 otherwise)	−103.3	−92.50	−	−
	(−8.17)	(−1.00)	−	−
SICK1 (1 if gynaecological or surgical case,	33.64	92.80[c]	−14.60	61.2
0 otherwise)	(2.97)	(1.76)	(−1.35)	(1.4)
SICK2 (1 if pneumonia, FMD or HS case,	−32.46	12.00	−14.90	2.4
0 otherwise)	(−0.92)	(0.27)	(−3.08)	(0.1)
Diarrhoea	−	−	−	−74.3
				(−5.0)
Mastitis	−	−	−	86.8
				(2.1)
SOLVED (1 if the problem was solved in	−0.48	−61.00[b]	8.83	−
that visit, 0 otherwise)	(−0.05)	(−2.07)	(2.01)	−
HOME (1 if home service, 0 otherwise)	67.62	172.60[b]	65.80	77.8
	(2.78)	(5.40)	(13.90)	(6.6)
Asset index	−	−	−	−19.3
	−	−	−	(−2.2)
POOR (1 if household belongs to bottom 40%,	0.58	−101.90	17.20	−
0 otherwise)	(0.05)	(−1.23)	(0.68)	−
GOV*POOR	−27.81	68.30	−15.05	−
	(−1.62)	(0.78)	(−0.56)	−
Adjusted R-squared	0.27	0.18	0.44	0.60
N (sample size)	356	340	612	297

[a]The design of the Orissa survey was slightly different than that of the other three states and hence not all variables are similarly defined.
[b]Significant at 1% level.
[c]Significant at 5% level.
Note: Figures in parentheses are t-statistics.

GOV and COOP, it is clear that, except in Gujarat, there was no significant difference in the fee charged by government and private veterinarians. In Gujarat, although the users paid prices that were higher than prescribed, these were still lower than the prices charged by private providers. Controlling for service quality as well as location-specific characteristics, the average difference between private and government doctors appeared to be in the range of Rs 60–70. Service from cooperative unions in Gujarat was still cheaper.[1]

_____

[1]The sample size for private veterinarians in both Kerala and Rajasthan was too small to allow meaningful testing of the differences. Thus, the finding of no significant difference in these two states is not very robust.

The interaction term between GOV and POOR helps us answer the question – did the poor receive government services at a relatively lower price? In all the three states, the coefficient on the interaction term is statistically insignificant. This implies that there is no targeting of relatively cheaper services towards the poor in any of the three states. It appears that the prevailing price in poorer areas was somewhat lower than that prevailing in richer areas. But, within the given area, both poor and rich paid the same price.

Demand for veterinary services

Regression results for demand for veterinary services are presented in Table 25.5. Primary variables of our concern in the table are the price of veterinary care, the wealth index and the interaction between price and wealth. The coefficient on price is negative and statistically significant in all the three states. This is consistent with economic theory and implies that a higher price does depress overall demand. Neither of the other two variables – wealth

Table 25.5. Demand functions for veterinary services in Indian states.

Explanatory variable	Department variable: number of veterinary visits during the reference period of the survey			
	Gujarat	Rajasthan	Kerala	Orissa
Intercept	0.938	−0.145	1.00	−2.60
	(1.04)[a]	(−0.157)	(0.65)	(1.08)
Milk price	0.002	0.005	0.262	0.247
	(0.003)	(0.05)	(1.92)	(2.35)
Price of veterinary service	−0.010	−0.003	−0.013	0.0008
	(−2.12)	(−1.59)	(−2.53)	(0.40)
Wealth index	−0.362	0.417	0.204	0.304
	(−1.40)	(1.49)	(0.76)	(1.32)
Veterinary service price × Wealth index	0.035	−0.002	−0.002	−0.003
	(1.23)	(−0.89)	(−0.56)	(−1.50)
Average education in the household	0.040	0.042	0.030	0.092
	(0.79)	(0.81)	(0.56)	(2.87)
Sickness dummy (1 if no animal sick during the reference period, 0 otherwise)	−8.770	−7.340	−11.680	–
	(−0.33)	(−0.24)	(−0.26)	–
Service time (min)	0.080	0.007	−0.051	–
	(2.65)	(3.06)	(−2.62)	–
Travel and waiting time (min)	−0.003	−0.002	−0.002	–
	(−0.76)	(−1.10)	(−0.28)	–
Number of buffaloes owned by the household	−0.020	0.047	−1.27	–
	(−0.25)	(1.79)	(−1.82)	–
Number of cows owned by the household	0.100	0.028	0.668	–
	(1.10)	(1.25)	(4.76)	–
Number of desi cows owned by the household	–	–	–	0.016
				(0.065)
Number of cross-bred cows owned by the household	–	–	–	0.265
				(0.146)
Number of bullocks owned by the household	–	–	–	0.096
				(0.049)
Number of small ruminants owned by the household	–	–	–	0.063
				(0.012)
Sample size	367	297	387	160
Log likelihood	−289.71	−296.11	−567.80	−189.0

[a] Figures in parentheses are Z values.

index and the interaction between wealth and price – is statistically significant. This implies that income is not a major determinant of service utilization. The sign on this parameter is positive in Rajasthan and Kerala, which is consistent with a priori expectations. In Gujarat, however, the analysis shows a negative wealth effect. One possible explanation for this result could be that the incidence of sickness in Gujarat may be lower for richer households compared to the poorer ones due to better diet and care, whereas such a relationship is not very strong in the other two states.[2]

Estimates of price elasticity of demand are presented in Table 25.6. Although the slope of demand function does not vary with income, we still calculated the elasticities for different income groups by valuing them at the mean price and visits for the respective income groups.

It is evident from the table that overall price elasticity of demand for these services is quite low – almost zero in Gujarat, Rajasthan and Orissa. In Kerala, on the other hand, the demand is relatively more elastic at –0.14, implying that an increase of 100% in the price could lead to a drop of 14% in use of veterinary services with not much difference across rich and poor. In other states, the price variation may not have much impact on the utilization rates.

To recapitulate, the analysis presented above establishes beyond a reasonable doubt that: (i) subsidized or free services are not reaching the farmers as intended; (ii) farmers are actually not looking for free or subsidized services as they consider the prices they are currently paying as 'reasonable'; (iii) the prices charged by government and private veterinarians are not significantly different; and (iv) the structure of 'economic demand' for these services is not very different across poor and non-poor. This would make a reasonably strong case for reducing/withdrawing these subsidies and putting this money into services such as disease prevention, reporting, control, awareness education and so on, for these are the services that are currently neglected due

Table 25.6. Price elasticity of demand for veterinary services.

State	Elasticity (%)
Gujarat	–0.016
Rajasthan	–0.040
Kerala	–0.140
Orissa	0.000

to fiscal pressures and are likely to generate a larger social good than simple treatment services. Disease prevention and control are also likely to result in reduced private cost of treatment by way of bringing down the incidence of those diseases that have serious livelihood implications for the poor. A number of models are now available around the world to organize effective and efficient service delivery in a wide variety of production, market and socio-economic contexts.

If policy choices are so clear, why does animal health policy in the region continue to encourage 'pervasive direct action by the government' in livestock service delivery rather than the government focusing more on delivery of public good services and playing a regulatory and market-enhancing role supported by targeted direct action? It is suggested that 'good economics' is only one of the many inputs in the choice of policy options. Indeed, policy has been described as a 'chaos of purpose and accidents' and not necessarily a matter of the rational implementation of the choices supported by economic analysis. It is therefore of critical importance to understand the processes that govern the choice of policy options and identify leverage points that can be used to influence choice of policy options in favour of intended beneficiaries, especially the poor. These processes depend heavily on the socio-politico-economic context and therefore vary greatly within and between countries.

In what follows, an attempt to understand and influence animal health policy in one of the southern Indian states, Andhra Pradesh, is described. Andhra Pradesh has many similarities to the states in the above study and therefore serves to illustrate the inherent complexity of policy-making processes.

---

[2] For lack of data on those variables, however, we are not able to test that hypothesis.

Assessment and Reflections on Livestock Services Delivery in Andhra Pradesh

In Andhra Pradesh, as in other Indian states, the government continues to be the largest provider of livestock services to farmers. Services are provided largely from stationary veterinary centres. It was observed that the government system of livestock service delivery is generally slow to catch up with changes in production systems or the resultant service needs. The economic sustainability of government service delivery is mostly through budgetary support, and not well focused on the needs of the receivers of services. Therefore, the receivers of services generally have little influence on such changes in service delivery. Similarly, veterinary services that generate public goods such as prevention, control and eradication of diseases, disease surveillance, quality enforcement of drugs, vaccines and biologicals did not receive their due priority from the government. In contrast the animal health systems under public–private partnership, NGOs and community-based organizations (CBOs) aim at economic viability, wider reach and home delivery of services.

To further assess the efficiency and effectiveness of livestock service delivery systems and to suggest appropriate reform measures a multi-tier consultative process was initiated. The initiative functioned under the overall guidance and supervision of a multistakeholder Steering Committee, which was chaired by the top bureaucrat from the Animal Husbandry Department. It was supported by the Pro-Poor Livestock Policy Initiative of the Food and Agriculture Organization in partnership with the 'Capitalization of Livestock Program Experiences India' project of SDC/IC and the Animal Husbandry Department of Government of Andhra Pradesh. Through detailed consultations and studies, service needs of the small livestock holders and the gaps and deficiencies in service delivery were identified. The results of the initial work led the people involved to demand further widening of the scope and coverage of the initiative. The resultant refinements included wider area and stakeholder coverage under the consultative process, additional studies to identify the gaps and weaknesses of the para-veterinary system and putting in place a legal framework for delivery of minor veterinary services. It also led to the development of an efficient and practical prevention and control strategy and an action plan for six animal diseases of economic importance to the poor.

The participatory process, in which the State Department of Animal Husbandry and the major stakeholder categories played an active role, improved the acceptability and implementability of the proposed reforms. Evolving a common agenda amid opposing views, striking a balance among strong divergent demands of stakeholder groups and maintaining strict neutrality of the consultative process have been major challenges. With refinements, the process demonstrates an effective model for service reforms elsewhere.

Summary

The process followed in the Andhra Pradesh could perhaps be described as an 'Inquiry Process'. This involved talking to a wide range of stakeholders to ascertain their views on effective livestock service delivery systems, discussing it with technical experts and people's representatives and conducting field studies to take an informed view on a policy intervention. This participatory process improved the acceptability and implementability of the proposed reforms. Evolving a common agenda against opposing views, striking a balance among strong divergent demands of stakeholder groups and maintaining strict neutrality of the consultative process are major challenges. In fact, the picture of conflicting interactions between politics, history, culture and ideologies is often far more complex than anticipated. Indeed, the lesson learned is that many animal health issues are about relationships between people.

Thus, it is critical that investment in 'economic analysis' of policy options is supplemented by a socio-political study of 'policy processes' and a long-term strategy of investment in 'relationship building'.

26 Approaches to Economic Analyses and Implications for Policy Issues in South-east Asia: Results from Three Case Studies in Crop–Animal Systems

C. Devendra

Introduction

Approaches to economic analyses in animal experiments per se are part and parcel of the protocols associated with materials and methods and statistical analyses of the results. However, the analyses become more discerning and complicated in farming systems research. The complexity stems from farming systems research owing its origin to cropping systems research from the early 1970s. It was only in 1984 that the animal component was added to cropping systems research, paving the way for farming systems research. This holistic approach provided a basis for economic analyses that could investigate the implications for emerging policy issues for crop–animal systems, and how these drive livestock development in Asia.

To illustrate the approaches to economic analyses, methods used and the implications for policy issues, discussion in this chapter will focus on three successful case studies in South-east Asia. All three projects have demonstrated efficiency in natural resource management, tangible socio-economic benefits and potential possibilities for the development of sustainable agriculture.

Case Studies

Indonesia has about 47 million hectares of land, of which about 85% is dry land and

is considered marginal. This includes Bali and the transmigration areas in Sumatra, Kalimantan and Irian Jaya, areas which relate to the two case studies referred to below. Soil fertility is inherently low, and the soils are acidic and prone to erosion. The annual rainfall ranges from 800 to 2000 mm/year, and long dry seasons are common, with resultant feed shortages and low productivity in animals. The farmers in these areas are very poor and have little or no access to improved technology and production resources.

Crop growth is therefore difficult, but both annual and perennial crops are grown. The annual crops include cereals, pulses and tubers, and the former meet the daily needs of households. Transmigrant farmers also grow grain legumes such as groundnuts and soybean. In the lowlands, where soil moisture is higher, rice is also grown. Within the annual cropping systems, ruminants are stall-fed during the cropping season and tethered or grazed during the off season. The perennial crops include coconuts, coffee, cloves, fruit trees such as citrus and cashew. In the transmigration areas, rubber was planted by the government and given to the settlers as a grant.

Three-strata forage system (Indonesia)

The three-strata forage system (TSFS) is a sustainable crop–animal system that was developed in Bali. It is a way of producing and conserving the food requirement of cattle and goats, without any degradation of the environment. For semi-arid dry land farming areas such as in eastern Indonesia and south Asia, the systems combine production of food crops, with shrubs and trees to produce food for all year-round feeding. Essentially, one unit of TSFS involves 0.25 ha of land comprising 0.16 ha of the core area of food crops (maize, groundnut, cassava and pigeon pea) for human use, surrounded by stratum 1 of 0.09 ha of pasture (*Cenchrus ciliaris* and *Stylosanthes guianensis*), stratum 2 with 2000 shrub legumes (*Gliricidia sepium* and *Leucaena leucocephala*) and stratum 3 with 42 fodder trees (*Ficus, Lannea* and *Hibiscus*). Cattle were introduced in the second year. A total of 26 farmers (12 with the project and 14 non-project, traditional) were involved over the period 1984–1993. The major highlights of the system are (Nitis *et al.*, 1990):

- Increased forage productions enabled higher stocking rates and live weight gains (3.2 animal units equivalent to 375 kg/ha/year in the TSFS compared to 2.1 animal units or 122 kg/ha/year in the non-TSFS).
- Cattle in the TSFS gained 19% more live weight and reached market weight 13% faster; farmers in the TSFS benefited by a 31% increase in farm income.
- The introduction of forage legumes into the TSFS reduced soil erosion by 57% in the TSFS compared to the non-TSFS. There was an associated increased soil fertility.
- The presence of 2000 shrubs and 112 trees logged twice a year produced 1.5 Mt/year of firewood, which met 64% of the farmers' annual firewood requirements.
- The integration of goats in addition to cattle into the system further increased the income of farmers.
- Institutionalization of the concept and technology.

Development of crop–animal system in transmigration areas (Indonesia)

In order to ease human population pressure in Jawa, the government of Indonesia has been encouraging relocation of families elsewhere to sparsely populated transmigration areas. The main economic activity envisaged was rubber production, but the role of food crops and animals in stabilizing the income of farmers in the early years was considered very important. The government provided 5.0 ha of land for each family, consisting of 2.0 ha of rubber, 2.0 ha of food crops and 1.0 ha for the home garden. Animals were introduced to develop an appropriate crop–animal system.

The research work was carried out in three phases, between 1985–1994, in four sites in south Sumatra. The first phase focused on the most appropriate farming system model, the second phase evaluated socio-economic factors, and the third phase was concerned with adoption of the model. A total of 80 farmers were involved in the overall assessment. The four treatments tested were as follows:

- Model A is a traditional system without animals (monitoring only).
- Model B is a traditional system with animals (monitoring only).
- Model C is integration with 1 cow, 3 goats and 11 chickens.
- Model D is integration with 2 cows, 5 goats and 23 chickens.

The results over the 9 years showed that increased incomes and improved livelihoods were associated with enhanced crop yields, animal production, the development of a revolving fund and self-reliance (CRIFC, 1995). During the last phase, between 1992 and 1994, net farm income in the three sites improved fourfold, in which the contributions to total farm income by animals, rubber and food crops were 10.0%, 17.3% and 72.7% respectively. Farmers in the project consistently enjoyed higher incomes than the traditional farmers and increased spending on better quality foods and investment on the education of their children.

Integrated oil palm–ruminants systems (Malaysia)

The third case study concerns integrated tree crops–ruminants systems. Tree crops refer mainly to coconuts, oil palm and rubber but can include other examples like citrus and coffee. Among these, the oil palm is especially important because of the expanding land area under it and the high demand and value of palm oil in international markets. The ruminant animals which have been used are buffaloes, cattle, goats and sheep; of these cattle are the most popular for economic reasons.

Integration with ruminants is justified by the presence of considerable availability of natural herbage under the canopy of the trees, various feed by-products from oil palm, potential economic benefits and increased total factor productivity due to the additive effects of trees and animals. Despite these advantages, however, and potential importance, this production system remains to be more fully explored. The benefits that have been demonstrated include increased yield of fresh fruit bunches, savings in the use of fertilizers and weedicides, transportation costs, development of *in situ* feeding systems and increased animal production and economic returns. A few studies have reported these benefits. These aspects, the potential future importance of the system and the need for expanded development have recently been reviewed (Devendra, 2004).

The main reasons why these integrated systems have not expanded significantly is because oil palm plantations are largely in the hands of plant individuals and planners, who see the integration with animals as a burdensome task, which requires additional capital investments, time and increased management responsibilities. Additionally, the task will require the expertise of animal scientists to oversee the operations. Despite these obstacles, the process of integration is gaining ground and the land area under such systems is expanding in both Malaysia and Indonesia.

The oil palm environment and large plantations under the crop offer major opportunities for on-farm research and development. With respect to feeds and their availability, the production system can vary from limited grazing plus stall-feeding to complete stall-feeding or zero-grazing. The latter aspects enable research into the whole area of types of feeds, availability and quality and feed mixtures. Component technology assessment includes, for example, effects of type and level of dietary supplements, complete feeds, inclusion of leguminous forages, effects of shade on animal performance and effects of grazing on soil fertility and compaction.

Economic Analyses and Methods Used

Together with the participatory methodologies that were used, an important prerequisite in the formulation of research activities was the design of the work, as well as how the results will be analysed. These were done through a series of meetings and workshops before as well as during the implementation of the project, which were very useful to sustain interest as well as ownership of the project. For the same reasons, the final results were shared and discussed with the participants, to ensure correct interpretation and confirmation.

With specific reference to the analyses of the results, the following methods were used in the projects:

- Partial-budget analysis to estimate anticipated profitability or loss due to a change in the farming system, usually a single intervention.
- The 'with and without' method was used due to the long duration of the work, and this enabled comparisons of the results in holistic terms between the participating farmers in the project and traditional farmers outside the project.
- The 'before and after' method was also used for treatments of a shorter duration of a few weeks. This was well suited for the component technology evaluations such as the effects of feeding different leguminous forages on performance in goats as in case study 3.
- Benefit/cost ratio, including discounted future costs and benefits, due to the long-term nature of the projects.

Implications for Policy Issues

Case study 1

- The demonstrable success of the project and the benefits resulted in a government directive to promote wider adoption of the system.
- Associated with the above, the timing of planting of cash crops, when and how to include tree legumes in the system were included in the Balinese calendar.

- The value of technology and the system have been recognized and replicated in similar environments in South Asia and in parts of Africa.

Case study 2

- The successful development of crop–animal systems combining annual and perennial crops and animals, including packages of improved technologies in the project sites, led to wider government promotion of the development of the system in other transmigration sites.
- The success of the system was also seen as providing important incentives for sedentarizing farmers and reducing shifting agriculture.
- The development of a farmer-managed revolving fund increased wider ownership and intensification of especially poultry production, and encouraged self-reliance. This promoted model was attractive to neighbouring villages and wider adoption followed.
- The approaches to, methods used in and experiences gained in the development of the improved crop–animal system led to these being applied in the development of the coastal areas elsewhere in Sumatra.

Case study 3

- The development of integrated oil palm–ruminant systems needs increased official support for its expansion, despite the economic benefits of added value and increased productivity. Policy interventions are required to stimulate more integration with animals, for use of the land area under oil palm through, e.g. tax incentives, and also to encourage increased private sector investments.

Conclusions

The changes in livestock production and their associated value chains are important in the challenges the State faces with animal disease prevention, control and eradication. In a developed country context, Professor M. Upton (personal communication, London, 2005) has commented that the issue of disease control and eradication could be considered more a *'club'* than a public good due to the reducing numbers of livestock producers. The smaller the number of livestock producers the stronger the argument for the State not to offer support to this 'club'. However, there are strong arguments for the need to regulate and monitor large industrial integrated livestock systems with the possibility of requiring them to put aside money in the event of animal health disaster. Some would argue for the need to separate diseases by their impact on human health, with the control of zoonotic diseases clearly creating a public good, whereas the control of non-zoonotic diseases may well create only private goods. The latter is very much dependent on the structure and governance of the value chains.

To balance this, Stott (2005) mentions that control and eradication of disease at farm level create *externalities* in terms of better-quality food and also lowering production costs that may be passed on to the food chain actors. These cannot be ignored and need to be recognized when devising support programmes for animal health problems. In a developing country context, the numbers of livestock producers are still large and require support and attention.

What is also of interest is that, as livestock value chains get more complex and there is greater separation between the producer and consumer, there are increased risks of *moral hazard* where the government has a role to regulate and monitor the activities of the different actors in the food value chain from the input provider to the processor and marketeer. Here, up-to-date information is needed on the food chains in order to determine the importance of each actor.

There are three aspects that require further examination. First, *if actions at farm level in disease control either increase quality and/or quantity of the products, then it is likely that the gains from these actions will be shared between the producer and the other actors further down the food chain.* The producer is unlikely to have the market power to retain all the benefits from the change in health status.[1] UK data clearly show that food price inflation is half that of other goods and, between 1988 and 2004, the farmer's share in the basket of food staples has fallen by 25% (DEFRA, 2005). A clear example is that externalities generated

_____

[1] For a discussion on value chain governance see Gereffi *et al.* (2003) and for a practical application see Velde *et al.* (2006).

by animal health changes at farm level need to be monitored by the State and, where necessary, actions need to be taken either through direct activities, subsidies or regulations to ensure that the producers are not disadvantaged in their endeavours that ultimately benefit society. To counter this view, there are arguments that food products as a whole have an inelastic demand, but livestock products may be highly elastic. The value added at the consumer level is due to processing and packaging of livestock products, and the link between farm-level revenues and externalities is not clear. There could in fact be a strong influence from the internationalization of livestock products markets and the international organizations such as the WTO and the OIE that regulate international trade. However, this suggests that a government with livestock value chains that are increasingly dominated by few buyers need to be aware that the governing actors in the value chain may utilize their power to squeeze farm-gate prices.

This leads into a second area of importance. An *ex ante* cost–benefit analysis for an animal disease control will focus on the costs and benefits to society of the control or eradication of that disease. Such an analysis can incorporate different levels of complexity to include the impact of changes on other sectors in society, consumer welfare, up to general equilibrium models, etc. (Rich *et al.*, 2005; Martin Upton, Chapter 11, this volume), but *a cost–benefit analysis is not a useful tool to consider the incentive structure of the different actors in the food chains.* Accurate description and understanding of the food chains are needed to identify which actors are important and who is likely to gain from the change in status. It is suggested that important actors need to have a further analysis to determine the institutional structure in which they work and to understand their incentives for cooperating in a disease control programme.[2] A clear understanding of the incentive structures for each actor will help the State to define its own

roles in supporting a programme and in turn improve the chance that such a programme will be successful. The added benefit is that actions that facilitate the roles of each actor should increase the profile of the State and hence improve their image within the production, processing and marketing community.

The third and important aspect of the development of the economics of animal health and production is recognizing the political economy context in which animal health decisions are made. *There is a need to recognize that the political economy affects: (i) whether public investments are made in animal health; and (ii) the institutional environment in which implementers of disease control measures operate.* It is recommended that at the outset of an animal health project or programme a political economy analysis is carried out in order to assess where the animal health actions and institutional development issues are best directed within existing organizations. In Bolivia, a project to strengthen the animal disease surveillance and epidemiology structures for the country ran into difficulties through having inadequate information on the political economy. This project could have been much more successful and sustainable if the initial implementation had included a political economy analysis (D. Muñoz, personal communication, La Paz, Bolivia, 2006). Vinod Ahuja's contribution (Chapter 25, this volume) demonstrates the need for dialogue at a local level in getting commitment from all stakeholders, and Hernán Rojas (Chapter 23, this volume) describes the development of the Chilean animal health system, which has strong public–private partnerships.

To conclude, a number of critical issues are highlighted for the economic analysis of animal health and production:

- Any analysis of animal health and production, even though it is based on technical interventions, should always be people-focused.
- Animal health and production interventions require thought and analysis at different levels and of different components of the livestock sector.

---

[2] See Ly (2003) for a practical application of estimating incentives in an African context.

- Economics of animal health and production can provide a better understanding of:
  - ongoing processes of change and development of the livestock sector and animal health status; and
  - the future developments of the sector with or without possible investments, policy or strategy change.
- Change is best facilitated and promoted where there is collaboration between the public and private sectors in terms of actions, strategies and policies.

Finally, it is concluded that the economics of animal health and production require a *holistic or systems perspective* which combines an analysis of the political economy, economic incentives, social acceptability and technical feasibility of disease control measures and programmes.

Bibliography

General

Ahuja, V. (2004) The economic rationale of public and private sector roles in the provision of animal health services. *Revue Scientifique et Technique Office International des Epizooties* 23(1), 33–45.

Ahuja, V., George, P.S., Ray, S., Kurup, M.P.G. and Gandhi, V. (2000) *Agricultural Services and the Poor: Case of Livestock Health and Breeding Services in India.* IIM Ahmedabad, The World Bank, and SDC, Bern, Switzerland.

Alguilar, S. and Rushton, J. (2005) *The Economics of Vicuña Capture and the Commercialization of Vicuña Fiber in Bolivia with a Focus on the Communities in the Apolobamba.* Final report for the project 'The conservation and economic management of vicuñas in Bolivia', financed by the University of South Florida, USA, 62 pp.

Alston, J.M., Norton, G.W. and Pardey, P.G. (1995) *Science Under Scarcity.* Cornell University Press, Ithaca, New York and London, 585 pp.

Anderson, R.M. and May, R.M. (1985) Vaccination and herd immunity to infectious diseases. *Nature* 318, 323–329.

Apple, J.L. (1978) Impact of plant disease on world food production. In: Pimentel, D. (ed.) *World Food, Pest Losses and the Environment. American Association for the Advancement of Science Symposium.* Westview Press, Boulder, Colorado, pp. 13, 39–49.

Ariza-Nino, E and Shapiro, K.H. (1984) Cattle as capital, consumables and cash: modelling age-of-sale decisions in African pastoral pr oduction. In: Simpson J.R. and Evangelou P. (eds) *Livestock Development in Subsaharan Africa: Constraints, Prospects and Policy.* Westview Press, Boulder, Colorado, pp. 317–333.

Arriaga-Jordan, C.M. and Pearson, R.A. (2004) The contribution of livestock to smallholder livelihoods: the situation in Mexico. In: Owen, E., Smith, T., Steele, M.A., Anderson, S., Duncan, A.J., Herrero, M., Leaver, J.D., Reynolds, C.K., Richards, J.I. and Ku-Vera, J.C. (eds) *Responding to the Livestock Revolution. The Role of Globalisation and Implications for Poverty Alleviation.* BSAS Publication 33, Nottingham, UK, pp. 99–115.

Arriaga-Jordan, C.M., Guadarrama-Estrada, J., Heredia-Nava, D., Garduño-Castro, Y., Espinoza-Ortega, A., González-Esquivel, C.E. and Castelán-Ortega, O.A. (2005) Inclusion of maize or oats–vetch silage in the feeding of milking dairy cows at grass in small-holder campesino systems in the highlands of Central Mexico. In: Rowlinson, P., Wachirapakorn, C., Pakdee, P. and Wanapat, M. (eds) *Proceedings of Integrating Livestock–Crop Systems to Meet the Challenges of Globalisation,* Vol. 2. AHAT/BSAS International Conference 14–18 November 2005, Khon Kaen, Thailand. AHAT, Bangkok, Thailand, p. P57.

Avilés-Nova, F., Espinoza-Ortega, A., Castelán-Ortega, O.A. and Arriaga-Jordan, C.M. (2005) Sheep performance under intensive continuous grazing of native grasslands of *Paspalum notatum* and *Axonopus compressus* in the subtropical region of the Highlands of Central Mexico. In: Rowlinson, P., Wachirapakorn, C., Pakdee, P. and Wanapat, M. (eds) *Proceedings of 'Integrating Livestock–Crop Systems to Meet the Challenges of Globalisation'*, Vol. 2. AHAT/BSAS International Conference, 14–18 November 2005, Khon Kaen, Thailand. AHAT, Bangkok, Thailand, p. T48.

Backhouse, R.E. (2002) *The Ordinary Business of Life. A History of Economics from the Ancient World to the Twenty-First Century*. Princeton University Press, Princeton, New Jersey, 369 pp.

Baptiste, R. (1987) Computer simulation of monitoring herd productivity under extensive conditions: sampling error of herd size and offtake rate. *Agricultural Systems* 24, 199–210.

Baptiste, R. (1992) Derivation of steady-state herd productivity. *Agricultural Systems* 39, 253–272.

Barnard, C.S and Nix, J.S. (1979) *Farming Planning and Control*, 2nd edn. Cambridge University Press, Cambridge, 600 pp.

Barnum, H.N. and Squire, L. (1979) *A Model of an Agricultural Household. Theory and Evidence*. World Bank Staff Occasional Papers, No. 27. Johns Hopkins University Press, Baltimore, Maryland, 107 pp.

Barrett, J. (1992) *The Economic Role of Cattle in Communal Farming Systems in Zimbabwe*. ODI Pastoral Development Network Paper 32b. ODI, London, 35 pp.

Beck, A.C. and Dent, J.B. (1987) A farm growth model for policy analysis in an extensive pastoral production system. *Australian Journal of Agricultural Economics* 31(1), 29–44.

Becker, G.S. (1965) A theory of the allocation of time. *Economic Journal* 5, 493–517.

Benito Gonzalez, P., Fernando Bas, M., Charif Tala, G. and Agustin Iriarte, W. (2000) *Manejo Sustentable de la Vicuña y el Guanaco*. SAG, Universidad Catolica de Chile y Fundacion para la Innovacion Agraria, Santiago, Chile, 276 pp.

Bennett, R.M. (1992) The use of 'economic' quantitative modelling techniques in livestock health and disease-control decision making: a review. *Preventive Veterinary Medicine* 13, 63–76.

Bennett, R.M. (2003) The 'direct' costs of livestock disease: the development of a system of models for the analysis of 30 endemic livestock diseases in Great Britain. *Journal of Agricultural Economics* 54, 55–72.

Bennett, R., Christiansen, K. and Clifton-Hadley, R. (1997) An economic study of the importance of non-notifiable diseases of farm animals in Great Britain. *Epidémiologie et Santé Animale* 31–32, 10.19.1–10.19.3.

Berdegue, J.A., Installe, M., Duque, Ch., Garcia, R. and Quezada, X. (1989) Application of a simulation software to the analysis of a peasant farming system. *Agricultural Systems* 30, 317–334.

Bernard, J.K., Mullen, M.D., Hathcock, B.R., Smith, R.A., Byford, J.L., Keisling, L.W., Thomsen, R.M. and Counce, E.W. (1992) Dairy production in Ecuador: problems and opportunities. *Journal of Dairy Science* 75(Supplement 1), xxi–xxv.

Bernet, T. (2000) The Peruvian dairy sector. Farmer perspectives, development strategies and policy options. PhD thesis, Swiss Federal Institute of Technology, Zurich, Switzerland, 131 pp.

Bhende, M.J. and Venkataram, J.V. (1994) Impact of diversification on household income and risk: a whole-farm modelling approach. *Agricultural Systems* 44, 301–312.

Boehlje, M.D. and Eidman, V.R. (1984) *Farm Management*. Wiley, New York, 806 pp.

Boserup, E. (1965) *The Conditions for Agricultural Growth. The Economics of Agrarian Change Under Population Pressure*. Earthscan, London, 124 pp.

Brockington, N.R., Gonzalez, C.A., Veil, J.M., Vera, R.R., Teixeira, N.M. and de Assis, A.G. (1983) A bio-economic modelling project for small-scale milk production systems in south-east Brazil. Part I. *Agricultural Systems* 12, 37–60.

Brockington, N.R., de Assis, A.G., Martinez, M.L. and Veil, J.M. (1986) A bio-economic modelling project for small-scale milk production systems in South-East Brazil: Part 2 – refinement and use of the model to analyse some short and long-term management strategies. *Agricultural Systems* 20, 53–81.

Brower, B. (1991) *Sherpa of Khumbu. People, Livestock and Landscape*. Oxford University Press, New Delhi, India, 202 pp.

Brown, M.L. (1979) *Farm Budgets from Farm Income Analysis to Agricultural Project Analysis*. World Bank Staff Occasional Papers, No. 29. The Johns Hopkins University Press, Baltimore, Maryland, 136 pp.

Burden, B. (2007) Public/private sector linkages: considerations in maintaining markets for large and small poultry operations. In: *Proceedings for Symposium for Markets and Trade Dimensions of Avian Influenza*. FAO, Rome, Italy, 13 November 2006. Available at: http://www.fao.org/es/ESC/en/20953/21014/21574/event_109566en.html

Byron Nelson, M. (2005) *International Rules, Food Safety and the Poor Developing Country Livestock Producer*. Pro-Livestock Policy Initiative Working Paper No. 25. FAO, Rome, Italy, 41 pp.

Cacho, O.J., Finlayson, J.D. and Bywater, A.C. (1995) A simulation model of grazing sheep: II. Whole farm model. *Agricultural Systems* 48, 27–50.

Caillavet, F., Guyomard, H. and Lifran, R. (eds) (1994) *Agricultural Household Modelling and Family Economics*. Elsevier, Amsterdam, The Netherlands.

Carabin, H., Budke, C.M., Cowan, L.D., Willingham III, A.L. and Torgerson, P. (2005) Methods for assessing the burden of parasitic zoonoses: echinococcosis and cysticercosis. *Trends in Parasitology* 21, 327–333.

Carney D. (ed.) (1998) *Sustainable Rural Livelihoods: What Contribution Can We Make?* Department for International Development, London, 213 pp.

Carpenter, T.E. (1980) Economic evaluation of *Mycoplasma meleagridis* infection in turkeys: I. Production losses. II. Feasibility of eradication. *Dissertation Abstracts International* 41B(2), 485.

Carpenter, T.E., Miller, K.F., Gentry, R.F., Schwartz, L.D. and Mallinson, E.T. (1979) Control of *Mycoplasma gallisepticum* in commercial laying chickens using artificial exposure to Connecticut F strain *Mycoplasma gallisepticum*. *Proceedings of the United States Animal Health Association* 83, 364–370.

Casley, D.J. and Kumar, K. (1987) *Project Monitoring and Evaluation in Agriculture*. Johns Hopkins University Press, Baltimore, Maryland.

Casley, D.J. and Lury, D.A. (1981) *Data Collection in Developing Countries*, 2nd edn. Clarendon Press, Oxford, 225 pp.

Catley, A. (1999) *Methods on the Move. A Review of Veterinary Uses of Participatory Approaches and Methods Focusing on Experiences in Dryland Africa*. IIED, London.

Catley, A. (2005) Animal health. In: Conroy, C. (ed.) *Participatory Livestock Research: A Guide*. ITDG Publishing, Bourton-on-Dunsmore, UK, pp. 57–72.

Central Bureau of Statistics (2002) *National Accounts of Nepal – 2002*. HMG Nepal, National Planning Commission Secretariat, Central Bureau of Statistics, Thapathali, Kathmandu, Nepal, 52 pp.

Collinson, M. (1981) A low cost approach to understanding small farmers. *Agricultural Administration* 8(6), 433–450.

Conroy, C. (ed.) (2005) *Participatory Livestock Research: A Guide*. ITDG Publishing, Bourton-on-Dunsmore, UK, 304 pp.

Chambers, R. (1983) *Rural Development: Putting the Last First*. Longman Scientific and Technical, London, UK.

Crotty, R. (1980) *Cattle Economics and Development*. CAB International, Wallingford, UK.

DANE (2002) *Encuesta nacional agropecuaria, resultados 2001*. DANE – Ministerio de Agricultura, Bogota, Colombia, 207 pp.

Dasgupta, A.K. and Pearce, D.W. (1978) *Cost–Benefit Analysis: Theory and Practice*. Macmillan, London, 270 pp.

De Alwis, M.C.L. (1982) Immune status of buffalo calves exposed to natural infection with haemorrhagic septicaemia. *Tropical Animal Health and Production* 14, 29–30.

Delforce, J.C. (1993) *Smallholder Agriculture in the Kingdom of Tonga: a Farm-Household Analysis*. Agricultural Economics Bulletin No. 40, Department of Agricultural Economics and Business Management. The University of New England, Armidale, Australia, 302 pp.

Delforce, J.C. (1994) Separability in farm-household economics: an experiment with linear programming. *Agricultural Economics* 10, 165–177.

Delgado, C., Rosegrant, M., Steinfeld, H., Ehui, S. and Courbois, C. (1999) *Livestock to 2020. The Next Food Revolution*. Food, Agriculture and the Environment Discussion Paper 28. IFPRI, Washington DC, 72 pp.

Delgado Santivañez, D.J. (2003) Perspectivas de la Producción de Fibra de Llama en Bolivia. Potencial y desarrollo de estrategias para mejorar la calidad de la fibra y su aptitud para la comercialización. PhD thesis, Hohenheim University, Germany, 198 pp.

Dent, J.B., Harrison, S.R. and Woodford, K.B. (1986) *Farm Planning with Linear Programming: Concept and Practice*. Butterworths, Sydney, Australia.

Dent, J.B., Edwards-Jones, G. and McGregor, M.J. (1995) Simulation of ecological, social and economic factors in agricultural systems. *Agricultural Systems* 49, 337–351.

Dessie, T. (1996) Studies in village poultry production in the Central Highlands of Ethiopia. MSc thesis, Swedish University of Agricultural Sciences, Department of Animal Nutrition and Management, Sweden.

Dijkhuizen, A.A., Huirne, R.B.M. and Jalvingh, A.W. (1995) Economic analysis of animal diseases and their control. *Preventive Veterinary Medicine* 25, 135–149.

Dillon, J.L. and Anderson, J.R. (1990) *The Analysis of Response in Crop and Livestock Production*, 3rd edn. Pergamon Press, Oxford, UK.

Doll, J.P. and Orazem, F. (1984) *Production Economics: Theory with Applications*, 2nd edn. Wiley, New York, 470 pp.

Doran, M.H., Low, A.R.C. and Kemp, R.L. (1979) Cattle as a store of wealth in Swaziland: implications for livestock development and overgrazing in Eastern and Southern Africa. *American Journal of Agricultural Economics* 61(1), 41–47.

Dorward, A.R. (1984) Farm management methods and their role in agricultural extension to smallholder farmers: a case study from Northern Malawi. Unpublished PhD thesis, University of Reading, Reading, UK.

Dorward, A. (1986a) Farm management and extension in smallholder agriculture: part 1 – the role of farm management in extension. *Agricultural Administration* 22, 21–37.

Dorward, A. (1986b) Farm management and extension in smallholder agriculture: part 2 – appropriate farm management skills and their use in extension. *Agricultural Administration* 22, 117–133.

Dorward, A. (1991) Integrated decision rules as farm management tools in smallholder agriculture in Malawi. *Journal of Agricultural Economics* 42(2), 146–160.

Dorward, A.R. (1995) Issues in farm management education in Africa. *Journal of International Farm Management* 1(4), 97–104.

Dorward, P.T., Shepherd, D.D. and Wolmer, W.L. (1996) *The Development of Farm Management Type Methodologies for Improved Needs Assessment: a Literature Review*. A paper commissioned by ODA from The University of Reading, Reading, UK.

Dubois, R. and Moura, J.A. (2004) La lutte contre la fièvre aphteuse au Bresil: la participation du secteur privé. *Revue Scientifique et Technique Office International des Epizooties* 23(1), 165–173. Available at: http://www.oie.int/fr/publicat/rt/2301/F_R23113.htm

Ellis, F. (1988) *Peasant Economics: Farm Households and Agrarian Development*. Cambridge University Press, Cambridge, 257 pp.

Ellis, F. (2000) *Rural Livelihoods and Diversity in Developing Countries*. Oxford University Press, Oxford, 273 pp.

Ellis, P.R. (1992) The epidemiology and economic assessment of poultry diseases. In: *Proceedings of International Seminar on Prevention and Control of Poultry Diseases, 7–13 September 1992*. Bangkok, Thailand, pp. 9–30.

Ellis, P.R., James, A.D. and Shaw, A.P.M. (1977) *Studies on the Epidemiology and Economics of Swine Fever Eradication in the EEC*. EUR 5738, Commission of the European Communities, Brussels, 90 pp.

Espinoza-Ortega, A. and Arriaga-Jordan, C.M. (2005a) Characterization of small dairy farms in highlands of central Mexico. In: Rowlinson, P., Wachirapakorn, C., Pakdee, P. and Wanapat, M. (eds) *Proceedings of Integrating Livestock–Crop Systems to Meet the Challenges of Globalisation*, Vol. 2. AHAT/BSAS International Conference 14–18 November 2005, Khon Kaen, Thailand. AHAT, Bangkok, Thailand, p. T120.

Espinoza-Ortega, A. and Arriaga-Jordan, C.M. (2005b) The economy of small dairy farms in highlands of central Mexico. In: Rowlinson, P., Wachirapakorn, C., Pakdee, P. and Wanapat, M. (eds) *Proceedings of Integrating Livestock–Crop Systems to Meet the Challenges of Globalisation*, Vol. 2. AHAT/BSAS International Conference 14–18 November 2005, Khon Kaen, Thailand. AHAT, Bangkok, Thailand, p. T5.

Falconi, C.A. (1993) Economic evaluation. In: Horton, D., Ballantyne, P., Peterson, W., Uribe, B., Gapasin, D. and Sheridan, K. (eds) *Monitoring and Evaluating Agricultural Research*. CAB International, Wallingford, UK, pp. 65–75.

FAO (2002) The vulnerability of mountain environments and mountain people. Available at: http://www.fao.org/docrep/005/y7352e

FAO (2005) *Livestock Policies and Poverty Reduction in Africa, Asia and Latin America*. Pro-Poor Livestock Policy Initiative Policy Brief. FAO, Rome, Italy.

FAO (2007) Pro poor livestock policy initiative. Available at: http://www.fao.org/ag/againfo/projects/en/pplpi

Fernández Baca, E. and Bojorquez, C. (1994) Milk production in the Valle del Mantaro [Peru]. 1. Resources available. (Produccion lechera en el Valle del Mantaro: 1. Recursos disponibles para la produccion.) *Revista de Investigaciones Pecuarias* 7(1), 45–53.

Ferrell, O.C., Hartline, M.D., Lucas, G.H. and Luck, D. (1998) *Marketing Strategy. The Dryden Press*, Harcourt Brace College Publishers, Orlando, Florida, 407 pp. Available at: http://www.dryden.com/mktng/ferrell

Finlayson, J.D., Cacho, O.J. and Bywater, A.C. (1995) A simulation model of grazing sheep: I. Animal growth and intake. *Agricultural Systems* 48, 1–25.

Fisher, J.R. (1980) The economic effects of cattle disease in Britain and its containment, 1850–1900. *Agricultural History* 54(2), 278–294.

Fisher, J.R. (1998) Cattle plagues past and present: the mystery of mad cow disease. *Journal of Contemporary History* 33(2), 215–228.

France, J. and Thornley, J.H.M. (1984) *Mathematical Models in Agriculture. A Quantitative Approach to Problems in Agriculture and Related Science*. Butterworth, London, UK, 335 pp.

Franzel, S. and Crawford, E.W. (1987) Comparing formal and informal survey techniques for farming systems research: a case study from Kenya. *Agricultural Administration and Extension* 27, 13–33.

Fricke, T.E. (1993) *Himalayan Households. Tamang Demography and Domestic Processes*. Book Faith India, Delhi, India, 227 pp.

Gardner, H. (2004) *Changing Minds. The Art and Science of Changing Our Own and Other People's Minds*. Harvard Business School Press, Boston, Massachusetts, 244 pp.

Geerts, S. and Holmes, P.H. (1998) *Drug Management and Parasite Resistance in Animal Trypanosomiasis in Africa*. PAAT (Programme Against African Trypanosomiasis) Technical and Scientific Series 1. FAO, Rome, 38 pp.

Gereffi, G., Humphrey, J. and Sturgeon, T. (2003) The governance of global value chains. *Review of International Political Economy* 12(1), 78–104.

Gitau, G.K., McDermott, J.J., Adams, J.E., Lissemore, K.D. and Waltner-Toews, D. (1994) Factors influencing calf growth and daily weight gain on smallholder dairy farms in Kiambu District, Kenya. *Preventive Veterinary Medicine* 21, 179–190.

Gittinger, J.P. (1982) *Economic Analysis of Agricultural Projects*, 2nd edn. Johns Hopkins University Press, Baltimore, Maryland.

Gonzalez, D.J.G., Arriaga-Jordan, C.M. and Sanchez, V.E. (1996) The role of cattle and sheep in campesino (peasant) production systems in the highlands of central Mexico. In: Dent, J.B., McGregor, M.J. and Sibbald, A.R. (eds) *Livestock Farming Systems: Research, Development, Socio-Economics and the Land Manager*. EAAP Publication No. 79, Wageningen, The Netherlands, pp. 103–108.

Greger, M. (2007) The human/animal interface: emergence and resurgence of zoonotic infectious diseases. *Reviews in Microbiology* 33, 243–299.

Grigg, D.B. (1974) *The Agricultural Systems of the World. An Evolutionary Approach*. Cambridge University Press, Cambridge, 358 pp.

Groenewald, P.C.N., Ferreira, A.V., van der Merwe, H.J. and Slippers, S.C. (1995) A mathematical model for describing and predicting the lactation curve of Merino ewes. *Animal Science* 61, 95–101.

Gulbenkian, M. (1993) The potentials for improvement of traditional sheep cheese production systems in Portugal. PhD thesis, University of Reading, Reading, UK.

Haan, C. de, Schillhorn van Veen, T., Brandenburg, B., Gauthier, J., Le Gall, F., Mearns, R. and Simeón, M. (2001) *Livestock Development: Implications for Rural Poverty, the Environment and Global Food Security*. The World Bank, Washington DC, 96 pp.

Habtemariam, T., Howitt, R., Ruppanner, R. and Riemann, H.P. (1984) Application of a linear programming model to the control of African trypanosomiasis. *Preventive Veterinary Medicine* 3, 1–14.

Hall, D.C., Kaiser, H.M. and Blake, R.W. (1998) Modelling the economics of animal health control programs using dynamic programming. *Agricultural Systems* 56, 125–144.

Hardaker, J.B., Huirne, R.B.M. and Anderson, J.R. (1997) *Coping with Risk in Agriculture*. CAB International, Wallingford, UK, 274 pp.

Hargraves, A. and Adasme, A. (2001) Manejo del ganado lechero. In: *Agenda del salitre*. Sociedad Química y Minera de Chile, Santiago, Chile, pp. 1047–1064.

Harris, M. (1975) *Cows, Pigs, Wars and Witches. Riddles of Culture*. Hutchinson, London.

Hazell, P.B.R. and Norton, R.D. (1986) *Mathematical Programming for Economic Analysis in Agriculture*. MacMillan Publishing Company, New York, 400 pp.

Heffernan, C. (2002) Livestock and the poor: issues in poverty focused development. In: Owen, E., Smith, T., Steele, M.A., Anderson, S., Duncan, A.J., Herrero, M., Leaver, J.D., Reynolds, C.K., Richards, J.I. and Ku-Vera, J.C. (eds) *Responding to the Livestock Revolution. The Role of Globalisation and Implications for Poverty Alleviation*. BSAS Publication 33, Nottingham, UK, pp. 229–245.

Heffernan, C., Misturelli, F., Nielsen, L. and Pilling, D. (2003) *The Livestock and Poverty Assessment Methodology: a Toolkit for Practitioners*. Livestock Development Group School of Agriculture, Policy and Development University of Reading, Reading, UK. Available at: http://www.livestockdevelopment. org/adobedocs/LPA%20Manual.PDF

Heffernan, C., Misturelli, F., Fuller, R. and Patnaik, S. (2005) The livestock and poverty assessment methodology: an overview. In: Owen, E., Kitalyi, A., Jayasuriya, N. and Smith, T. (eds) *Livestock and Wealth Creation. Improving the Husbandry of Animals Kept By Resource-Poor People in Developing Countries*. Nottingham University Press, Nottingham, UK, pp. 53–69.

Henson, S. (2006) The role of public and private standards in regulating international food markets. In: *Proceedings of the International Agricultural Trade and Research Consortium Summer Symposium Held in Bonn, Germany 28–30 May 2006*.

Holden, S.T. (1993) Peasant household modelling: farming systems evolution and sustainability in northern Zambia. *Agricultural Economics* 9, 241–267.

Houben, E.H.P. (1995) Economic optimization of decisions with respect to dairy cow health management. PhD thesis, Landbouwuniversiteit, Wageningen, The Netherlands, 146 pp.

House of Commons (2008) *Foot and Mouth Disease 2007: A Review and Lessons Learned*. Crown Copyright, Crown, London, 139 pp.

Hoyos, G., Rushton, J. and Angus, S. (2000) *The economic impact of foot and mouth disease in extensive beef systems of Bolivia*. Poster presentation at The Society of Veterinary Epidemiology and Preventive Medicine meeting in Edinburgh, Scotland.

Hugh-Jones, M.E., Ellis, P.R. and Felton, M.R. (1975) *An Assessment of the Eradication of Bovine Brucellosis in England and Wales.* Department of Agriculture and Horticulture, University of Reading, Reading, UK, viii + 75 pp.

Hunt, D. (1991) Farm system and household economy as frameworks for prioritising and appraising technical research: a critical appraisal of current approaches. In: Haswell, M. and Hunt, D. (eds) *Rural Households in Emerging Societies: Technology and Change in Sub-Saharan Africa.* Pergamon Press, Oxford, pp. 49–75.

INDEC (Instituto Nacional de Estadística y Censo) (1999) *Encuesta nacional agropecuaria. Resultados generales*, Vol. 1, Santiago, Chile, pp. 9–18.

INE (1997) *VI Censo Nacional Agropecuario. Resultados Preliminares.* INE, Santiago, Chile, 443 pp.

INE (2002a) *Anuario de estadísticas agropecuarias,* 1991–2001. INE, Santiago, Chile, 103 pp.

INE (2002b) *Bolivia: Distribución de la Población.* Publicaciones y Datos Censo 2001. Serie 1 Resultados Nacionales Volumen 1. INE, La Paz, Bolivia, pp. 32, 81.

INEC-MAG-SICA (2002) *Censo del Sector Agropecuario.* Quito, Ecuador.

Informal Sector Research and Study Centre (2002) *District Demographic Profile of Nepal.* Informal Sector Research and Study Centre, PO Box No. 94, Kamaladi, Kathmandu, Nepal, 735 pp.

Jahnke, H.E. (1982) *Livestock Production Systems and Livestock Development in Tropical Africa.* Wissenschaftsverlag Vauk, Kiel, Germany.

Jalvingh, A.W. (1993) Dynamic livestock modelling for on-farm decision support. PhD thesis, Landbouwuniversiteit, Wageningen, The Netherlands.

James, A.D. (1995) Systems simulation in animal health and production. Unpublished lecture notes. VEERU, University of Reading, Reading, UK.

James, A.D. and Carles, A. (1996) Measuring the productivity of grazing and foraging livestock. *Agricultural Systems* 52(2/3), 271–291.

James, A.D. and Ellis, P.R. (1978) Benefit–cost analysis in foot-and-mouth disease control programmes. *British Veterinary Journal* 134(1), 47–52.

Jarvis, L.S. (1974) Cattle as capital goods and ranchers as portfolio managers: an application to the Argentine cattle sector. *Journal of Political Economy* 82, 489–520.

Jarvis, L.S. (1980) Cattle as a store of wealth: comment. *American Journal of Agricultural Economics* 62, 606–613.

Johnston, J. and Cumming, R. (1991) *Control of Newcastle Disease in Village Chickens with Oral V4 Vaccine.* ACIAR Economic Assessment Series 7. Australian Centre for International Agricultural Research, Canberra, Australia, 23 pp.

Jolly, C.M. (1988) The use of action variables in determining recommendation domains: Senegalese farmers for research and extension. *Agricultural Administration and Extension* 30, 253–267.

Joshi, B.R. (2002) The role of large ruminants. Available at: www.fao/docrep

Kaplinsky, R. and Morris, M. (2000) *A Handbook for Value Chain Research.* IDS working paper, IDS, Sussex, UK, 109 pp.

Kennedy, J.O.S. (1986) *Dynamic Programming: Applications to Agriculture and Natural Resources.* Elsevier, London.

Kirsopp-Reed, K. (1994) A review of PRA methods for livestock research and development. In: *RRA Notes Issue 21.* IIED, London, pp. 11–36 (PDF file).

Kletke, D. (1989) Enterprise budgets. In: Tweeten, L. (ed.) *Agricultural Policy Analysis Tools for Economic Development.* Westview Press, Boulder, Colorado, pp. 189–211.

Koirala, G.P. (1998) *Clogs in Shallow Groundwater Use.* Winrock International, Policy Analysis in Agriculture and Related Resource Management, Research Report No. 39. Winrock International/Nepal, Kathmandu, Nepal, 50 pp.

Kral, K., Maclean, M. and San, S. (1993) Cambodia. In: Patten, B.E., Spencer, T.L., Johnson, R.B., Hoffmann, D. and Lehane, L. (eds) *Pasteurellosis in Production Animals.* ACIAR Proceedings 43, 246–248.

Kristjanson, P.M. (1997) *Measuring Returns to ILRI's Research.* Systems Analysis and Impact Assessment Working Paper 97–1, ILRI, Nairobi, Kenya, 65 pp.

Kristjanson, P.M., Swallow, B.M., Rowlands, G.J., Kruska, R.L. and de Leeuw, P.N. (1999) Measuring the potential benefits to control African animal trypanosomosis and the returns to research. *Agricultural Systems* 59, 79–98.

Kuit, H.G., Traore, A. and Wilson, R.T. (1986) Livestock production in central Mali: ownership, management and productivity of poultry in the traditional sector. *Tropical Animal Health and Production* 18, 222–231.

Kumar, K. (ed.) (1993) *Rapid Appraisal Methods.* World Bank, Washington, DC, 218 pp.

Leonard, D.K. (2000) The new institutional economics and the restructuring of animal health services in Africa. In: Leonard, D.K. (ed.) *Africa's Changing Markets for Health and Veterinary Services. The New Institutional Issues.* Macmillan Press, London, pp. 1–40.

Leonard, D.K. (2004) Tools from the new institutional economics for reforming the delivery of veterinary services. *Revue Scientifique et Technique Office International des Epizooties* 23(1), 47–57.

Lescano Rivero, J.L. (1988) Farming systems in the Lake Titicaca area. (Los sistemas agricolas en el anillo lacustre.) *Boletin Genetico (Castelar)* 15, 3–8.

Lopes, G.M.B. (1990) The constraints to production by the small farmers in the Agresti region of Pernambulo, Brazil. PhD thesis, University of Reading, Reading, UK.

Low, A.R.C. (1986) *Agricultural Development in Southern Africa: Farm Household Theory and the Food Crisis.* James Currey, London, 215 pp.

Ly, C. (2003) The economics of community based animal health workers. Part 1: Economic theory and CBAHWs. In: *Community Based Animal Health Workers – Threat or Opportunity?* The IDL Group, Crewkerne, Somerset, UK, pp. 91–99.

Mace, R. and Houston, A. (1989) Pastoralist strategies for survival in unpredictable environments: a model of herd composition that maximises household viability. *Agricultural Systems* 31, 185–204.

MAFF (1980) *Definition of Terms Used in Agricultural Business Management.* Booklet 2269. MAFF, Pinner, UK, 39 pp.

Mandip, R., Rushton, J., Anderson, S. and Tuluchan, P. (2004) *A Review Paper on Livestock Technology and Policy.* Output from the LTIP project. Imperial College, London.

Mangen, M.J.J. (2002) Economic welfare analysis of simulated control strategies for Classical Swine Fever epidemics. PhD thesis, Wageningen University, Wageningen, The Netherlands, 188 pp.

Mangen, M.J.J., Jalvingh, A.W., Nielen, M., Mourits, M.C.M., Klinkenberg, D. and Dijkhuizen, A.A. (2001) Spatial and stochastic simulation to compare two emergency-vaccination strategies with a marker vaccine in the 1997/1998 Dutch Classical Swine Fever epidemic. *Preventive Veterinary Medicine* 48(3), 177–200.

Mariner, J.C. (2001) *Manual on Participatory Epidemiology – Method for the Collection of Action-Oriented Epidemiological Intelligence.* FAO Animal Health Manual 10. FAO, Rome, Italy.

Marshall, A. (1920) *Principles of Economics,* 8th edn. Originally published by Macmillan, London. Prometheus Books, New York, 319 pp.

Matthewman, R.W. (1977) *A Survey of Small Livestock Production at the Village Level in the Derived Savannah and Lowland Forest Zones of Southwest Nigeria.* Study No. 24. Department of Agriculture and Horticulture, University of Reading, Reading, UK.

Matthewman, R.W. and Perry, B.D. (1985) Measuring the benefits of disease control: relationship between herd structure, productivity and health. *Tropical Animal Health and Production* 17, 39–51.

McCracken, J.A., Pretty, J.N. and Conway, G.R. (1988) *An Introduction to Rapid Rural Appraisal for Agricultural Development.* IIED, London.

McGregor, M., Dent, B. and Cropper, M. (1994) The role of multi-criteria decision making methods in guiding grazing systems development. Paper presented at the International Livestock Systems Symposium, Aberdeen, September, 1994.

McInerney, J.P. (1988) The economic analysis of livestock disease: the developing framework. *Acta Veterinaria Scandinavica* 84(Supplement), 66–74.

McInerney, J.P. (1996) Old economics for new problems – livestock disease: presidential address. *Journal of Agricultural Economics* 47(3), 295–314.

McInerney, J.P., Howe, K.S. and Schepers, J.A. (1992) A framework for the economic analysis of disease in farm livestock. *Preventive Veterinary Medicine* 13(2), 137–154.

McIntire, J., Bourzat, D. and Pingali, P. (1992) *Crop–Livestock Interaction in Sub-Saharan Africa.* The World Bank, Washington DC.

McLeod, A. (1993) A model for infectious diseases of livestock. PhD thesis, University of Reading, Reading, UK.

McLeod, R.S. (1995) Costs of major parasites to the Australian livestock industries. *International Journal for Parasitology* 25, 1363–1367.

McLeod, R.S. (1998) TICKCOST. Available at: http://www.esys.com.au/tickcost.htm

Meininger, H. (1997) Working cattle in the Cotacachi region in the Andes north of the equator. (Les bovins laboureurs à Cotacachi (Andes septentrionales de l'Equateur).) *Ethnozootechnie* 60, 67–73.

Ministerio de Desarrollo Humano (1993) *Mapa de Pobreza. Una Guia para la Accion Social.* UDAPSO, INE, UPP, UDAPE, La Paz, Bolivia.

Moris, J. and Copestake, J. (1993) *Qualitative Enquiry for Rural Development: A Review.* Intermediate Technology Publications, London, 117 pp.

Morris, R.S. (1997) How economically important is animal disease and why? In: Dijkhuizen, A.A. and Morris, R.S. (eds) *Animal Health Economics: Principles and Applications.* Post Graduate Foundation in Veterinary Science, University of Sydney, Sydney South, Australia, pp. 1–12.

Morrison, D.A., Kingwell, R.S. and Pannell, D.J. (1986) A mathematical programming model of a crop–livestock farm system. *Agricultural Systems* 20, 243–268.

Mortimore, M. and Turner, B. (1993) *Crop–Livestock Farming Systems in the Semi-arid Zone of Sub-Saharan Africa. Ordering Diversity and Understanding Change*. ODI Agricultural Administration (Research and Extension) Network, No. 46, ODI, London.

Muchena, M.E. (1993) Cattle in mixed farming systems in Zimbabwe: an economic analysis. Unpublished PhD thesis, University of Reading, Reading, UK, 370 pp.

Mukhebi, A.W., Perry, B.D. and Kruska, R.L. (1992) Estimated economics of theileriosis control in Africa. *Preventive Veterinary Medicine* 12, 73–85.

Mukherjee, N. (1994) Livestock, livelihood and drought: a PRA exercise in Botswana. In: *RRA Notes Number 20 – Special Issue on Livestock*. IIED, London, pp. 127–131.

Nakajima, C. (1986) *Subjective Equilibrium Theory of the Farm Household*. Elsevier, Amsterdam, The Netherlands, 302 pp.

Narayan, D. (1996) *Toward Participatory Research*. World Bank Technical Paper No. 307. World Bank, Washington, DC, 265 pp.

Nicholson, C.F., Lee, D.R., Boisvert, R.N., Blake, R.W. and Urbina, C.I. (1994) An optimization model of the dual-purpose cattle production system in the humid lowlands of Venezuela. *Agricultural Systems* 46, 311–334.

Nix, J. (1994) *Farm Management Pocketbook*. 25th edn (1995). Wye College, University of London, UK, 219 pp.

Nix, J. (2001) *Farm Management Pocketbook*. 32nd edn (2002). Imperial College, Wye, UK, 256 pp.

Nyangito, H.O., Richardson, J.W., Mukhebi, A.W., Mundy, D.S., Zimmel, P., Namken, J. and Perry, B.D. (1994) Whole farm economic analysis of East Coast fever immunization strategies in Kilifi District, Kenya. *Preventive Veterinary Medicine* 21, 215–235.

Nyangito, H.O., Richardson, J.W., Mukhebi, A.W., Mundy, D.S., Zimmel, P. and Namken, J. (1995) Whole farm economic evaluation of East Coast fever immunization strategies on farms in the Uasin Gishu District of Kenya. *Computers and Electronics in Agriculture* 12, 19–33.

Nyangito, H.O., Richardson, J.W., Mukhebi, A.W., Mundy, D.S., Zimmel, P., Namken, J. and Perry, B.D. (1996a) Whole farm simulation analysis of economic impacts of east coast fever immunization strategies on mixed crop–livestock farms in Kenya. *Agricultural Systems* 51, 1–27.

Nyangito, H.O., Richardson, J.W., Mundy, D.S., Mukhebi, A.W., Zimmel, P. and Namken, J. (1996b) Economic impacts of East Coast Fever immunization strategies on smallholder farms, Kenya: a simulation analysis. *Agricultural Economics* 13, 163–177.

Olavarria, H.R. (1994) An assessment of an animal disease control policy in Chilean peasant agriculture: the case of brucellosis. Unpublished MSc dissertation, University of Reading, Reading, UK.

Omamo, S.W. (2003) *Policy Research on African Agriculture: Trends, Gaps, and Challenges*. ISNAR Research Report 21. International Service for National Agricultural Research, The Hague.

Ott, S.L., Seitzinger, A.H. and Hueston, W.D. (1995) Measuring the national economic benefits of reducing livestock mortality. *Preventive Veterinary Medicine* 24, 203–211.

Otte, M.J., Roland-Holst, D., Pfeiffer, D., Soares-Magalhaes, R., Rushton, J., Graham, J. and Silbergeld, E. (2007) *Industrial Livestock Production and Global Health Risks*. Research Report, FAO-PPLPI, Rome, Italy, with Johns Hopkins School of Public Health, Maryland, University of California, California and RVC, London.

Owen, E., Best, J., Devendra, C., Ku-Vera, J., Mtenga, L., Richards, W., Smith, T. and Upton, M. (2005) Introduction – the need to change the 'mind-set'. In: Owen, E., Kitalyi, A., Jayasuriya, N. and Smith, T. (eds) *Livestock and Wealth Creation. Improving the Husbandry of Animals Kept by Resource-poor People in Developing Countries*. Nottingham University Press, Nottingham, UK, pp. 1–11.

PAN Livestock Services (1991) *The Livestock Production Efficiency Calculator. User Guide*. PAN Livestock Services, Dept. of Agriculture, Earley Gate, PO Box 236, Reading RG6 6AT, UK.

Peeler, E. (1996) *Manual of Livestock Production Systems in Kenya*. KARI/ODA Livestock Socio-Economics and Epidemiology Project, KARI, Nairobi, Kenya.

Perry, B.D., Kalpravidh, W., Coleman, P.G., Mcdermott, J.J., Randolph, T.F. and Gleeson, L.J. (1999) The economic impact of foot and mouth disease and its control in South-East Asia: a preliminary assessment with special reference to Thailand. *Revue Scientifique et Technique Office International des Epizooties* 2, 478–497.

Perry, B.D., McDermott, J. and Randolph, T. (2001) Can epidemiology and economics make a meaningful contribution to national animal-disease control? *Preventive Veterinary Medicine* 48, 231–260.

Perry, B., Randolph, T.F., McDermott, J.J., Sones, K.R. and Thornton, P.K. (2002) *Investing in Animal Health Research to Alleviate Poverty*. ILRI, Nairobi, Kenya, 140 pp.

Perry, B.D., Randolph, T.F., Asheley, S., Chimedza, R., Forman, T., Morrison, J., Poulton, C., Sibanda, L., Stevens, C., Tebele, N. and Yngstrom, I. (2003) *The Impact and Poverty Reduction Implications of Foot and Mouth Disease Control in Southern Africa with Special Reference to Zimbabwe*. ILRI, Nairobi, Kenya, 137 pp.

Perry, B.D., Nin Pratt, A., Sones, K. and Stevens, C. (2005) *An Appropriate Level of Risk: Balancing the Need for Safe Livestock Products with Fair Market Access for the Poor*. Pro-Livestock Policy Initiative Working Paper No. 23. FAO, Rome, Italy, 53 pp.

Pingali, P., Bigot, Y. and Binswanger, H. (1987) *Agricultural Mechanization and the Evolution of Farming Systems in Sub-Saharan Africa*. Johns Hopkins University Press, Baltimore, Maryland.

Poate, C.D. and Daplyn, P.F. (1993) *Data for Agrarian Development*. Wye Studies in Agricultural and Rural Development. Cambridge University Press, Cambridge, 387 pp.

Power, A.P. and Harris, S.A. (1973) A cost–benefit evaluation of alternative control policies for foot-and-mouth disease in Great Britain. *Journal of Agricultural Economics* 24, 573–596.

Pritchard, D.G. (2004) Animal welfare. How much can you afford? Bill Snowden Lecture presented in Australia in September 2004.

Putt, S.N.H., Shaw, A.P.M., Woods, A.J., Tyler, L. and James, A.D. (1988) *Veterinary Epidemiology and Economics in Africa. A Manual for Use in the Design and Appraisal of Livestock Health Policy*. ILCA Manual No. 3. Publication produced by ILCA (now ILRI), Addis Ababa, Ethiopia and VEERU, University of Reading, Reading, UK, 130 pp.

Rabinovich, J.E., Capurro, A.F. and Pessina, L.L. (1991) Vicuña use and the bio-economics of an Andean peasant community in Catamarca, Argentina. In: Robinson, J.G. and Redford, K.H. (eds) *Neotropical Wildlife Use and Conservation*. University of Chicago Press, Chicago, Illinois, pp. 337–358.

Rae, A.N. (1994) *Agricultural Management Economics. Activity Analysis and Decision Making*. CAB International, Wallingford, UK, 358 pp.

Rich, K.M. and Winter-Nelson, A. (2007) An integrated epidemiological-economic analysis of foot and mouth disease: applications to the southern cone of South America. *American Journal of Agricultural Economics* 89(3), 682–697.

Rich, K.M., Winter-Nelson, A. and Miller, G.Y. (2005) A review of economic tools for the assessment of animal disease outbreaks. *Revue Scientifique et Technique Office International des Epizooties* 24(3), 833–845.

Richardson, J.W., Mukhebi, A.W., Zimmel, P.T., Nyangito, H.O., Moehring, C.A. and Numken, J. (1993) *Technical Description of TIES: A Farm Level Technology Impact Evaluation System*. ILRAD, Nairobi, Kenya.

Rocha, A., Starkey, P. and Dionisio, A. (1991) Cattle production and utilisation in smallholder farming systems in Southern Mozambique. *Agricultural Systems* 37, 55–75.

Rogers, C. (2004) *Secrets of Manang. The Story Behind the Phenomenal Rise of Nepal's Famed Business Community*. Mandala Publications, Kathmandu, Nepal, 204 pp.

Romero, C. and Rehman, T. (1984) Goal programming and multiple criteria decision-making in farm planning: an expository analysis. *Journal of Agricultural Economics* 35(2), 177–190.

Romero, C. and Rehman, T. (1989) *Multiple Criteria Analysis for Agricultural Decisions*. Elsevier, Amsterdam, The Netherlands.

Roth, F., Zinsstag, J., Orkhon, D., Chimed-Ochir, G., Hutton, G., Cosivi, O., Carrin, G. and Otte, J. (2003) Human health benefits from livestock vaccination for brucellosis: case study. *Bulletin of the World Health Organization* 81, 867–876.

Rushton, J. (1995) An anthrax outbreak in a South India village. In: *The Society of Veterinary Epidemiology and Preventive Medicine Poster Display Booklet*, SVEPM, UK, pp. 160–163.

Rushton, J. (1996) Quantitative methods for the economic assessment of livestock in smallholder crop–livestock systems. PhD thesis, University of Reading, Reading, UK.

Rushton, J. (2002) The economic impact of livestock diseases. In: *CABI Animal Health and Production Compendium*, 2002 edition. CAB International, Wallingford, UK. CD and the Internet.

Rushton, J. (2003) *Methods for the Assessment of Livestock Development Interventions in Smallholder Livestock Systems*. FAO, Pro-Poor Livestock Policy Initiative, Working Paper No. 4. Available at: http://www.fao.org/ag/againfo/projects/en/pplpi/project_docs.html

Rushton, J. (2004) *Desarrollo de modelos de evaluación de impacto económico de las campañas de sanidad de la Alianza para el Campo*. Informe para el Proyecto UTF/MEX/053/MEX: Evaluación de la Alianza para el Campo, México DF, México, 82 pp.

Rushton, J. (2006) Animal health systems and status – Are they trade barriers or mechanisms to improve global animal disease control? In: *Proceedings of the International Agricultural Trade and Research Consortium Summer Symposium Held in Bonn, Germany 28–30 May 2006*. Available at: http://www.ilr1.uni-bonn.de/iatrc/iatrc_program/Session%202/J%20Rushton.pdf

Rushton, J. and Ellis, P.R. (1996) The changing role of cattle in the mixed farm systems around Bangalore, India. In: Dent, J.B., McGregor, M.J. and Sibbald, A.R. (eds) *Livestock Farming Systems: Research, Development, Socio-economics and the Land Manager*. EAAP Publication No. 79. Wageningen, The Netherlands.

Rushton, J. and Ngongi, S.N. (1998) Poultry, women and development: old ideas, new applications and the need for more research. *World Animal Review* 91(2), 43–49.

Rushton, J. and Viscarra, R.E. (2003) *The Use of Participatory Methodologies in Veterinary Epidemiology.* CEVEP, La Paz, Bolivia, 60 pp.

Rushton, J. and Viscarra, R.E. (2006) *A Guide for Concerted Action on Livestock and Livelihoods (CALL).* DfID–Livestock Production Programme, NRI, UK (in English and Spanish), La Paz, Bolivia.

Rushton, J. and Viscarra, R.E. (Forthcoming) *Livestock Production Systems in South America: Issues and Trends.* FAO, Rome, Italy.

Rushton, J., Thornton, P. and Otte, M.J. (1999) Methods of economic impact assessment. In: *The Economics of Animal Disease Control. OIE Revue Scientifique et Technique* 18(2), 315–338.

Rushton, J., Hoyos, G. and Sonco, M. (2001a) *Análisis de la Economía Pecuaria en Bolivia.* MAGDR, La Paz, Bolivia.

Rushton, J., Viscarra, R., Baptista, R. and Lucuy, M. (2001b) *Estudio Epidemiológico y Socio Económico en Sanidad y Nutrición Animal en los Seis Municipios de las Provincias Nor Y Sud Cinti del Departamento de Chuquisaca.* PASACH, Camargo, Bolivia.

Rushton, J., Taylor, N., Wilsmore, T., Shaw, A. and James, A. (2002) *Economic analysis of vaccination strategies for foot and mouth disease in the UK.* Royal Society, London, 95 pp. http://www.royalsociety.ac.uk/inquiry/566.pdf

Rushton, J., McLeod, A. and Lubroth, J. (2006a) *Managing Transboundary Animal Disease.* World Livestock, FAO, Rome, Italy, pp. 29–44.

Rushton, J., Mercado, R., Viscarra, R.E. and Nair, S. (2006b) Western Caribbean and Central America (Honduras, Nicaragua, Cuba, Yucatan peninsula, Belize, Guatemala). Regional Scan for an IDRC study on 'Productive Strategies for Poor Rural Households to Participate Successfully in Global Economic Processes' Coordinated by ODI, London, p. 45.

Rushton, J., Upton, M., Ayala, G. and Velasco, R. (2006c) Balancing active and passive policies for the prevention of transboundary diseases. In: *Proceedings of the International Society for Veterinary Epidemiology and Economics 6–11 August 2006.*

Rushton, J., Viscarra, R.E., Mercado, R. and Barrance, A. (2006d) Country report for Honduras. IDRC study on 'Productive Strategies for Poor Rural Households to Participate Successfully in Global Economic Processes'. Coordinated by ODI, London, p. 39.

Rushton, J., Viscarra, R.E., Otte, J., McLeod, A. and Taylor, N. (2007) *Animal Health Economics. Where have we Come from and Where do we Go Next? Perspectives in Agriculture, Veterinary Science, Nutrition and Natural Resources.* CABI 2007 1 No. 031. Wallingford, UK.

Ruthenberg, H. (1980) *Farming Systems in the Tropics*, 3rd edn. Clarendon Press, Oxford, 424 pp.

Saatkamp, H.W., Huirne, R.B.M., Geers, R., Dijkhuizen, A.A., Noordhuizen, J.P.T.M. and Goedseels, V. (1996) State-transition modelling of classical swine fever to evaluate national identification and recording systems: general aspects and model description. *Agricultural Systems* 51, 215–236.

SAGPyA (1996) *Argentina Agropecuaria, Agroindustrial y pesquera.* SAGPyA, Buenos Aires, Argentina.

Sahley, C.T., Torres Vargas, J. and Sachez Valdivia, J. (2006) Community ownership and live shearing of Vicuñas in Peru. Evaluating management strategies and their sustainability. In: Silvius, K., Bodmer, R. and Fragoso, J. (eds) *People in Nature: Wildlife Conservation in South and Central America.* Columbia University Press, New York.

Sanders, J.O. and Cartwright, T.C. (1979a) A general cattle production systems model. I: structure of the model. *Agricultural Systems* 4, 217–227.

Sanders, J.O. and Cartwright, T.C. (1979b) A general cattle production systems model. II: procedures used for simulating animal performance. *Agricultural Systems* 4, 289–309.

Schlecht, E., Mahler, F., Sangare, M., Susenbeth, A. and Becker, K. (1993) Quantitative and qualitative estimation of nutrient intake and faecal excretion of zebu cattle grazing natural pasture in semi-arid Mali. In: *Livestock and Sustainable Nutrient Cycling in Mixed Farming Systems of Sub-Saharan Africa, Conference Proceedings.* Addis Ababa, Ethiopia, November, 1993. ILCA, Addis Ababa, Ethiopia.

Schulte, M. (1999) *Llameros y Caseros. La economia regional kallawaya.* PIEB, La Paz, Bolivia, 323 pp.

Scoones I. (1998) *Sustainable Rural Livelihoods: a Framework for Analysis.* IDS Working Paper 72, Institute of Development Studies at the University of Sussex, Brighton, UK, 72 pp.

Scoones, I. and Wolmer, W. (2006) *Livestock Disease, Trade and Markets: Policy Choices for the Livestock Trade in Africa.* IDS Working Paper 269, Institute of Development Studies, Brighton, UK, 52 pp.

SENASA (2002) Estadisticas. Available at: http://www.senasa.gov.ar/estadisticas

Sere, C. and Steinfeld, H. (1996) *World Livestock Production Systems – Current Status, Issues and Trends.* Animal Production and Health Paper No. 127. FAO, Rome, Italy, 89 pp.

Shapiro, B.I. and Staal, S.J. (1995) The policy analysis matrix applied to agricultural commodity markets. In: Scott, G.J. (ed.) *Prices, Products, and People. Analyzing Agricultural Markets in Developing Countries.* Lynne Rienner Publishers, Boulder, Colorado, pp. 73–98.

Shaw, A.P.M. (1989) *CLIPPER. Computerised Livestock Project planning Exercise. User Notes.* AP Consultants, Andover, UK.

Shaw, A.P.M., Hendrickx, G., Gilbert, M., Mattioli, R., Codjia, V., Dao, B., Diall, O., Mahama, C., Sibibé, I. and Wint, W. (2006) *Mapping the Benefits: a New Decision Tool for Tsetse and Trypanosomias Interventions.* Research Report. Department for International Development, Animal Health Programme, Centre for Tropical Veterinary Medicine, University of Edinburgh, UK and Programme Against African Trypanosomiasis, FAO, Rome, Italy, 154 pp.

SIAP (2003) *Anuario Estadístico de la producción agrícola por Municipioe.* CD ROM. SAGARPA, Mexico DF República de México.

Simpson, J.R. (1988) *The Economics of Livestock Systems in Developing Countries. Farm and Project Level Analysis.* Westview Press, Boulder, Colorado.

Singh, I., Squire, L. and Strauss, J. (1986) *Agricultural Household Models. Extensions, Applications and Policy.* John Hopkins University Press, Baltimore, Maryland, p. 335.

Sloman, J. (1991) *Economics.* Harvester Wheatsheaf, London, 1021 pp.

Snow, W.F., Norton, G.A. and Rawlings, P. (1996) Application of a systems approach to problem analysis of African animal trypanosomiasis in The Gambia. *Agricultural Systems* 51, 339–356.

Spadbrow, P.B. (1993) Newcastle disease in village chickens. *Poultry Science Review* 5, 57–96.

Speirs, M. and Olsen, O. (1992) *Indigenous Integrated Farming Systems in the Sahel.* World Bank Technical Paper No. 179. World Bank, Washington, DC, 80 pp.

Stegeman, A., Bouma, A., Elbers, A.R., de Jong, M.C., Nodelijk, G., de Klerk, F., Koch, G. and van Boven, M. (2004) Avian influenza A virus (H7N7) epidemic in The Netherlands in 2003: course of the epidemic and effectiveness of control measures. *Journal of Infectious Diseases* 190(12), 2088–2095.

Steinfeld, H. (1988) *Livestock Development in Mixed Farming Systems. A Study of Smallholder Livestock Production Systems in Zimbabwe.* Farming Systems and Resource Economics in the Tropics, Vol. 3, Wissenschaftsverlag Vauk, Kiel, Germany, 244 pp.

Steinfeld, H. and Mäki-Hokkonen, J. (1995) A classification of livestock production systems. *World Animal Review* 84/85, 83–94.

Steinfeld, H., Gerber, P., Wassenaar, T., Castel, V., Rosales, M. and de Haan, C. (2006) *Livestock's Long Shadow: Environmental Issues and Options.* FAO, Rome, Italy, 390 pp.

Stevens, S.F. (1996) *Claiming the High Ground. Sherpas, Subsistence and Environmental Change in the Highest Himalya.* Motilal Banarsidass Publishers, Delhi, India, 537 pp.

Stott, A.W. (2005) Costs and benefits of preventing animal diseases: a review focusing on endemic diseases. Report to SEERAD under Advisory Activity 211. Available at: http://www.scotland.gov.uk/library5/environment/cbpad-00.asp

Theis, J. and Grady, H.M. (1991) *Participatory Rapid Appraisal for Community Development. A Training Manual Based on Experiences in the Middle East and North Africa.* IIED and Save the Children Fund, London.

Thomas, T.H. (1991) A spreadsheet approach to the economic modelling of agroforestry systems. *Forest Ecology and Management* 45, 207–235.

Thompson, D., Muriel, P., Russell, D., Osborne, P., Bromley, A., Rowland, M., Creigh-Tyte, S. and Brown, C. (2002) Economic costs of the foot and mouth disease outbreak in the United Kingdom in 2001. *Revue Scientifique et Technique Office International des Epizooties* 21(3), 675–688.

Thomson, E.F. and Bahhady, F.A. (1995) A model-farm approach to research on crop–livestock integration – I. Conceptual framework and methods. *Agricultural Systems* 49, 1–16.

Thomson, E.F., Bahhady, F.A., Nordblom, T.L. and Harris, H.C. (1995) A model-farm approach on crop–livestock integration – III. Benefits of crop–livestock integration and a critique of the approach. *Agricultural Systems* 49, 31–44.

Tisdell, C. (1995) *Assessing the Approach to Cost–Benefit Analysis of Controlling Livestock Diseases of McInerney and Others.* Paper No. 3 of Research Papers and Reports in Animal Health Economics, University of Queensland, Australia, 22 pp.

Tisdell, C. (1996) *Economics of Investing in the Health of Livestock: New Insights?* Paper No. 29 of Research Papers and Reports in Animal Health Economics, University of Queensland, Australia, 9 pp.

Tulachan, P.M. (2004) Demand and supply changes in the dairy sector in Kathmandu city: impact on smallholders. In: Owen, E., Smith, T., Steele, M.A., Anderson, S., Duncan, A.J., Herrero, M., Leaver, D., Reynolds, C.K., Richards, J.L. and Ku-Vera, J.C. (eds) *Responding to the Livestock Revolution: the Role of Globalisation and Implications for Poverty Alleviation.* BSAS Publication 33, Nottingham, UK, pp. 333–346.

Tweeten, L. (ed.) (1989) *Agricultural Policy Analysis Tools for Economic Development.* Westview Press, Boulder, Colorado and IT Publications, London.

Udo, H.M.J. and Brouwer, B.O. (1993) A computerised method for systematically analysing the livestock component of farming systems. *Computers and Electronics in Agriculture* 9, 335–356.

Umali, D.L., Feder, G. and de Haan, C. (1992) *The Balance Between Public and Private Sector Activities in the Delivery of Livestock Services.* World Bank Discussion Paper No. 163. The World Bank, Washington, DC.

UNEPCA (1997) *Censo Nacional Llamas y Alpacas Bolivia.* UNEPCA, Oruro, Bolivia, 174 pp.

Upton, M. (1987) *African Farm Management.* Cambridge University Press, Cambridge, 190 pp.

Upton, M. (1989) Livestock productivity assessment and herd growth models. *Agricultural Systems* 29, 149–164.

Upton, M. (1993) Livestock productivity assessment and modelling. *Agricultural Systems* 43, 459–472.

Urioste, M. (2005) *Los Nietos de la Reforma Agraria acceso, tenencia y uso de la tierra en el altiplano de Bolivia.* Fundación Tierra, La Paz, Bolivia, 56 pp.

van Elderen, E. (1987) *Scheduling Farm Operations: a Simulation Model.* Pudoc, Wageningen, The Netherlands, 218 pp.

Van Keulen, H. and Veeneklaas, F.R. (1993) Options for agricultural development: a case study for Mali's fifth region. In: Penning de Vries, F.W.T., Teng, P.S. and Metselaar, K. (eds), *Systems Approaches for Agricultural Development.* Kluwer, Dordrecht, The Netherlands, pp. 367–380.

van Schaik, G. (1995) An economic study of smallholder dairy farms in Murang'a District Kenya. A thesis for the Department of Farm Management, Wageningen Agricultural University, The Netherlands in collaboration with the International Laboratory for Research on Animal Diseases, Nairobi, Kenya.

Vinding, M. (1998) *The Thakali. A Himalayan Ethnography.* Serindia Publications, London, UK, 470 pp.

von Fürer-Haimendorf, C. (1984) *The Sherpas Transformed.* Sterling Publishers, New Delhi, India, 197 pp.

Waddington, K. (2002) Safe meat and healthy animals: BSE and bovine TB. History and policy. Available at: http://www.historyandpolicy.org/papers/policy-paper-04.html accessed March 2008.

Waters-Bayer, A. and Bayer, W. (1994) *Planning with Pastoralists: PRA and More. A Review of Methods Focused on Africa.* German Agency for Technical Cooperation, Eschborn, Germany, 153 pp.

Weiers, R.M. (1986) *Investigación de Mercados.* Prentice-Hall-Hispanoamericana, S.A., Mexico, 540 pp.

Whittlesey, D. (1936) Major agricultural regions of the earth. *Annals of the Association of American Geographers* 26, 199–240.

Williams, T.O. (1994) Identifying target groups for livestock improvement research: the classification of sedentary livestock producers in Western Niger. *Agricultural Systems* 46, 227–237.

Wilson, R.T. (1979) Studies on the livestock of southern Darfur, Sudan: VII. Production of poultry under simulated traditional conditions. *Tropical Animal Health and Production* 11, 143–150.

Wilson, R.T. (1995) *Livestock Production Systems.* CTA/Macmillan, London, 141 pp.

Winpenny, J.T. (1991) *Values for the Environment. A Guide to Economic Appraisal.* HMSO, London, 277 pp.

Winrock International (1992) *Assessment of Animal Agriculture in Sub-Saharan Africa.* Winrock International Institute for Agricultural Development, Arkansas.

Wint, W. and Robinson, T. (2007) *Gridded Livestock of the World 2007.* FAO, Rome, Italy, 131 pp.

Winter-Nelson, A. and Rich, K.M. (2008) Mad cows and sick birds: financing international responses to animal disease in developing countries. *Development Policy Review* 26(2), 211–226.

Wood, P.D.P. (1967) Algebraic model of the lactation curve in cattle. *Nature* 216, 164–165.

World Bank (1996) *The World Bank Participation Sourcebook.* World Bank, Washington DC, 259 pp.

Wright, A. (1971) Farming systems, models and simulation. In: Dent, J.B. and Anderson, J.R. (eds) *Systems Analysis in Agricultural Management.* Wiley, Sydney, Australia, pp. 17–33.

Young, J., Dijkema, H., Stoufer, H., Ojha, N., Shrestha, G. and Thapa, L. (1994) Evaluation of an animal health improvement programme in Nepal. In: *RRA Notes Number 20 – Special issue on Livestock.* IIED, London, pp. 59–66.

Zessin, K.-H. and Carpenter, T.E. (1985) Benefit–cost analysis of an epidemiologic approach to provision of veterinary service in the Sudan. *Preventive Veterinary Medicine* 3(4), 323–337.

Zuckerman, P.S. (1973) Yoruba smallholders' farming systems. Unpublished PhD thesis, University of Reading, Reading, UK.

Tisdell Chapter

Baumol, W.J. and Quandt, R.E. (1964) Rules of thumb and optimally imperfect decisions. *American Economic Review* 54, 23–46.

McInerney, J.P. (1991) Cost–benefit analysis of livestock diseases: a simplified look at its economics foundations. In: Martin, S.W. (ed.) *Proceedings of the International Symposium on Veterinary Epidemiology and Economics.* Department of Population Medicine, Ontario Veterinary College, University of Guelph, Guelph, Canada, pp. 149–153.

McInerney, J.P., Howe, K.S. and Scheper, J.A. (1992) A framework for economic analysis of disease in farm livestock. *Preventative Veterinary Medicine* 13, 137–154.

Ramsay, G., Harrison, S.R. and Tisdell, C. (1999) Assessing the value of additional animal health information. In: Sharma, P. and Baldock, C. (eds) *Understanding Animal Health in Southeast Asia.* Australian Centre for International Agricultural Research, Canberra, Australia, pp. 260–281.

Tisdell, C. (1968) *The Theory of Price Uncertainty, Production and Profit.* Princeton University Press, Princeton, New Jersey.

Tisdell, C. (1995) *Assessing the Approach to Cost–Benefit Analysis of Controlling Livestock Diseases of McInerney and Others.* Animal Health Economics Research Paper No. 3. School of Economics, The University of Queensland, Brisbane, 4072, Australia.

Tisdell, C.A. (1996) *Bounded Rationality and Economic Evolution.* Edward Elgar, Cheltenham, UK and Northampton, Massachusetts.

von Neumann, J. and Morgenstern, O. (1953) *Theory of Games and Economic Behavior.* Princeton University Press, Princeton, New Jersey.

James Chapter

Ferguson, N.M., Donnelly, C.A. and Anderson, R.M. (2001) The foot-and-mouth epidemic in Great Britain: pattern of spread and impact of interventions. *Science* 292, 1155–1160.

Gupta, S. (2001) Avoiding ambiguity. Scientists sometimes use mathematics to give the illusion of certainty. *Nature* 412, 589 (9 August 2001).

Hugh-Jones, M.E. (1976) A model of bovine brucellosis in UK dairy herds. In: *Proceedings of the First International Symposium on Veterinary Epidemiology and Economics.* Reading University, Reading, UK.

Risk Solutions (2003) *FMD Epidemiological Modelling Project Report – The Silent Spread Model.* A report for DEFRA, February 2003. Risk Solutions, London, UK.

Taylor, N.M. (2003) Review of the use of models in informing disease control policy development and adjustment. A report to DEFRA. Available at: http://www.defra.gov.uk/science/Publications/2003/UseofModelsinDiseaseControlPolicy.pdf, 98 pp.

Taylor, N.M. and James, A.D. (2003) Comparison of two cases where epidemiological modelling was used to support decisions regarding FMD control in UK. In: *Proceedings of the Tenth International Symposium on Veterinary Epidemiology and Economics.* ISVEE, Santiago, Chile.

Stott Chapter

Bellman, R. (1957) *Dynamic Programming.* Princeton University Press, Princeton, New Jersey.

Bennett, R.M. (2003) The 'direct' costs of livestock disease: the development of a system of models for the analysis of 30 endemic livestock diseases in Great Britain. *Journal of Agricultural Economics* 54(1), 55–72.

Boehlje, M.D. and Eidman, V.R. (1984) *Farm Management.* Wiley, New York.

Chi, J.W., Weersink, A., VanLeeuwen, J.A. and Keefe, G.P. (2002) The economics of controlling infectious diseases on dairy farms. *Canadian Journal of Agricultural Economics* 50(3), 237–256.

Garnsworthy, P. (2004) The environmental impact of fertility in dairy cows: a modelling approach to predict methane and ammonia emissions. *Animal Feed Science and Technology* 112, 211–223.

Gunn, G.J., Stott, A.W. and Humphry, R.W. (2004) Modelling and costing BVD outbreaks in beef herds. *Veterinary Journal* 167(2), 143–149.

Holden, S. (1999) The economics of the delivery of veterinary services. *Revue Scientifique et Technique Office International des Epizooties* 18(2), 425–439.

Jalvingh, A.W., Dijkhuizen, A.A. and Renkema, J.A. (1997) Linear programming to meet management targets and restrictions. In: Dikhuizen, A.A and Morris, R.S. (eds) *Animal Health Economics Principles and Applications.* Post Graduate Foundation in Veterinary Science, University of Sydney, Sydney, Australia, pp. 69–82.

MacKenzie, D. (2004) The big, bad wolf and the rational market: portfolio insurance, the 1987 crash and the proformativity of economics. *Economy and Society* 33(3), 303–334.

Marsh, W. (1999) The economics of animal health in farmed livestock at the herd level. *Revue Scientifique et Technique Office International des Epizooties* 18(2), 357–366.

McInerney, J. (1996) Old economics for new problems – livestock disease: presidential address. *Journal of Agricultural Economics* 47, 295–314.

McInerney, J.P., Howe, K.S. and Schepers, J.A. (1992) A framework for the economic analysis of disease in farm livestock. *Preventive Veterinary Medicine* 13, 137–154.

Milne, C.E. (2005) The economic modelling of sheep ectoparasite control in Scotland. Unpublished PhD thesis, University of Aberdeen, Aberdeen, UK.

Ngategize, P.K., Kaneene, J.B., Harsh, S.B., Bartlett, P.C. and Mather, E.L. (1986) Decision analysis in animal health programs: merits and limitations. *Preventive Veterinary Medicine* 4, 187–197.

Santarossa, J.M., Stott, A.W., Woolliams, J.A., Brotherstone, S., Wall, E. and Coffey, M.P. (2004) An economic evaluation of long-term sustainability in the dairy sector. *Animal Science* 79, 315–325.

Santarossa, J.M., Stott, A.W., Humphry, R.W. and Gunn, G.J. (2005) Optimal risk management vs willingness to pay for BVDV control options. *Preventive Veterinary Medicine* 4, 183–187.

Stinespring, J.R. (2002) *Mathematica for Microeconomics.* Academic Press, San Diego, California.

Stott, A.W. (2005) Costs and benefits of preventing animal diseases: a review focusing on endemic diseases. Report to SEERAD under Advisory Activity 211. Available at: http://www.scotland.gov.uk/library5/environment/cbpad-00.asp

Stott, A.W., Veerkamp, R.F. and Wassell, T.R. (1999) The economics of fertility in the dairy herd. *Animal Science* 68, 49–57.

Stott, A.W., Jones, G.M., Gunn, G.J., Chase-Topping, M., Humphry, R.W., Richardson, H. and Logue, D.N. (2002) Optimum replacement policies for the control of subclinical mastitis due to *S. aureus* in dairy cows. *Journal of Agricultural Economics* 53(3), 627–644.

Stott, A.W., Lloyd, J., Humphry, R.W. and Gunn, G.J. (2003) A linear programming approach to estimate the economic impact of bovine viral diarrhoea (BVD) at the whole-farm level in Scotland. *Preventive Veterinary Medicine* 59(1–2), 51–66.

Stott, A.W., Jones, G.M., Humphry, R.W. and Gunn, G.J. (2005a) The financial incentive to control paratuberculosis (Johne's disease) on UK dairy farms. *Veterinary Record* 156, 825–831.

Stott, A.W., Milne, C.E., Goddard, P. and Waterhouse, A. (2005b) Projected effect of alternative farm management strategies on profit and animal welfare in extensive sheep production systems in Great Britain. *Livestock Production Science* 97, 161–171.

Stott, A.W., Brotherstone, S. and Coffey, M.P. (2005c) Including lameness and mastitis in a profit index for dairy cattle. *Animal Science* 80(1), 41–52.

Tisdell, C. (1995) *Assessing the Approach to Cost–Benefit Analysis of Controlling Livestock Diseases of McInerney and Others.* Research papers and reports in animal health economics No. 3. An ACIAR-Australian project. The University of Queensland, Brisbane, Australia, 22 pp.

Yalcin, C., Stott, A.W., Logue, D.N. and Gunn, J. (1999) The economic impact of mastitis-control procedures used in Scottish dairy herds with high bulk-tank somatic cell counts. *Preventive Veterinary Medicine* 41, 135–149.

Upton Chapter

Delgado, C., Rosegrant, M., Steinfeld, H., Ehui, S. and Courbois, C. (1999) *Livestock to 2020: The Next Food Revolution.* IFPRI, Washington, DC, FAO, Rome, and ILRI, Nairobi.

Ellis, F. (1992) *Agricultural Policies in Developing Countries.* Cambridge University Press, Cambridge.

FAO (1991) *Working with CAPPA Series.* FAO, Rome.

Hallam, D. (1984) A quantitative framework for livestock development planning: part 2 – the determination of livestock requirements. *Agricultural Systems* 14(1), 45–59.

Hallam, D., Gartner, J.A. and Hrabovszky, J.P. (1983) A quantitative framework for livestock development planning: part 1 – the planning context and an overview. *Agricultural Systems* 12(4), 231–249.

Rushton, J., Duran, N. and Anderson, S. (2004) Demand and supply side changes in the Santa Cruz, Bolivia, milk sector 1985–2002: impact on small-scale producers and poor consumers. In: Owen, E., Smith, T., Steele, M.A., Anderson, S., Duncan, A.J., Herrero, M., Leaver, J.D., Reynolds, C.K., Richards, J.I. and Ku-Vera, J.C. (eds) *Responding to the Livestock Revolution: the Role of Globalisation and Implications for Poverty Alleviation.* BSAS Publication 33, Nottingham University Press, Nottingham, UK, pp. 315–322.

Sadoulet, E. and de Janvry, A. (1995) *Quantitative Development Policy Analysis.* Johns Hopkins University Press, Baltimore, Maryland.

Staal, S.J., Waithaka, M.M., Owour, G.A.and Herrero, M. (2004) Demand and supply changes in the livestock sector and their impact on smallholders: the case of dairying in Kenya: a summary. In: Owen, E., Smith, T., Steele, M.A., Anderson, S., Duncan, A.J., Herrero, M., Leaver, J.D., Reynolds, C.K., Richards, J.I. and Ku-Vera, J.C. (eds) *Responding to the Livestock Revolution: the Role of Globalisation and Implications for Poverty Alleviation.* BSAS Publication 33, Nottingham University Press, Nottingham, UK, pp. 323–327.

Tulachan, P.M. (2004) Demand and supply changes in the dairy sector in Kathmandu city: impact on smallholders. In: Owen, E., Smith, T., Steele, M.A., Anderson, S., Duncan, A.J., Herrero, M., Leaver, J.D., Reynolds, C.K., Richards, J.I. and Ku-Vera, J.C. (eds) *Responding to the Livestock Revolution: the Role of Globalisation and Implications for Poverty Alleviation.* BSAS Publication 33, Nottingham University Press, Nottingham, UK, pp. 328–332.

Tweeten, L. (ed.) (1989) *Agricultural Policy Analysis Tools for Economic Development.* Westview Press, Boulder, Colorado and San Francisco, California, IT Publications, London.

Rushton and Leonard Chapter

Ahuja, V. (2004) The economic rationale of public and private sector roles in the provision of animal health services. *Revue Scientifique et Technique Office International des Epizooties* 23(1), 33–45.

Leonard, D.K. (2000) The new institutional economics and the restructuring of animal health services in Africa. In: Leonard, D.K. (ed.) *Africa's Changing Markets for Health and Veterinary Services. The New Institutional Issues.* Macmillan Press, London, pp. 1–40.

Leonard, D.K. (2004) Tools from the new institutional economics for reforming the delivery of veterinary services. *Revue Scientifique et Technique Office International des Epizooties* 23(1), 47–57.

North, D.C. (1990) *Institutions, Institutional Change and Economic Performance.* Cambridge University Press, Cambridge, UK, 152 pp.

Pratt, J.W. and Zeckhauser, R.J. (eds) (1985) *Principals and Agents: The Structure of Business.* Harvard Business School Press, Boston, Massachusetts, 241 pp.

Shaw Chapter

Budke, C.M., Deplazes, P. and Torgerson, P.R. (2006) Global socioeconomic impact of cystic echinococcosis. *Emerging Infectious Diseases* 12(2), 296–303. Available at: http://www.cdc.gov/ncidod/EID/vol12no02/05-0499.htm

Carabin, H., Budke, C.M., Cowan, L.D., Willingham, III, A.L. and Torgerson, P. (2005) Methods for assessing the burden of parasitic zoonoses: echinococcosis and cysticercosis. *Trends in Parasitology* 21, 327–333.

Cleaveland, C., Fèvre, E.M., Kaare, M. and Coleman, P.G. (2002) Estimating human rabies mortality in the United Republic of Tanzania from dog bite injuries. *Bulletin of the World Health Organization* 83, 360–368.

Cleaveland, S., Kaare, M., Knobel, D. and Laurenson, M.K. (2006) Canine vaccination – providing broader benefits for disease control. *Veterinary Microbiology* 117(1), 43–50.

Coleman, P. (2002) Zoonotic diseases and their impact on the poor. In: Perry, B.D., Randolph, T.F., McDermott, J.J., Sones, K.R. and Thornton, P.K. (eds) *Investing in Animal Health Research to Alleviate Poverty.* International Livestock Research Institute (ILRI), Nairobi, Kenya.

Drummond, M.F., Sculpher, M.J., Torrance, G.W., O'Brien, B. and Stoddart, G.L. (2005) *Methods for the Economic Evaluation of Health Care,* 3rd edn. Oxford University Press, Oxford.

Fèvre, E.M., Odiit, M., Coleman, P.G., Welburn, S.C. and Woolhouse, M.E.J. (2008) Estimating the burden of *rhodesiense* sleeping sickness during an outbreak in Serere, eastern Uganda. *BMC Public Health* 8, 96.

Gittinger, J.P. (1982) *Economic Analysis of Agricultural Projects.* Johns Hopkins University Press – EDI Series on Economic Development, Baltimore, Maryland.

Haydon, D.T., Randall, D.A., Matthews, L., Knobel, D.L., Tallents, L.A., Gravenor, M.B., Williams, S.D., Pollilnger, J.P., Cleaveland, S., Woolhouse, M.E., Sillero-Zubirfi, C., Marino, J., Macdonald, D.W. and Laurenson, M.K. (2006) Low-coverage vaccination strategies for the conservation of endangered species. *Nature,* 443(7112), 692–695.

Knobel, D.L., Cleaveland, S., Coleman, P.G., Fèvre, E.M., Meltzer, M.I., Miranda, E.G., Shaw, A., Zinsstag, J. and Meslin, F.X. (2005) Re-evaluating the burden of rabies in Africa and Asia. *Bulletin of the World Health Organization* 85, 360–368.

Kunda, J., Fitzpatrick, J., Kazwala, R., French, N.P., Shirima, G., Macmillan, A., Kambarage, D., Bronsvoort, M. and Cleaveland, S. (2007) Health-seeking behaviour of human brucellosis cases in rural Tanzania. *BMC Public Health* 3(147), 315.

Meltzer, M.I. (2001) An introduction to health economics for physicians. *The Lancet* 358, 993–998.

Murray, C.J.L. (1994) Quantifying the burden of disease: the technical basis for disability adjusted life years. *Bulletin of the World Health Organisation* 72, 429–445.

Odiit, M., Shaw, A., Welburn, S.C., Fèvre, E.M., Coleman, P.G. and McDermott, J.J. (2004) Assessing the patterns of health-seeking behaviour and awareness among sleeping-sickness patients in eastern Uganda. *Annals of Tropical Medicine and Parasitology* 98, 339–348.

Odiit, M., Coleman, P.G., Liu, W.-C., McDermott, J., Fèvre, E.M., Welburn, S.C. and Woolhouse, M.E.J. (2005) Quantifying the level of under-detection of *Trypanosoma brucei rhodesiense* sleeping sickness cases. *Tropical Medicine and International Health* 10, 840–849.

Roth, F., Zinsstag, J., Orkhon, D., Chimed-Ochir, G., Hutton, G., Cosivi, O., Carrin, G. and Otte, J. (2003) Human health benefits from livestock vaccination for brucellosis: case study. *Bulletin of the World Health Organization* 81, 867–876.

Schelling, E., Grace, D., Willingham, A.L. and Randolph, T. (2007) Research approaches for improved pro-poor control of zoonoses. *Food and Nutrition Bulletin* 28(2-supplement), S345-S356.

Schwabe, C.W. (1984) *Veterinary Medicine and Human Health,* 3rd edn. Williams and Wilkins, Baltimore, Maryland.

Serra, I., García, V., Pizarro, A., Luzoro, A., Cavada, G. and López, J. (1999) A universal method to correct underreporting of communicable diseases. Real incidence of hydatidosis in Chile, 1985–1994. *Review of Medicine Chile* 127(4), 485–492.

WHO/DfID (2006) The control of neglected zoonotic diseases – a route to poverty alleviation. Report of a joint WHO/DfID Animal Health Programme meeting with the participation of FAO and OIE, Geneva 20 and 21 Sept. 2005. WHO, Geneva. Available at: http://www.who.int/zoonoses/Report_Sept06.pdf

Woolhouse, M.E.J. and Gowtage-Sequeria, S. (2005) Host range and emerging and re-emerging pathogens. *Emerging Infectious Diseases* 11, 1842–1847. Available at: http://www.cdc.gov/ncidod/EID/vol11no12/05–0997.htm

Zinsstag, J., Schelling, E., Roth, F., Bonfoh, B., de Savigny, D. and Tanner, M. (2007) Human benefits of animal interventions for zoonosis control. *Emerging Infectious Diseases* 13(4), 527–531. Available at: http://www.cdc.gov/EID/content/13/4/06–0381.htm

Rojas Chapter

Cancino, R. (1988) *Erradicación del Brote de Fiebre Aftosa en Chile en 1987.* Servicio Agrícola y Ganadero, Santiago, Chile.

Cancino, P. and Rivera, A. (2006) *Brote de Loque Americana en Chile.* Boletín Veterinario Permanente, Servicio Agrícola y Ganadero, Santiago, Chile.

Cancino, R. and Vidal, M. (1984) *Erradicación del Foco de Fiebre Aftosa en la comuna de Santa Barbara, Provincia del Bio-Bio, VIII Región.* Servicio Agrícola y Ganadero, Santiago, Chile.

Espejo, G. (2006) *Programa de Prevención de para Fiebre Aftosa en Zonas Fronterizas 2000–2005.* Servicio Agrícola y Ganadero, Santiago, Chile.

Estrada, A. (2007) *Vigilancia en PRRS en Chile (Resúmen 2007).* Servicio Agrícola y Ganadero, Santiago, Chile.

Rojas, H. and Moreira, R. (2006) *Influenza Aviar en Chile: Una sinopsis.* Boletín Veterinario Permanente, Servicio Agrícola y Ganadero, Santiago, Chile.

Rojas, H., Naranjo, J., Pinto, J and Rosero, J. (2002) Risk management for FMD with neighboring countries: the case of Chile. In: *Proceeding of the Annual Meeting of the British Society for Veterinary Epidemiology and Preventive Medicine*. SVEPM, Cambridge, UK.
Verdugo, C., Rojas, H. and Urcelay, S. (2004) Evaluación del impacto económico de un brote de influenza aviar altamente patógena en planteles de producción avícola en Chile. In: Congreso Nacional de Medicina Veterinaria, Chillán.

Bonnet and Lesnoff Chapter

Anselin, L. (1995) Local indicators of spatial association LISA. *Geographical Analysis* 27(2), 93–115.
Bonnet, P. (2005) *The Use of Spatial Autocorrelation toward Accurate Identification of Epidemiological and Socio-economic Zones at Risk in Animal Health. A Case Study on Contagious Bovine Pleuropneumonia (CBPP) and Cattle Mobility in the Ethiopian Highlands.* Université Montpellier III – Paul Valéry, UFR III Sciences humaines et sciences de l'environnement, Montpellier, France, 487 pp. (in French).
Bonnet, P., Lesnoff, M., Workalemahu, A. and Jean-Baptiste, S. (2003) Social and geographical accessibility to service, concepts and indicators on animal health care systems. An application to a farmer census data set in highlands of Ethiopia. In: *Tenth International Symposium for Veterinary Epidemiology and Economics, 17–21 November 2003*, Viña del mar, Chile.
Bonnet, P., Lesnoff, M., Thiaucourt, F., Workalemahu, A. and Kifle, D. (2005) Seroprevalence of Contagious Bovine Pleuropneumonia in Ethiopian highlands (West Wellega zone, Bodji district). *Ethiopian Veterinary Journal* 9(2), 14.
Drummond, M., O'Brien, B. and Stoddart, G.G.W.T. (1998) *Methods For the Economic Evaluation of Health Care Programmes.* Oxford Medical Publications, London, 305 pp.
Grignon, M. (2002) *La Prévention: approches économiques.* Assemblée générale de l'IGAS (Inspection générale des affaires sociales), 28 Mars 2002, Paris, France, 21 pp.
Haggett, P. (2000) *The Geographical Structure of Epidemics.* Oxford Clarendon Press, New York (The Clarendon Lectures in Geography and Environmental Studies), 149 pp.
Laval, G. and Workalemahu, A. (2002) Traditional Horro cattle production in Boji district, West Wellega (Ethiopia). *Ethiopian Journal of Animal Productions* 2, 97–114.
Leonard, D.K. (1993) Structural reform of the veterinary profession in Africa and the new institutional economics. *Development and Change* 24, 227–267.
Lesnoff, M., Diedhiou, M.L., Laval, G., Bonnet, P., Workalemahu, A. and Kifle, D. (2002) Demographic parameters of domestic cattle in a contagious-bovine-pleuropneumonia infected area of Ethiopian highlands. *Revue d'Elevage et de Médecine Vétérinaire des Pays Tropicaux* 55(2), 139–147.
Lesnoff, M., Laval, G., Bonnet, P., Chalvet-Monfrey, K., Lancelot, R. and Thiaucourt, F. (2004a) A mathematical model of the effects of chronic carriers on the within-herd spread of contagious bovine pleuropneumonia in an African mixed crop–livestock system. *Preventive Veterinary Medicine* 62(2), 101–117.
Lesnoff, M., Laval, G., Bonnet, P. and Workalemahu, A. (2004b) A mathematical model of contagious bovine pleuropneumonia (CBPP) within-herd outbreaks for economic evaluation of local control strategies: an illustration from a mixed crop–livestock system in Ethiopian highlands. *Animal Research* 53, 429–438.

Ahuja Chapter

Ahuja, V., Morrenhof, J. and Sen, A. (2003a) Veterinary services delivery and the poor: case of rural Orissa, India. *OIE Scientific and Technical Review* 22(3), 931–948.
Ahuja, V., Umali-Deininger, D. and de Haan, C. (2003b) Market structure and the demand for veterinary services in India. *Agricultural Economics* 29, 27–42.

Devendra Chapter

CRIFC (Central Research Institute for Food Crops) (1995) *Final Report on Crop–Animal Systems Research.* CRIFC, Bogor, Indonesia, 61 pp.

Devendra, C. (2004) Integrated tree crops – ruminants systems. The potential importance of the oil palm. *Outlook on Agriculture* 33, 157–166.

Nitis, I.M., Lana, K., Sukanten, W., Suarna, M. and Putra, S. (1990) The concept and development of the three strata forage system. In: Devendra, C. (ed.) *Shrubs and Tree Fodders for Farm Animals*, 22–24 July 1989, International Development Research Centre, IDRC-276e, Ottawa, Canada, pp. 92–102.

For the Section on History and Diseases

Ellis

Appleby, E.C. and Ellis, P.R. (1973) A progress report on the international zoo data scheme (V.R.Z.A.). In: Ippen, R. and Schroder, H.-D. (eds) *Erkrankungen der Zootiere. Verhandlungsbericht des XV. Internationalen Symposiums, Kolmarden 1973*. Akademie-Verlag, Berlin, German Democratic Republic, pp. 389–393.

Asby, C.B., Ellis, P.R., Griffin, T.K. and Kingwill, R.G. (1974) Mastitis control is good business. *Dairy Farmer* 21(4), 36–39, 44.

Asby, C.B., Ellis, P.R., Griffin, T.K. and Kingwill, R.G. (1975) *The Benefits and Costs of a System of Mastitis Control in Individual Herds*. Department of Agriculture and Horticulture, University, Reading, UK, vi + 14 pp.

Brander, G.C. and Ellis, P.R. (1976) *The Control Oof Disease*. Baillière Tindall, London, UK, vi + 136 pp.

Crom, R.J., Worden, G., Riemenschneider, R., Friend, R.E., Pope, F. Jr, Ellis, P.R. and Hall, H.L. (1979) *Proceedings of International Symposium on Animal Health and Disease Data Banks. 4–6 December 1978, Washington, DC. Section V. Animal Production and Economic Data*. USDA, Washington, DC.

Done, J.T. and Ellis, P.R. (1988) Aujeszky's disease: need for economic review. *Veterinary Record* 122(25), 615–616.

Ellis, P.R. (1972a) *An Economic Evaluation of the Swine Fever Eradication Programme in Great Britain, Using Cost–Benefit Analysis Techniques*. Study No. 11, Department of Agriculture, Reading University, Reading, UK, 77 pp.

Ellis, P.R. (1972b) The veterinarian's contribution to the task of increasing world beef supplies. *Veterinary Record* 91(22), 530–532.

Ellis, P.R. (1972c) International and domestic major disease eradication programmes. In: *Environmental and Economic Features of Animal Health*. Agricultural Club, Department of Agriculture, University of Reading, Reading, UK, pp. 14–20.

Ellis, P.R. (1975a) The movement of live animals: health aspects of world trade in animals and animal products. *World Animal Review* 16, 6–12.

Ellis, P.R. (1975b) The economics of animal health. Economic factors affecting egg production. In: *Proceedings of the Tenth Poultry Science Symposium, 18–20th September 1974*. British Poultry Science, Edinburgh, UK, pp. 71–82.

Ellis, P.R. (1976a) Disease as a constraint upon animal production in developing countries. *Journal of the Science of Food and Agriculture* 27(9), 889.

Ellis, P.R. (1976b) The economics of swine fever control and eradication. In: *Seminar on Diagnosis and Epizootiology of Classical Swine Fever 30 April –2 May 1974, Amsterdam, The Netherlands*. Directorate-General Scientific and Technical Information and Information Management, Luxembourg, pp. 236–248.

Ellis, P.R. (1978) Aspects of integrated disease control planning. In: Ellis, P.R., Shaw, A.P.M. and Stephens, A.J. (eds) *New Techniques in Veterinary Epidemiology and Economics*. Department of Agriculture, University, Reading, UK, pp. 168–173.

Ellis, P.R. (1979a) Management, health control and recording systems for improved dairy breeds. Dairy cattle breeding in the humid tropics. In: *Working Papers Presented at the FAO/GAO Expert Consultation held in Hissar, India, 12–17 February*. Haryana Agricultural University, Hissar, India, pp. 257–264.

Ellis, P.R. (1979b) Epidemiology of disease and the effects of increasing size of the E.E.C.: swine fever. In: *The Pig Veterinary Society Proceedings*. Volume 5. c/o R.H.C. Penny, Royal Veterinary College Field Station, Hatfield, Herts, UK, pp. 41–44.

Ellis, P.R. (1980) International aspects of animal disease surveillance. In: *Proceedings of the Second International Symposium on Veterinary Epidemiology and Economics, 7–11 May 1979*. ISVEE, Canberra, Australia, pp. 11–15.

Ellis, P.R. (1981a) Animal health – information, planning and economics. *Bulletin de l'Office International des Epizooties* 93(5/6), 775–782.

Ellis, P.R. (1981b) Animal health: information, planning and economics. Review of papers. *Bulletin de l'Office International des Epizooties* 93(5/6), 763–774.

Ellis, P.R. (1982a) Epidemiology, economics and decision making. Epidemiology in animal health. In: *Proceedings of a Symposium Held at the British Veterinary Association's Centenary Congress, Reading 22–25 September 1982.* Society for Veterinary Epidemiology and Preventive Medicine, SVEPM, Reading, UK, pp. 17–30.

Ellis, P.R. (1982b) Informe sobre salud animal: planification y economia (Animal health information: planning and economics). In: *III Reunion Interamericana de Directores de Salud Animal, Buenos Aires, 5–8 Agosto de 1981.* Instituto Interamericano de Cooperacion para la Agricultura, San Jose, Costa Rica, pp. 121–132.

Ellis, P.R. (1984) Health control in relation to livestock production. In: Nestel, B. (ed.) *Development of Animal Production Systems.* Elsevier Science Publishers, Amsterdam, The Netherlands, pp. 63–77.

Ellis, P.R. (1986) Interactions between parasite and vector control, animal productivity and rural welfare. In: Howell, M.J. (ed.) *Parasitology – Quo vadit?* Proceedings of the 6th International Congress of Parasitology, 24–29 August 1986, Brisbane, Queensland, Australia. Australian Academy of Science, Canberra, ACT 2601, Australia, pp. 577–585.

Ellis, P.R. (1988) Multilevel training activities in veterinary epidemiology and economics in developing countries. *Acta Veterinaria Scandinavica* 84(Supplement), 507–509.

Ellis, P.R. (1989) OIE/ADB follow-up to the Manila Workshop on Animal Disease Information Systems in Asia. In: *Proceedings of the 16th Conference of the OIE Regional Commission for Asia, the Far East and Oceania.* Office International des Epizooties (OIE), Paris, France, pp. 3–8.

Ellis, P.R. (1994a) Information systems in disease control programs. In: Copland, J.W., Gleeson, L.J. and Chamnanpood, C. (eds) *Diagnosis and Epidemiology of Foot-and-Mouth Disease in Southeast Asia. Proceedings of an International Workshop, Lampang, Thailand, 6–9 September 1993.* Australian Centre for International Agricultural Research (ACIAR), Canberra, Australia, pp. 111–115.

Ellis, P.R. (1994b) The economics of foot-and-mouth disease control. In: Copland, J.W., Gleeson, L.J. and Chamnanpood, C. (eds) *Diagnosis and Epidemiology of Foot-and-mouth Disease in Southeast Asia. Proceedings of an International Workshop, Lampang, Thailand, 6–9 September 1993.* Australian Centre for International Agricultural Research (ACIAR), Canberra, Australia, pp. 57–63. 4 refs.

Ellis, P.R. and Asby, C.B. (1975) The economics of mastitis control. In: *Proceedings of the IDF Seminar on Mastitis Control 1975.* International Dairy Federation, Brussels, Belgium, pp. 453–457.

Ellis, P.R. and Hugh-Jones, M.E. (1977) Economics of infection during pregnancy in farm livestock. In: Coid, C.R. (ed.) *Infections and Pregnancy.* Academic Press, London, New York, pp. 565–589.

Ellis, P.R. and James, A.D. (1978) Foot and mouth disease, India: disease control strategy in developing countries. In: Ellis, P.R., Shaw, A.P.M. and Stephens, A.J. (eds) *New Techniques in Veterinary Epidemiology and Economics.* Department of Agriculture, Reading University, Reading, UK, pp. 168–173.

Ellis, P.R. and James, A.D. (1979a) The economics of animal health. (2) Economics in farm practice. *Veterinary Record* 105(23), 523–526.

Ellis, P.R. and James, A.D. (1979b) The economics of animal health – (1) major disease control programmes. *Veterinary Record* 105(22), 504–506.

Ellis, P.R. and Stephens, A.J. (1979) Recent advances in preventative medicine in the United Kingdom. In: Cooper, M.G. (ed.) *Australian Advances in Veterinary Science, 1979.* Australian Veterinary Association, 134–136 Hampden Road, Artarmon, NSW 2064, Australia, pp. 81–82.

Ellis, P.R., James, A.D. and Shaw, A.P. (1977a) A review of the epidemiology and economics of swine fever eradication in the EEC. In: *Agricultural Research Seminar on Hog Cholera/Classical Swine Fever and African Swine Fever, Held at the Tierarztliche Hochschule, Hannover, 6–11 September, 1976.* Directorate-General XIII, Luxembourg, pp. 448–465.

Ellis, P.R., James, A.D. and Shaw, A.P. (1977b) *Studies on the Epidemiology and Economics of Swine Fever Eradication in the EEC.* Commission of the European Communities, Luxembourg, v + 90 pp.

Ellis, P.R., Esslemont, R.J. and Stephens, A.J. (1983) COSREEL. *Veterinary Record* 12(12), 285.

Ellis, P.R., James, A.D., Otte, J. and Hanks, J. (1997) Approaches to the establishment of veterinary epidemiology and economic services in developing countries. *Epidémiologie et Santé Animale* 31/32, 02.A.23.

Esslemont, R.J. and Ellis, P.R. (1974) Components of a herd calving interval. *Veterinary Record* 5(14), 319–320.

Esslemont, R.J. and Ellis, P.R. (1975) *The Melbread Dairy Herd Health Recording Scheme. A Report on the Economic, Reproductive and Husbandry Changes in 22 Herds over Three Seasons.* Reading University, Reading, UK, 42 pp.

Esslemont, R.J., Eddy, R.G. and Ellis, P.R. (1977) Planned breeding in autumn-calving dairy herds. *Veterinary Record* 100(20), 426–427.

Esslemont, R.J., Stephens, A.J. and Ellis, P.R. (1982) The design of DAISY the dairy information system. In: *Proceedings of the XIIth World Congress on Diseases of Cattle, The Netherlands,* Volume I. Utrecht, The Netherlands, pp. 643–646.

Felton, M.R. and Ellis, P.R. (1978) *Studies on the Control of Rinderpest in Nigeria.* Study No. 23, Veterinary Epidemiology Unit, Department of Agriculture, Reading University, Reading, Berkshire, UK, 40 pp.

Hugh-Jones, M.E., Ellis, P.R. and Felton, M.R. (1978) The use of a computer model of brucellosis in the dairy herd. In: Ellis, P.R., Shaw, A.P.M., and Stephens, A.J. (eds) *New Techniques in Veterinary Epidemiology and Economics.* Department of Agriculture, Reading University, Reading, UK, pp. 168–173.

James, A.D. and Ellis, P.R. (1978) Benefit–cost analysis in foot and mouth disease control programmes. *British Veterinary Journal* 134(1), 47–52.

James, A.D. and Ellis, P.R. (1980) The evaluation of production and economic effects of disease. In: *Proceedings of the Second International Symposium on Veterinary Epidemiology and Economics, 7–11 May 1979.* ISVEE, Canberra, Australia, pp. 363–372. 8 refs.

Otte, M.J., Gonzalez, C.A., Abuabara, Y. and Ellis, P.R. (1986) The effect of haemoparasite infections on weight gains in calves. In: *Anaplasma and Babesia in Colombia.* ISVEE, Singapore, pp. 297–299.

Putt, S.N.H., Shaw, R.W., Bourn, D.M., Underwood, M., James, A.D., Hallam, M.J. and Ellis, P.R. (1980) *The Social and Economic Implications of Trypanosomiasis Control. A Study of its Impact on Livestock Production and Rural Development in Northern Nigeria.* Source Study, No. 25, Department of Agriculture and Horticulture, Veterinary Epidemiology and Economics Research Unit, University of Reading, Reading, xx + 549 pp.

Shavulimo, R.S., Rurangirwa, F., Ruvuna, F., James, A.D., Ellis, P.R. and McGuire, T. (1988a) Evaluation of resistance against *Haemonchus contortus* in three breeds of goats. In: *Premières Journées Vétérinaires Africaines, Hammamet, Tunisie, 31 mai–2 juin 1987.* Office International des Epizooties (OIE), Paris, France, pp. 287–300.

Shavulimo, R.S., Rurangirwa, F., Ruvuma, F., James, A.D., Ellis, P.R. and McGuire, T. (1988b) Genetic resistance to gastrointestinal nematodes, with special reference to *Haemonchus contortus,* in three breeds of goats in Kenya. *Bulletin of Animal Health and Production in Africa* 36(3), 233–241.

Stephens, A.J., Esslemont, R.J., Ellis, P.R. and James, A.D. (1977) A feasibility study of a national herd fertility control scheme. In: *An Approach to Improving the Fertility of Dairy and Beef Herds in Great Britain. A working group's report to the Chief Veterinary Officer.* Ministry of Agriculture, Fisheries and Food, Tolworth, Surrey, UK, pp. 1–19.

Stephens, A.J., Esslemont, R.J. and Ellis, P.R. (1980) The evolution of a health and productivity monitoring system for dairy herds in the UK. In: *Proceedings of the Second International Symposium on Veterinary Epidemiology and Economics, 7–11 May 1979.* Canberra, Australia, pp. 53–58.

Stephens, A.J., Esslemont, R.J. and Ellis, P.R. (1982) DAISY in veterinary practice – Planned animal health and production services and small computers. *Veterinary Annual* 22, 6–17.

Vaz, Y. and Ellis, P.R. (1997) Problems of eradicating *Brucella melitensis* from small ruminant flocks in mountain areas of Portugal. *Epidémiologie et Santé Animale* 31/32 04.10.1–04.10.3.2.

Hugh-Jones

Cowen, P., Hugh-Jones, M.E. and Bailey, J.W. (1997) Zoonosis surveillance using the internet: how the ProMED-mail system works and a description of disease communications in 1996. *Epidémiologie et Santé Animale* 31/32, 04.21.1–04.21.3.

Enright, F.M. and Hugh-Jones, M.E. (1984) Effects of reactor retention on the spread of brucellosis in strain 19 adult vaccinated herds. *Preventive Veterinary Medicine* 2, 505–514.

Holmes, R.A., Smith, R.D., Dunavent, B., Hugh-Jones, M.E. and Kearney, M.E. (1995) Computerized decision analysis for the diagnosis and treatment of canine heartworm disease. In: Soll, M.D. and Knight, D.H. (eds) *Proceedings of the Heartworm Symposium '95, Auburn, Alabama, USA 31 March–2nd April, 1995.* American Heartworm Society, Batavia, Illinois, pp. 157–163. 8 refs.

Hugh-Jones, M.E. (1972a) Anomalous distribution of bovine mesothelioma. *Veterinary Record* 91(25), 632.

Hugh-Jones, M.E. (1972b) The uses and limitations of animal disease surveillance. *Veterinary Record* 92(1), 11–15.

Hugh-Jones, M.E. (1972c) Causes of death diagnosed during 1971 at veterinary investigation centres in Great Britain. In: *VII International Meeting on Diseases of Cattle, London 1972.* World Association of Buiatrics, pp. 1–15a.

Hugh-Jones, M.E. (1972d) Epidemiological studies on the 1967–68 foot and mouth epidemic: attack rates and cattle density. *Research in Veterinary Science* 13(5), 411–417.

Hugh-Jones, M.E. (1976a) Epidemiological studies on the 1967–1968 foot-and-mouth disease epidemic: the reporting of suspected disease. *Journal of Hygiene* 77(3), 299–306.

Hugh-Jones, M.E. (1976b) A simulation spatial model of the spread of foot-and-mouth disease through the primary movement of milk. *Journal of Hygiene* 77(1), 1–9.

Hugh-Jones, M.E. (1978) An assessment of the eradication of bovine brucellosis in England and Wales. In: Ellis, P.R., Shaw, A.P.M. and Stephens, A.J. (eds) *New Techniques in Veterinary Epidemiology and Economics.* Department of Agriculture, Reading University, Reading, UK, pp. 175–177.

Hugh-Jones, M.E. (1981) A simple vaccination model. *Bulletin de l'Office International des Epizooties* 93(1/2), 1–8.

Hugh-Jones, M.E. (1983) Surveillance for respiratory disease in Louisiana beef herds. In: *Third International Symposium on Veterinary Epidemiology and Economics, Arlington, Virginia, USA, 6–10 September 1982.* Veterinary Medicine Publishing Co., Edwardsville, Kansas, pp. 604–611.

Hugh-Jones, M.E. (1984) A systems approach to the economic assessment of disease control and eradication and a discussion of some control costs and benefits. *Preventive Veterinary Medicine* 2, 493–503.

Hugh-Jones, M.E. (1994a) Livestock: management and decision making. In: Griffiths, J.F. (ed.) *Handbook of Agricultural Meteorology.* Oxford University Press, New York, pp. 290–298.

Hugh-Jones, M.E. (1994b) Remote sensing, wetlands, and health. In: Mitsch, W.J. (ed.) *Global Wetlands: Old World and New.* Elsevier Science Publishers, Amsterdam, The Netherlands, pp. 833–837.

Hugh-Jones, M.E. and Hubbert, W. (1988) Seroconversion rates to bovine leukosis virus, bluetongue virus, *Leptospira hardjo* and *Anaplasma marginale* infections in a random series of Louisiana beef cattle. *Acta Veterinaria Scandinavica* 84(Supplement), 107–109.

Hugh-Jones, M.E. and Hussaini, S.N. (1974) An anthrax outbreak in Berkshire. *Veterinary Record* 94(11), 228–232.

Hugh-Jones, M.E. and Hussaini, S.N. (1975) Anthrax in England and Wales 1963–1972. *Veterinary Record* 97(14), 256–261.

Hugh-Jones, M.E. and Samui, K.L. (1993) Epidemiology of eastern equine encephalitis in Louisiana and Mississippi. *Journal of the Florida Mosquito Control Association* 64(2), 112–118.

Hugh-Jones, M.E. and Tinline, R.R. (1976) Studies on the 1967–68 foot and mouth disease epidemic: incubation period and herd serial interval. *Journal of Hygiene* 77(2), 141–153.

Hugh-Jones, M.E., Harvey, R.W.S. and McCoy, J.H. (1975) A *Salmonella* California contamination of a turkey feed concentrate. *British Veterinary Journal* 131(6), 673–680.

Hugh-Jones, M.E., Moorhouse, P. and Seger, C.L. (1984) Serological study of the incidence and prevalence of antibodies to bovine leukemia virus in aged sera. *Canadian Journal of Comparative Medicine* 48(4), 422–424.

Hugh-Jones, M.E., Moorhouse, P.D. and Fulton, R.W. (1985) Retrospective serological study on bluetongue antibody prevalence in a Louisiana herd. *Tropical Animal Health and Production* 317(3), 180–182.

Hugh-Jones, M.E., Broussard, J.J., Stewart, T.B., Raby, C. and Morrison, J.E. (1986a) Prevalence of *Toxoplasma* antibodies in southern Louisiana swine. *International Journal of Zoonoses* 13(1), 25–31.

Hugh-Jones, M.E., Broussard, J.J., Stewart, T.B., Raby, C. and Morrison, J.E. (1986b) Prevalence of *Toxoplasma gondii* antibodies in southern Louisiana swine in 1980 and 1981. *American Journal of Veterinary Research* 47(5), 1050–1051.

Hugh-Jones, M.E., Scotland, K., Applewhaite, L.M. and Alexander, F.M. (1988a) Seroprevalence of anaplasmosis and babesiosis in livestock on St. Lucia, 1983. *Tropical Animal Health and Production* 20(3), 137–139.

Hugh-Jones, M.E., Busch, D., Raby, C. and Jones, F. (1988b) Seroprevalence survey for *Anaplasma* card-test reactors in Louisiana, USA, cattle. *Preventive Veterinary Medicine* 6(2), 143–153.

Hugh-Jones, M.E., Taylor, W.P., Jones, F., Luther, G., Miller, J., Karns, P. and Hoyt, P. (1989) Serological observations on the epidemiology of bluetongue infections in Louisiana cattle. *Preventive Veterinary Medicine* 7(1), 11–18.

Hugh-Jones, M.E., Turnbull, P.C.B., Jones, M.N., Hutson, R.A., Quinn, C.P. and Kramer, J.M. (1991) Re-examination of the mineral supplement associated with a 1972 anthrax outbreak. *Veterinary Record* 128(26), 615–616.

Hugh-Jones, M.E., Hubbert, W.T. and Hagstad, H.V. (1995) *Zoonoses: Recognition, Control, and Prevention,* 1st edn. Iowa State University Press, Ames, Iowa, xiii + 369 pp.

Hugh-Jones, M.E., Hubbert, W.T. and Hagstad, H.V. (2000) *Zoonoses: Recognition, Control and Prevention.* Iowa State University Press, Ames, Iowa, xiii + 369 pp.

Jackson, P.J., Walthers, E.A., Kalif, A.S., Richmond, K.L., Adair, D.M., Hill, K.K., Kuske, C.R., Andersen, G.L., Wilson, K.H., Hugh-Jones, M.E. and Keim, P. (1997) Characterization of the variable-number of tandem repeats in vrrA from different *Bacillus anthracis* isolates. *Applied and Environmental Microbiology* 63(4), 1400–1405.

Jemal, A. and Hugh-Jones, M.E. (1995) Association of tsetse control with health and productivity of cattle in the Didessa Valley, western Ethiopia. *Preventive Veterinary Medicine* 22(1/2), 29–40.

Jemal, A., Justic, D. and Hugh-Jones, M.E. (1995) The estimated long-term impact of tsetse control on the size of the population of cattle in the Didessa Valley, western Ethiopia. *Veterinary Research Communications* 19(6), 479–485.

Johnachan, P.M., Smith, G.S., Grant, G. and Hugh-Jones, M.E. (1990) Serological survey for leptospiral antibodies in goats in St Elizabeth Parish, Jamaica, 1985–1986. *Tropical Animal Health and Production* 22(3), 171–177.

Keim, P., Klevytska, A.M., Price, L.B., Schupp, J.M., Zinser, G., Smith, K.L., Hugh-Jones, M.E., Okinaka, R., Hill, K.K. and Jackson, P.J. (1999) Molecular diversity in *Bacillus anthracis*. *Journal of Applied Microbiology* 87(2), 215–217.

Knoke, M.A.R., Rice, D.A. and Hugh-Jones, M.E. (1983) A serological survey of bovine brucellosis in El Salvador. In: *Third International Symposium on Veterinary Epidemiology and Economics, Arlington, Virginia, USA, 6–10 September 1982*. Veterinary Medicine Publishing, Edwardsville, Kansas, pp. 612–619.

Malone, J.B., Loyacano, A., Hugh-Jones, M.E., Armstrong, D.A. and Archbald, L.F. (1983) Liver fluke control in the United States with albendazole. In: *XXII World Veterinary Congress, Abstracts Booklet*. World Veterinary Congress, Perth, Australia, p. 141.

Malone, J.B., Loyacano, A.F., Hugh-Jones, M.E. and Corkum, K.C. (1984) A three-year study on seasonal transmission and control of *Fasciola hepatica* of cattle in Louisiana. *Preventive Veterinary Medicine* 3(2), 131–141.

McGinnis, B., Zingeser, J., Grant, G. and Hugh-Jones, M.E. (1988) Bovine anaplasmosis in Jamaica. *Tropical Animal Health and Production* 20(1), 42–44.

Moorhouse, P.D. and Hugh-Jones, M.E. (1981) Serum banks. *The Veterinary Bulletin* 51(5), 277–290.

Moorhouse, P.D. and Hugh-Jones, M.E. (1983) The results of retesting bovine sera stored at –18 deg C for twenty years, with lessons for future serum banks. In: *Third International Symposium on Veterinary Epidemiology and Economics, Arlington, Virginia, USA, 6–10 September 1982*. Veterinary Medicine Publishing, Edwardsville, Kansas, pp. 44–51.

Moorhouse, P.D., Hugh-Jones, M.E., Barta, O. and Swann, A.I. (1982) Leptospiral and brucellar titers in frozen bovine sera after 20 years of storage. *American Journal of Veterinary Research* 43(11), 2031–2034.

Morley, R.S. and Hugh-Jones, M.E. (1989a) Seroepidemiology of *Anaplasma marginale* in white-tailed deer (*Odocoileus virginianus*) from Louisiana. *Journal of Wildlife Diseases* 25(3), 342–346.

Morley, R.S. and Hugh-Jones, M.E. (1989b) The effect of management and ecological factors on the epidemiology of anaplasmosis in the Red River plains and south-east areas of Louisiana. *Veterinary Research Communications* 13(5), 359–369.

Morley, R.S. and Hugh-Jones, M.E. (1989c) The cost of anaplasmosis in the Red River plains and south-east areas of Louisiana. *Veterinary Research Communications* 13(5), 349–358.

Morley, R.S. and Hugh-Jones, M.E. (1989d) Incidence of clinical anaplasmosis in cattle in the Red River plains and south-east areas of Louisiana. *Veterinary Research Communications* 13(4), 297–305.

Morley, R.S. and Hugh-Jones, M.E. (1989e) Seroprevalence of anaplasmosis in the Red River plains and south-east areas of Louisiana. *Veterinary Research Communications* 13(4), 287–296.

Olcott, B.M., Strain, G.M., Hugh-Jones, M.E., Aldridge, B.M., Cho, D.Y., Kim, H.N., Olcott, B.M., Strain, G.M., Hugh-Jones, M.E., Aldridge, B.M., Cho, D.Y. and Kim, H.N. (1986) Suckling problem calves: definition, clinical and pathological findings. In: *Proceedings of 14th World Congress on Diseases of Cattle, Dublin*, Vol. 2. Dublin, Ireland, pp. 1201–1206.

Olcott, B.M., Strain, G.M., Hugh-Jones, M.E., Aldridge, B.M., Cho, D.Y. and Kim, H.N. (1987) Suckling problem calves. *Irish Veterinary News* 9(11), 13–17.

Reyes Knoke, M.A., Rice, D.A. and Hugh-Jones, M.E. (1984) Case study of estimation of prevalence of bovine brucellosis in El Salvador. *Preventive Veterinary Medicine* 2, 473–480.

Samui, K.L. and Hugh-Jones, M.E. (1988a) The financial cost of bovine dermatophilosis in Zambia. *Acta Veterinaria Scandinavica* 84(Supplement), 369–370.

Samui, K.L. and Hugh-Jones, M.E. (1988b) The prevalence of bovine dermatophilosis in Zambia. *Acta Veterinaria Scandinavica* 84(Supplement), 98–100.

Samui, K.L. and Hugh-Jones, M.E. (1990a) The financial and production impacts of bovine dermatophilosis in Zambia. *Veterinary Research Communications* 14(5), 357–365.

Samui, K.L. and Hugh-Jones, M.E. (1990b) The epidemiology of bovine dermatophilosis in Zambia. *Veterinary Research Communications* 14(4), 267–278.

Sen, S., Shane, S.M., Scholl, D.T., Hugh-Jones, M.E. and Gillespie, J.M. (1998) Evaluation of alternative strategies to prevent Newcastle disease in Cambodia. *Preventive Veterinary Medicine* 35(4), 283–295.

Smith, K.L., de Vos, V., Bryden, H.B., Hugh-Jones, M.E., Klevytska, A., Price, L.B., Keim, P. and Scholl, D.T. (1999) Meso-scale ecology of anthrax in southern Africa: a pilot study of diversity and clustering. *Journal of Applied Microbiology* 87(2), 204–207.

Smith, K.L., DeVos, V., Bryden, H., Price, L.B., Hugh-Jones, M.E. and Keim, P. (2000) *Bacillus anthracis* diversity in Kruger National Park [South Africa]. *Journal of Clinical Microbiology* 38(10), 3780–3784.

Smith, L.P., Hugh-Jones, M.E. and Jackson, O.F. (1972) Weather conditions and disease. *Veterinary Record* 91(25), 642.

Turnbull, P.C.B., Hugh-Jones, M.E. and Cosivi, O. (1999) World Health Organization activities on anthrax surveillance and control. *Journal of Applied Microbiology* 87(2), 318–320.

Turnwald, G.H., Shires, P.K., Turk, M.A.M., Cox, H.U., Pechman, R.D., Kearney, M.T., Hugh-Jones, M.E., Balsamo, G.A. and Helouin, C.M. (1986) Diskospondylitis in a kennel of dogs: clinicopathologic findings. *Journal of the American Veterinary Medical Association* 188(2), 178–183.

Whitney, J.C., Blackmore, D.K., Townsend, G.H., Parkin, R.J., Hugh-Jones, M.E., Crossman, P.J., Graham-Marr, T., Rowland, A.C., Festing, M.F.W. and Krzysiak, D. (1976) Rabbit mortality survey. *Laboratory Animals* 10(3), 203–207.

Zingeser, J., Daye, Y., Lopez, V., Grant, G., Bryan, L., Kearney, M. and Hugh-Jones, M.E. (1991) National survey of clinical and subclinical mastitis in Jamaican dairy herds, 1985–1986. *Tropical Animal Health and Production* 23(1), 2–10.

James

Awan, M.A., Otte, M.J. and James, A.D. (1994) The epidemiology of Newcastle disease in rural poultry: a review. *Avian Pathology* 23(3), 405–423.

Boneschanscher, J., James, A.D., Stephens, A.J. and Esslemont, R.J. (1982) The costs and benefits of pregnancy diagnosis in dairy cows: a simulation model. *Agricultural Systems* 9(1), 29–34.

Chema, S. and James, A.D. (1984) An approach to the information needs of a Ministry of Livestock. In: Hawksworth, D.L. (ed.) *Advancing Agricultural Production in Africa. Proceedings of CAB's First Scientific Conference, Arusha, Tanzania, 12–18 February 1984.* Commonwealth Agricultural Bureaux, Farnham Royal, Slough, UK, pp. 282–285.

Chema, S., Waghela, S., James, A.D., Dolan, T.T., Young, A.S., Masiga, W.N., Irvin, A.D., Mulela, G.H.M. and Wekesa, L.S. (1986) Clinical trial of parvaquone for the treatment of East Coast fever in Kenya. *Veterinary Record* 118(21), 588–589.

Chema, S., Chumo, R.S., Dolan, T.T., Gathuma, J.M., Irvin, A.D., James, A.D. and Young, A.S. (1987) Clinical trial of halofuginone lactate for the treatment of East Coast fever in Kenya. *Veterinary Record* 120(24), 575–577.

Davies, F.G., Linthicum, K.J. and James, A.D. (1985) Rainfall and epizootic Rift Valley fever. *Bulletin of the World Health Organization* 63(5), 941–943.

de Castro, J.J., James, A.D., Minjauw, B., di Giulio, G.U., Permin, A., Pegram, R.G., Chizyuka, H.G.B. and Sinyangwe, P. (1997) Long-term studies on the economic impact of ticks on Sanga cattle in Zambia. *Experimental and Applied Acarology* 21(1), 3–19.

Gettinby, G. and James, A.D. (1986) Data management for the evaluation of performance and productivity of cattle immunized against East Coast fever. In: Irvin, A.D. (ed.) *Immunization Against East Coast Fever. Report of a Workshop on Collection, Handling and Analysis of Performance and Productivity Data, Nairobi, Kenya, 23–25 September 1985.* International Laboratory for Research on Animal Diseases, PO Box 30709, Nairobi, Kenya, pp. 16–24.

Hanks, J.D., Bedard, B.G., Navis, S., Akoso, B.T., Putt, S.N.H., James, A.D. and Heriyanto, A. (1994) DIAG, a laboratory information management system development for regional animal disease diagnostic laboratories in Indonesia. *Tropical Animal Health and Production* 26(1), 13–19.

James, A.D. (1978) Epidemiological models and systems simulation. In: Ellis, P.R., Shaw, A.P.M. and Stephens, A.J. (eds) *New Techniques in Veterinary Epidemiology and Economics.* Department of Agriculture, Reading University, Reading, UK, pp. 52–54.

James, A.D. (1985) Data management aspects of an East Coast fever immunization network. In: Irvin, A.D. (ed.) *Immunization Against Theileriosis in Africa. Proceedings of a Joint Workshop, 1–5 October 1984, Nairobi, Kenya, ILRAD and FAO.* International Laboratory for Research on Animal Diseases, P.O. Box 30709, Nairobi, Kenya, pp. 133–139.

James, A.D. (1987) Principles and problems of benefit–cost analysis for disease control schemes. In: *EUR Report*. Commission of the European Communities. EUR 11285, Brussels, Belgium, pp. 69–77.

James, A.D. (1997) How do we integrate economics into the policy development and implementation process? In: Dijkhuizen, A.A. and Morris, R.S. (eds) *Animal Health Economics: Principles and Applications*. University of Sydney, Post-Graduate Foundation in Veterinary Science, Sydney South, Australia, pp. 187–231.

James, A.D. (1998) Guide to epidemiological surveillance for rinderpest. *Revue Scientifique et Technique Office International des Epizooties* 17(3), 796–824.

James, A.D. and Esslemont, R.J. (1979) The economics of calving intervals. *Animal Production* 29(2), 157–162.

James, A.D. and Rossiter, P.B. (1986) A simulation model of the epidemiology of rinderpest. In: *Proceedings of the 4th International Symposium for Veterinary Epidemiology and Economics, Singapore*, ISVEE, Singapore, pp. 268–271.

James, A.D. and Rossiter, P.B. (1989) An epidemiological model of rinderpest. I. Description of the model. *Tropical Animal Health and Production* 21(1), 59–68.

Minjauw, B., Otte, M.J. and James, A.D. (1997a) Incidence of clinical and sub-clinical *Theileria parva* infection in Sanga cattle kept under different ECF control strategies in Zambia. *Epidémiologie et Santé Animale* 31/32, 02.18.1–02.18.3.

Minjauw, B., Otte, J., James, A.D., de Castro, J.J. and Sinyangwe, P. (1997b) Effect of different East Coast fever control strategies on fertility, milk production and weight gain of Sanga cattle in the Central Province of Zambia. *Experimental and Applied Acarology* 21(12), 715–730.

Minjauw, B., Otte, M.J. and James, A.D. (1998a) Epidemiology and control of East Coast fever in Zambia. A field trial with traditionally managed Sanga cattle. *Annals of the New York Academy of Sciences* 849, 219–225.

Minjauw, B., Otte, M.J., James, A.D., de Castro, J.J., Permin, A. and di Giulo, G. (1998b) An outbreak of East Coast fever in a herd of Sanga cattle in Lutale, Central Province of Zambia. *Preventive Veterinary Medicine* 35(2), 143–147.

Minjauw, B., Otte, M.J., James, A.D., de Castro, J.J. and Sinyangwe, P. (1998c) Effect of different East Coast fever control strategies on disease incidence in traditionally managed Sanga cattle in Central Province of Zambia. *Preventive Veterinary Medicine* 35(2), 101–113.

Minjauw, B., Rushton, J., James, A.D. and Upton, M. (1999) Financial analysis of East Coast fever control strategies in traditionally managed Sanga cattle in Central Province of Zambia. *Preventive Veterinary Medicine* 38(1), 35–45.

Pegram, R.G., James, A.D., Oosterwijk, G.P.M. and Chizyuka, H.G.B. (1991a) The economic impact of cattle tick control in Central Africa. In: Chaudhury, M.F.B. (ed.) *Insect Science and Its Application* 12(1/2/3), 139–146.

Pegram, R.G., James, A.D., Oosterwijk, G.P.M., Killorn, K.J., Lemche, J., Ghirotti, M., Tekle, Z., Chizyuka, H.G.B., Mwase, E.T. and Chizhuka, F. (1991b) Studies on the economics of ticks in Zambia. *Experimental and Applied Acarology* 12(1,2), 9–26.

Pegram, R.G., James, A.D., Bamhare, C., Dolan, T.T., Hove, T., Kanhai, G.K. and Latif, A.A. (1996) Effects of immunisation against *Theileria parva* on beef cattle productivity and economics of control options. *Tropical Animal Health and Production* 28(1), 99–111.

Pflug, W. and James, A.D. (1989) Herdengesundheit-Herdenmanagement eine neue Chance fur das Verhaltnis Tierarzt – Landwirt (Herd health-herd management. A new view of cooperation between veterinarian and farmer.) *Tierarztliche Umschau* 44(6), 339–344, 347–348.

Purvis, G.M., Ostler, D.C., Starr, J., Baxter, J., Bishop, J., James, A.D., Dunn, P.G.C., Lyne, A.R., Ould, A. and McClintock, M. (1979) Lamb mortality in a commercial lowland sheep flock with reference to the influence of climate and economics. *Veterinary Record* 104(11), 241–242.

Putt, S.N.H., Shaw, A.P.M., Woods, A.J., Tyler, L. and James, A.D. (1988) *Veterinary Epidemiology and Economics in Africa. A Manual for Use in the Design and Appraisal of Livestock Health Policy*. ILCA Manual No. 3, ILCA, Addis Ababa, Ethiopia, 130 pp.

Rossiter, P.B. and James, A.D. (1989) An epidemiological model of rinderpest. II. Simulations of the behaviour of rinderpest virus in populations. *Tropical Animal Health and Production* 21(1), 69–84.

Villamil, L.C. and James, A.D. (1986) The assessment of the efficiency of cattle production. In: *Proceedings of the 4th International Symposium on Veterinary Epidemiology and Economics, Singapore, 18–22 November 1985*. Singapore Veterinary Association, Singapore, pp. 241–243.

Shaw

Griffin, T., Shaw, A.P.M., Topik, J.H., Wilkes, K., Miller, S.L. and Shapiro, P. (1982) Report on development alternatives in the Dilly Pastoral Zone. *AIDS Research and Development Abstracts* 10(1/2), 10.

Hoste, C. and Shaw, A.P.M. (1988a) International exchanges of trypanotolerant cattle in West and Central Africa – evaluation and future prospects. *Publication – International Scientific Council for Trypanosomiasis Research and Control* 114, 319–320.

Hoste, C.H. and Shaw, A.P.M. (1988b) Trypanotolerant cattle and livestock development in West and Central Africa. In: *Proceedings, IV World Conference on Animal Production, Helsinki, 1988.* Finnish Animal Breeding Associations, Helsinki, Finland, p. 485.

Putt, S.N.H. and Shaw, A.P.M. (1983) The socio-economic effects of the control of tsetse transmitted trypanosomiasis in Nigeria. In: *Third International Symposium on Veterinary Epidemiology and Economics. Arlington, Virginia, United States of America, 6–10 September 1982.* Veterinary Medicine Publishing, Edwardsville, Kansas, pp. 515–523.

Shaw, A.P.M. (1985) The use of spread-sheet models in assessing economic implications of disease control policy. In: *Proceedings of the Society for Veterinary Epidemiology and Preventive Medicine, 27–29 March 1985, Reading, UK,* SVEPM, Reading, UK, pp. 104–111.

Shaw, A.P.M. (1987) Epidémiologie et économie en Grande-Bretagne: le rôle des modèles de production animale dans l'analyse économique du contrôle des maladies animales (Epidemiology and economics in Great Britain: role of models of animal production in economic analysis of the control of animal diseases.) *Epidémiologie et Santé Animale* 11, 37–51.

Shaw, A.P.M. (1988a) The economics of trypanosomiasis control in the Sudan and northern Guinea zones of West Africa: a study based on examples from Nigeria and Mali. *Index to Theses Accepted for Higher Degrees in the Universities of Great Britain and Ireland* 36(3), 1255.

Shaw, A.P.M. (1988b) Teaching economics to post-experience veterinarians. In: Thrusfield, M.V. (ed.) *Proceedings of a Meeting held at the University of Edinburgh, 13–15 April 1988.* Socity for Veterinary Epidemiology and Preventive Medicine, University of Edinburgh, Roslin, Midlothian EH25 9RG, UK, pp. 1–12.

Shaw, A.P.M. (1989a) Comparative analysis of the costs and benefits of alternative disease control strategies: vector control versus human case finding and treatment. *Annales de la Société Belge de Médecine Tropicale* 69(1), 237–253.

Shaw, A.P.M. (1990) A spreadsheet model for the economic analysis of tsetse control operations benefitting cattle production. *Insect Science and Its Application* 11(3), 449–453. 7 refs.

Shaw, A.P.M. (1991) Mathematical models of trypanosomiasis control. *Publication – International Scientific Council for Trypanosomiasis Research and Control* 115, 106–114.

Shaw, A.P.M. (1995) Evaluation micro-économique analyse d'une action au niveaux des troupeaux (Economical analysis of disease control at the herd level.) *Epidémiologie et Santé Animale* 28, 27–38.

Shaw, A.P.M. and Hoste, C.H. (1989) *Trypanotolerant Cattle and Livestock Development in West and Central Africa. Vol. 1. The International Supply and Demand for Breeding Stock.* FAO Animal Production and Health Paper, No. 67/1, Rome, Italy, viii + 184 pp.

Shaw, A.P.M. and Hoste C.H. (1991a) Les échanges internationaux de bovins trypanotolérants. I. Historique et synthese (International exchanges of trypanotolerant cattle. 1. Historical analysis.) *Revue d'Elevage et de Médecine Vétérinaire des Pays Tropicaux* 44(2), 221–228.

Shaw, A.P.M. and Hoste, C.H. (1991b) Les échanges internationaux de bovins trypanotolérants. II. Tendances et perspectives (International exchanges of trypanotolerant cattle. 2. Tendencies and prospects.) *Revue d'Elévage et de Médecine Vétérinaire des Pays Tropicaux* 44(2), 229–237.

Shaw, A.P.M. and Kamate, C. (1982) An economic evaluation of the trypanosomiasis problem in Zone 1. *AIDS Research and Development Abstracts* 10(1/2), 9.

McLeod

McLeod, A. (1991) Management of PARC sero-monitoring data. The sero-monitoring of rinderpest throughout Africa. Phase one. In: *Proceedings of a Final Research Co-ordination Meeting of the FAO/IAEA/SIDA/OAU/IBAR/PARC Co-ordinated Research Programme held in Bingerville, Côte d'Ivoire, 19–23 November 1990.* International Atomic Energy Authority, A1400 Vienna, Austria, pp. 81–83.

McLeod, A. and Tyler, L. (1991) Steps in the implementation of a micro-computer approach to the management of animal disease information. *Revue Scientifique et Technique Office International des Epizooties* 10(1), 25–49.

Ndiritu, C.G. and McLeod, A. (1996) Institutionalisation of veterinary epidemiology and economics: the Kenyan experience. *Preventive Veterinary Medicine* 25(2), 93–106.

Okuthe, S., Otte, J., McLeod, A., Peeler, E. and Omore, A. (1997) Assessment of livestock constraints in the smallholder mixed farming systems in the Western Kenya highlands. *Epidémiologie et Santé Animale* 31/32, 02.08.1–02.08.3.

Oruko, L.O., Upton, M. and McLeod, A. (2000) Restructuring of animal health services in Kenya: constraints, prospects and options. *Development Policy Review* 18(2), 123–138.

Otieno, L., Upton, M., Mukhebi, A. and McLeod, A. (1997) Animal health services delivery in two dairy production systems in Kenya. *Epidémiologie et Santé Animale* 31/32, 02.A.20.

Leslie

Lawrence-Jones, W., Leslie, J., Pozo, M. and Serrate, J. (1983) *Un estudio de las fincas en Murillo con enfasis en el manejo de cerdos en el area de colonizacion del norte de Santa Cruz* (A study of farms in Murillo, concentrating on pig management in the colonization area to the north of Santa Cruz.) Documento de Trabajo No. 36. Centro de Investigacion Agricola Tropical, Bolivia. iii + 36 pp.

Leslie, J. (2000) Newcastle disease: outbreak losses and control policy costs. *Veterinary Record* 146(21), 603–606.

Leslie, J. and Upton, M. (1999) The economic implications of greater global trade in livestock and livestock products. *Revue Scientifique et Technique Office International des Epizooties* 18(2), 440–457.

Leslie, J., Barozzi, J. and Otte, J. (1997) The economic implications of a change in FMD policy: a case study in Uruguay. *Epidémiologie et Santé Animale* 31/32, 10.21.1–10.21.3.

Putt, S.N.H., Leslie, J. and Willemse, L. (1988) The economics of trypanosomiasis in Western Zambia. *Acta Veterinaria Scandinavica* 84(Supplement), 394–397.

Carpenter

Carpenter, T.E. (1978) Linear programming as a tool for disease control planning (brucellosis in beef cattle in California). In: Ellis, P.R., Shaw, A.P.M. and Stephens, A.J. (eds) *New Techniques in Veterinary Epidemiology and Economics*. Department of Agriculture, University of Reading, Reading, UK, p. 95.

Carpenter, T.E. (1979) Animal health economics: a course taught in the Master's in Preventive Veterinary Medicine program at Davis, California. In: *Proceedings of the Second International Symposium on Veterinary Epidemiology and Economics, 7–11 May 1979*. Canberra, Australia, pp. 328–330.

Carpenter, T.E. (1980) Economic evaluation of *Mycoplasma meleagridis* infection in turkeys: I. Production losses. II. Feasibility of eradication. *Dissertation Abstracts International* 41B(2), 485.

Carpenter, T.E. (1983) A microeconomic evaluation of the impact of *Mycoplasma meleagridis* infection in turkey production. *Preventive Veterinary Medicine* 1(4), 289–301.

Carpenter, T.E. (1994) Veterinary economics – tips, tricks, and traps. *Preventive Veterinary Medicine* 18(1), 27–31.

Carpenter, T.E. and Howitt, R. (1980) A linear programming model used in animal disease control. In: *Proceedings of the Second International Symposium on Veterinary Epidemiology and Economics, 7–11 May 1979, Canberra, Australia*. ISVEE, Canberra, Australia, pp. 483–489.

Carpenter, T.E. and Howitt, R.E. (1982) A model to evaluate the subsidization of governmental animal disease control programs. *Preventive Veterinary Medicine* 1(1), 17–25.

Carpenter, T.E. and Howitt, R.E. (1988) Dynamic programming approach to evaluating the economic impact of disease on (broiler) production. *Acta Veterinaria Scandinavica* 84(Supplement), 356–359.

Carpenter, T.E. and Norman, B.B. (1983) An economic evaluation of metabolic and cellular profile testing in calves to be raised in a feedlot. *Journal of the American Veterinary Medical Association* 183(1), 72–75.

Carpenter, T.E. and Thieme, A. (1980) A simulation approach to measuring the economic effects of foot-and-mouth disease in beef and dairy cattle. In: *Proceedings of the Second International Symposium on Veterinary Epidemiology and Economics, 7–11 May 1979, Canberra, Australia*. ISVEE, Canberra, Australia, pp. 511–516.

Carpenter, T.E., Miller, K.F., Gentry, R.F., Schwartz, L.D. and Mallinson, E.T. (1979) Control of *Mycoplasma gallisepticum* in commercial laying chickens using artificial exposure to Connecticut F strain *Mycoplasma gallisepticum*. *Proceedings of the United States Animal Health Association* 83, 364–370.

Carpenter, T.E., Howitt, R., McCapes, R., Yamamoto, R. and Riemann, H.P. (1981a) Formulating a control program against *Mycoplasma meleagridis* using economic decision analysis. *Avian Diseases* 25(2), 260–271.

Carpenter, T.E., Edson, R.K. and Yamamoto, R. (1981b) Decreased hatchability of turkeys eggs caused by experimental infection with *Mycoplasma meleagridis*. *Avian Diseases* 25(1), 151–156.

Carpenter, T.E., Berry, S.L. and Glenn, J.S. (1987) I. Economics of *Brucella ovis* control in sheep: epidemiological simulation model. II. Economics of *Brucella ovis* control in sheep: computerized decision-tree analysis. *Journal of the American Veterinary Medical Association* 190(8), 977–987.

Carpenter, T.E., Snipes, K.P., Wallis, D. and McCapes, R. (1988) Epidemiology and financial impact of fowl cholera in turkeys: a retrospective analysis. *Avian Diseases* 32(1), 16–23.

Christiansen, K.H. and Carpenter, T.E. (1983) Linear programming as a planning tool in the New Zealand brucellosis eradication scheme. In: *Third International Symposium on Veterinary Epidemiology and Economics, Arlington, Virginia, USA, 6–10 September 1982*. Veterinary Medicine Publishing, Edwardsville, Kansas, pp. 369–376.

Davidson, J.N., Carpenter, T.E. and Hjerpe, C.A. (1981) An example of an economic decision analysis approach to the problem of thromboembolic meningoencephalitis (TEME) in feedlot cattle. *Cornell Veterinarian* 71(4), 383–390.

Kimsey, S.W., Carpenter, T.E., Pappaioanou, M. and Lusk, E. (1985) Benefit–cost analysis of bubonic plague surveillance and control at two campgrounds in California, USA. *Journal of Medical Entomology* 22(5), 499–506.

Mohammed, H.O., Carpenter, T.E. and Yamamoto, R. (1987) Economic impact of *Mycoplasma gallisepticum* and *M. synoviae* in commercial layer flocks. *Avian Diseases* 31(3), 477–482.

Mousing, J., Vagsholm, I., Carpenter, T.E., Gardner, I.A. and Hird, D.W. (1988) Financial impact of transmissible gastroenteritis in pigs. *Journal of the American Veterinary Medical Association* 192(6), 756–759.

Rodrigues, C.A., Gardner, I.A. and Carpenter, T.E. (1990) Financial analysis of pseudorabies control and eradication in swine. *Journal of the American Veterinary Medical Association* 197(10), 1316–1323.

Ruegg, P.L. and Carpenter, T.E. (1989) Decision-tree analysis of treatment alternatives for left displaced abomasum. *Journal of the American Veterinary Medical Association* 195(4), 464–467.

Sischo, W.M., Hird, D.W., Gardner, I.A., Utterback, W.W., Christiansen, K.H., Carpenter, T.E., Danaye-Elmi, C. and Heron, B.R. (1990) Economics of disease occurrence and prevention on California dairy farms: a report and evaluation of data collected for the National Animal Health Monitoring system, 1986–87. *Preventive Veterinary Medicine* 8(2–3), 141–156.

Thorburn, M.A., Carpenter, T.E. and Plant, R.E. (1987) Perceived vibriosis risk by Swedish rainbow trout net-pen farmers: its effect on purchasing patterns and willingness-to-pay for vaccination. *Preventive Veterinary Medicine* 4(5/6), 419–434.

Vagsholm, I., Carpenter, T.E. and Jasper, D.E. (1988) Impact of a mastitis control program in Valdres, Norway, during 1982–1985. *Preventive Veterinary Medicine* 6(3), 223–234.

Vagsholm, I., Carpenter, T.E. and Howitt, R.E. (1991) Shadow costs of disease and its impact on output supply and input demand: the dual estimation approach. *Preventive Veterinary Medicine* 10(3), 195–212. 20 refs.

Zessin, K.H. and Carpenter, T.E. (1985) Benefit–cost analysis of an epidemiologic approach to provision of veterinary service in the Sudan. *Preventive Veterinary Medicine* 3(4), 323–337.

McInerney and Howe

Beynon, V.H. and Howe, K.S. (1975) Losses incurred in pig, cattle and sheep production in the United Kingdom. In: *The Committee of Inquiry into the Veterinary Profession*. Volume II. *Appendices to Report*. HM Stationery Office, London, pp. 56–81.

Bourne, J., Donnelly, C.A., Cox, D.R., Gettinby, G., McInerney, J.P., Morrison, I. and Woodroffe, R. (2000) Bovine tuberculosis: towards a future control strategy. *Veterinary Record* 146(8), 207–210.

Howe, K. (1985) The economics of disease control. *Veterinary Record* 117(15), 375.

Howe, K. and Christiansen, K.H. (2004) The state of animal health economics: a review. In: *The Proceedings of SVEPM, 2004*. SVEPM, London.

Howe, K., McInerney, J. and Schepers, J. (1989) Disease losses and research priorities. *Veterinary Record* 125(9), 244.

McInerney, J.P. (1986) Bovine tuberculosis and badgers – technical, economic and political aspects of a disease control programme. *Journal of the Agricultural Society*, University College of Wales 67, 136–167.

McInerney, J.P. (1987) Assessing the policy of badger control and its effects on the incidence of bovine tuberculosis. In: *Proceedings of the Society for Veterinary Epidemiology and Preventive Medicine*, pp. 133–147.

McInerney, J.P. (1988) The economic analysis of livestock disease: the developing framework. *Acta Veterinaria Scandinavica* 84(Supplement), 66–74.

McInerney, J.P. (1991) Assessing the benefits of farm animal welfare. In: Carruthers, S.P. (ed.) *Cas Paper* 22. Centre for Agricultural Strategy, University of Reading, Reading, UK, pp. 15–31.

McInerney, J.P. (1994) Animal welfare: an economic perspective. In: Bennett, R.M. (ed.) *Occasional Paper* 3. Department of Agricultural Economics and Management, University of Reading, Reading, UK, pp. 9–25.

McInerney, J.P. (1999) Livestock disease as an economic problem. In: Bennett, R.M. and Marshall, B.J. (eds) *Economic Assessment of Livestock Disease Problems*. Proceedings of a conference and workshops organized by the Department of Agricultural and Food Economics and the Centre for Agricultural Strategy, The University of Reading, March 1999. University of Reading, Reading, UK, pp. 25–40.

McInerney, J.P. and Turner, M.M. (1989) Assessing the economic effects of mastitis at the herd level using farm accounts data. In: *Proceedings, Society for Veterinary Epidemiology and Preventive Medicine, 12–14 April 1989, Exeter, UK.* Society for Veterinary Epidemiology and Preventive Medicine, Roslin, Midlothian, UK, pp. 46–59.

McInerney, J.P., Howe, K.S. and Schepers, J.A. (1992) A framework for the economic analysis of disease in farm livestock. *Preventive Veterinary Medicine* 13(2), 137–154.

Morrison, W.I., Bourne, F.J., Cox, D.R., Donnelly, C.A., Gettinby, G., McInerney, J.P. and Woodroffe, R. (2000) Pathogenesis and diagnosis of infections with *Mycobacterium bovis* in cattle. *Veterinary Record* 146(9), 236–242.

Willeberg, P., Leontides, L., Ewald, C., Mortensen, S., McInerney, J.P., Howe, K.S. and Kooij, D. (1996) Effect of vaccination against Aujeszky's disease compared with test and slaughter programme: epidemiological and economical evaluations. *Acta Veterinaria Scandinavica Supplement* 90, 25–51.

Dijkhuizen

Barkema, H.W., Heeres, A.A., Dijkhuizen, A.A., Schukken, Y.H. and Brand, A. (1995) Economic aspects of mastitis management in three cohorts of Dutch dairy farms. In: Saran, A. and Soback, S. (eds) *Proceedings of the Third IDF International Mastitis Seminar Tel-Aviv, Israel, 28 May–1 June 1995. Book 2.* National Mastitis Reference Center, Bet-Dagan, Israel, pp. s-4, 88–89.

Benedictus, G., Dijkhuizen, A.A. and Stelwagen, J. (1985) Economic losses due to paratuberculosis in cattle. [Dutch] Bedrijfseconomische schade van paratuberculose bij het rund. *Tijdschrift voor Diergeneeskunde* 110(8), 310–319.

Benedictus, G., Dijkhuizen, A.A. and Stelwagen, J. (1986) The economic losses due to clinical paratuberculosis in cattle. In: *Proceedings of 14th World Congress on Diseases of Cattle, Dublin,* Vol. 1. Dublin, Ireland, pp. 288–291.

Benedictus, G., Dijkhuizen, A.A. and Stelwagen, J. (1987) Economic losses due to paratuberculosis in dairy cattle. *Veterinary Record* 121(7), 142–146.

Berentsen, P.B.M., Dijkhuizen, A.A. and Oskam, A.J. (1990a) Cost–benefit analysis of foot and mouth disease control, with special attention to the effects of potential export bans. In: Noort, P.C. van den (ed.) *Costs and Benefits of Agricultural Policies and Projects. Proceedings of the 22nd Symposium of the European Association of Agricultural Economists (EAAE), 12–14 October 12th-14th, 1989, Amsterdam, The Netherlands.* Wissenschaftsverlag Vauk Kiel KG, Kiel, Germany, pp. 173–191.

Berentsen, P.B.M., Dijkhuizen, A.A. and Oskam, A.J. (1990b) *Foot-and-mouth Disease and Export, an Economic Evaluation of Preventive and Control Strategies for The Netherlands.* Wageningse Economische Studies 20, Wageningen University, Wageningen, The Netherlands, 89 pp.

Berentsen, P.B.M., Dijkhuizen, A.A. and Oskam, A.J. (1991) Economic analysis of veterinary regulations in partly integrated markets: the case of foot and mouth disease. *Tijdschrift voor Sociaal Wetenschappelijk Onderzoek van de Landbouw* 6(2), 89–112.

Berentsen, P.B.M., Dijkhuizen, A.A. and Oskam, A.J. (1992a) A dynamic model for cost–benefit analyses of foot-and-mouth disease control strategy. *Preventive Veterinary Medicine* 12(3–4), 229–243.

Berentsen, P.B.M., Dijkhuizen, A.A. and Oskam, A.J. (1992b) A critique of published cost–benefit analyses of foot-and-mouth disease. *Preventive Veterinary Medicine* 12(3–4), 217–227.

Breukink, H.J. and Dijkhuizen, A.A. (1982) Cost–benefit analysis of surgical correction of left abomasal displacement. [Dutch] De lebmaagdislocatie naar links in economisch perspectief. *Tijdschrift voor Diergeneeskunde* 107(7), 264–270.

Buijtels, J.A.A.M., Huirne, R.B.M., Dijkhuizen, A.A., Renkema, J.A. and Noordhuizen, J.P.T.M. (1996) Basic framework for the economic evaluation of animal health control programmes. *Revue Scientifique et Technique Office International des Epizooties* 15(3), 775–795.

Dijkhuizen, A.A. (1977) Economic aspects of disease and disease controls in particular mastitis in Netherlands dairy farming. [Dutch] *Economische aspecten van ziekten en ziektebestrijding, in het bijzonder de mastitis, in de Nederlandse melkveehouderij.* Publikatie No. 2, Fakulteit der Diergeneeskunde, Vakgroep Zootechniek, Afdeling Agrarische Economie, Rijksuniversiteit Utrecht, Utrecht, The Netherlands, 87 pp.

Dijkhuizen, A.A. (1983a) Economic aspects of diseases and their control in dairy cattle. [Dutch] *Economische aspecten van ziekten en ziektebestrijding bij melkvee.* Faculteit der Diergeneeskunde, Rijksuniversiteit Utrecht, Utrecht, The Netherlands, 166 + 27 pp.

Dijkhuizen, A.A. (1983b) Economic aspects of diseases, and of the prevention and treatment of disease, in dairy cattle. [Dutch] *Economische aspecten van ziekten en ziektebestrijding bij melkvee.* Rijksuniversiteit Utrecht, Utrecht, The Netherlands (Bedrijfsontwikkeling 14, 10, 779).

Dijkhuizen, A.A. (1987) Economic aspects of disease for the individual pig producer: a farm management view. In: *EUR Report.* EUR 11285, Commission of the European Communities, Brussels, pp. 123–136.

Dijkhuizen, A.A. (1988) Epidemiological and economic evaluation of foot and mouth disease control strategies, using a Markov Chain spreadsheet model [Netherlands]. *Acta Veterinaria Scandinavica* 84(Supplement), 350–352.

Dijkhuizen, A.A. (1989a) Economic aspects of common health and fertility problems for the individual pig producer: an overview. *Veterinary Quarterly* 11(2), 116–124.

Dijkhuizen, A.A. (1989b) Epidemiological and economic evaluation of foot-and-mouth disease control strategies in the Netherlands. *Netherlands Journal of Agricultural Science* 37(1), 1–12.

Dijkhuizen, A.A. (1998) Economic and social aspects of animal health, animal welfare and food safety: basic framework and some examples. *Tijdschrift voor Sociaalwetenschappelijk Onderzoek van de Landbouw* 13(3), 147–156.

Dijkhuizen, A.A. (1999) The 1997/98 outbreak of classical swine fever in The Netherlands: lessons to be learned from an economic perspective. In: Goodall, E.A. and Thursfield, M.V. (eds) *Society for Veterinary Epidemiology and Preventive Medicine. Proceedings of a Meeting Held at the University of Bristol, UK, on the 24–26 March, 1999.* Society for Veterinary Epidemiology and Preventive Medicine, Roslin, UK, pp. xi–xx.

Dijkhuizen, A.A. and Morris, R.S. (eds) (1997) *Animal Health Economics: Principles and Applications.* University of Sydney, Postgraduate Foundation in Veterinary Science, Sydney, Australia.

Dijkhuizen, A.A. and Renkema, J.A. (1977) Economic aspects of diseases and dairy herd health programmes in the Netherlands with special reference to mastitis. [Dutch] Economische aspecten van ziekten en ziektebestrijding, in het bijzonder mastitis, in de Nederlandse melkveehouderij. *Tijdschrift voor Diergeneeskunde* 102(21), 1239–1248.

Dijkhuizen, A.A. and Renkema, J.A. (1983) Economic importance of mastitis and its control in the Netherlands. [German] Wirtschaftliche Bedeutung der Mastitis und ihre Bekampfung in den Niederlanden. *Der Tierzuchter* 35(2), 64–66.

Dijkhuizen, A.A. and Stelwagen, J. (1981) The economic significance of mastitis under existing and modified agricultural policies. [Dutch] De economische betekenis van mastitis bij huidig en gewijzigd landbouwbeleid. *Tijdschrift voor Diergeneeskunde* 106(10), 492–496.

Dijkhuizen, A.A. and Stelwagen, J. (1982) The economic significance of mastitis in the Netherlands. *Netherlands Milk and Dairy Journal* 36(3), 267–269.

Dijkhuizen, A.A. and Valks, M.M.H. (1997) Economic evaluation of porcilis APP in fattening pigs. *Epidémiologie et Santé Animale* 31/32, 10.24.1–10.24.3.

Dijkhuizen, A.A., Renkema, J.A. and Stelwagen, J. (1984) Economic evaluation of the culling of cows because of infertility. [Dutch] De vervangingsbeslissing bij melkvee in geval van moeilijk te verkrijgen dracht: een economische evaluatie. *Tijdschrift voor Diergeneeskunde* 109(12), 485–493, 506.

Dijkhuizen, A.A., Stelwagen, J. and Renkema, J.A. (1985) Economic aspects of reproductive failure in dairy cattle. I. Financial loss at farm level. II. The decision to replace animals. *Preventive Veterinary Medicine* 3(3), 251–276.

Dijkhuizen, A.A., Hardaker, J.B. and Huirne, R.B.M. (1994) Risk attitude and decision making in contagious disease control. *Preventive Veterinary Medicine* 18(3), 203–212.

Dijkhuizen, A.A., Huirne, R.B.M. and Jalvingh, A.W. (1996) Economic analysis of animal diseases and their control. *Preventive Veterinary Medicine* 25(2), 135–149.

Dijkhuizen, A.A., Horst, H.S. and Jalvingh, A.W. (1997a) A new approach to integrate risk analysis and economics. *Epidémiologie et Santé Animale* 31/32, 06.08.1–06.08.3.

Dijkhuizen, A.A., Huirne, R.B.M. and Jalving, A.W. (1997b) Economics of reproduction and replacement in sows. [Italian] Aspetti economici della riproduzione e della rimonta nelle scrofe. In: *Atti della Societa Italiana di Patologia ed Allevamento dei Suini 1997 XXIII Meeting Annuale*. Societa Italiana di Patologia ed Allevamento dei Suini, Brescia, Italy, pp. 269–281.

Dijkhuizen, A.A., Jalvingh, A.W. and Huirne, R.B.M. (1998) Cost–benefit analysis in animal disease control. In: *Towards Livestock Disease Diagnosis and Control in the 21st Century: Proceedings of an International Symposium on Diagnosis and Control of Livestock Diseases Using Nuclear and Related Techniques, Vienna, Austria, 7–11 April 1997*. International Atomic Energy Agency (IAEA), Vienna, Austria, pp. 457–473.

Enting, H., Kooij, D., Dijkhuizen, A.A., Huirne, R.B.M. and Noordhuizen-Stassen, E.N. (1997) Economic losses due to clinical lameness in dairy cattle. *Livestock Production Science* 49(3), 259–267.

Fels-Klerx, H.J. van der, Jalvingh, A.W., Huirne, R.B.M. and Dijkhuizen, A.A. (1999) An economic model to estimate farm-specific losses due to bovine respiratory diseases in dairy heifers. In: Thrusfield, M.V. and Goodall, E.A. (eds) *Society for Veterinary Epidemiology and Preventive Medicine. Proceedings of a Meeting Held at the University of Edinburgh on the 29th, 30th and 31st of March 2000*. Society for Veterinary Epidemiology and Preventive Medicine, Roslin, UK, pp. 163–171.

Geurts, J.A.M.M., Burrell, A.M. and Dijkhuizen, A.A. (1997) An empirical modelling approach to estimate the economic effects of BSE for livestock industries. In: Goodall, E.A. and Thursfield, M.V. (eds) *Society for Veterinary Epidemiology and Preventive Medicine. Proceedings, University College, Chester, UK 9th, 10th and 11th April 1997*. Society for Veterinary Epidemiology and Preventive Medicine, Roslin, UK, pp. 76–84.

Horst, H.S., Dijkhuizen, A.A. and Huirne, R.B.M. (1996) Outline for an integrated modelling approach concerning risks and economic consequences of contagious animal diseases. *Netherlands Journal of Agricultural Science* 44(2), 89–102.

Horst, H.S., Huirne, R.B.M. and Dijkhuizen, A.A. (1997a) Risks and economic consequences of introducing classical swine fever into the Netherlands by feeding swill to swine. *Revue Scientifique et Technique Office International des Epizooties* 16(1), 207–214.

Horst, H.S., Dijkhuizen, A.A., Huirne, R.B.M. and Meuwissen, M.P.M. (1997b) Reducing the risk of introducing exotic animal disease into a country: computer simulation to help set priorities in policy making. *Epidémiologie et Santé Animale* 31/32, 06.02.1–06.02.3.

Horst, H.S., Dijkhuizen, A.A., Huirne, R.B.M. and Meuwissen, M.P.M. (1999) Monte Carlo simulation of virus introduction into the Netherlands. *Preventive Veterinary Medicine* 41(2/3), 209–229.

Houben, E.H.P., Thelosen, J.G.M., Huirne, R.B.M. and Dijkhuizen, A.A. (1990) Economic comparison of insemination and culling policies in commercial sow herds, assessed by stochastic simulation. *Netherlands Journal of Agricultural Science* 38(2), 201–204.

Houben, E.H.P., Dijkhuizen, A.A., Arendonk, J.A.M. and Huirne, R.B.M. (1993) Short- and long-term production losses and repeatability of clinical mastitis in dairy cattle. *Journal of Dairy Science* 76(9), 2561–2578.

Houben, E.H.P., Huirne, R.B.M., Dijkhuizen, A.A. and Kristensen, A.R. (1994) Optimal replacement of mastitic cows determined by a hierarchic Markov process. *Journal of Dairy Science* 77(10), 2975–2993.

Jalvingh, A.W., Vonk Noordegraaf, A., Nielen, M., Maurice, H. and Dijkhuizen, A.A. (1998) Epidemiological and economic evaluation of disease control strategies using stochastic and spatial simulation: general framework and two applications. In: Thursfield, M.V. and Goodall, E.A. (eds) *Society for Veterinary Epidemiology and Preventive Medicine. Proceedings of a Meeting Held on 25–27 March 1998*. Veterinary Field Station, Roslin EH25 9RG, UK, pp. 86–99.

Joosten, I., Stelwagen, J. and Dijkhuizen, A.A. (1988) Economic and reproductive consequences of retained placenta in dairy cattle. *Veterinary Record* 123(2), 53–57.

Klink, E.G.M. van, Sande, W.J.H. van der, Komijn, R.E., Cromwijk, W.A.J., Schukken, Y.H., Jong, M.C. de and Dijkhuizen, A.A. (1991) Diagnostic methods, spread and economic impact of the porcine reproductive and respiratory syndrome in the Netherlands. [French] Approches diagnositques, diffusion et impact économique du syndrome dysgénésique et respiratoire du porc aux Pays-Bas. *Epidémiologie et Santé Animale* 20, 61–69.

Mangen, M.J.J., Jalvingh, A.W., Nielen, M., Mourits, M.C.M., Klinkenberg, D. and Dijkhuizen, A.A. (2001) Spatial and stochastic simulation to compare two emergency-vaccination strategies with a marker vaccine in the 1997/1998 Dutch Classical Swine Fever epidemic. *Preventive Veterinary Medicine* 48(3), 177–200.

Meuwissen, M.P.M., Horst, H.S., Huirne, R.B.M. and Dijkhuizen, A.A. (1997) Insurance against losses from contagious animal disease. *Epidémiologie et Santé Animale* 31/32, 10.13.1–10.13.3.

Meuwissen, M.P.M., Horst, S.H., Huirne, R.B.M. and Dijkhuizen, A.A. (1999) A model to estimate the financial consequences of classical swine fever outbreaks: principles and outcomes. *Preventive Veterinary
Medicine* 39(4), 249–270.

Nielen, M., Jalvingh, A.W., Meuwissen, M.P.M., Horst, S.H. and Dijkhuizen, A.A. (1999) Spatial and stochastic simulation to evaluate the impact of events and control measures on the 1997–1998 classical
swine fever epidemic in the Netherlands. II. Comparison of control strategies. *Preventive Veterinary
Medicine* 39(4), 297–317.

Noordegraaf, A.V., Jalvingh, A.W., Nielen, M., Franken, P. and Dijkhuizen, A.A. (1999) Simulation mod-
elling to support policy making in the control of bovine herpes virus type 1. In: Goodall, E.A. and
Thursfield, M.V. (eds) *Society for Veterinary Epidemiology and Preventive Medicine. Proceedings of a Meeting
Held at the University of Bristol, UK, on the 24–26 March, 1999*. Society for Veterinary Epidemiology and
Preventive Medicine, Roslin, UK, pp. 18–29.

Noordegraaf, A.V., Jalvingh, A.W., de Jong, M.C.M., Franken, P. and Dijkhuizen, A.A. (2000) Evaluating
control strategies for outbreaks in BHV1-free areas using stochastic and spatial simulation. *Preventive
Veterinary Medicine* 44(1/2), 21–42.

Pasman, E.J., Dijkhuizen, A.A. and Wentink, G.H. (1994) A state-transition model to simulate the economics of bovine virus diarrhoea control. *Preventive Veterinary Medicine* 20(4), 269–277.

Renkema, J.A. and Dijkhuizen, A.A. (1979) Economic aspects of disease in animals, with special reference
to dairy cattle. [Dutch] Economische aspecten van dierziekten, in het bijzonder bij melkvee. *Tijdschrift
voor Diergeneeskunde* 104(24), 977–985. (*Veterinary Bulletin* 50(7), 4182.)

Renkema, J.A. and Dijkhuizen, A.A. (1985) Economic aspects of animal diseases with special reference
to preventive veterinary measures in dairy farming. [German] Betriebswirtschaftliche Aspekte von
Tierkrankheiten unter besonderer Berucksichtigung von tiergesundheitliche Vorbeugemassnahman
in der Milchviehhaltung. *Zuchtungskunde* 57(4), 225–236. 7 refs.

Renkema, J.A., Sol, J. and Dijkhuizen, A.A. (1981) Some further contributions to the economic evaluation of
preventive health programmes. *Bulletin de l'Office International des Epizooties* 93(5/6), 1023–1037.

Rougoor, C.W., Dijkhuizen, A.A., Barkema, H.W. and Schukken, Y.H. (1994) The economics of caesarian
section in dairy cattle. *Preventive Veterinary Medicine* 19(1), 27–37.

Rougoor, C.W., Dijkhuizen, A.A., Huirne, R.B.M. and Marsh, W.E. (1996) Impact of different approaches to
calculate the economics of disease in pig farming. *Preventive Veterinary Medicine* 26(3/4), 315–328.

Rougoor, C.W., Hanekamp, W.J.A., Dijkhuizen, A.A., Nielen, M. and Wilmink, J.B.M. (1999) Relationships
between dairy cow mastitis and fertility management and farm performance. *Preventive Veterinary
Medicine* 39(4), 247–264.

Schakenraad, M.H.W. and Dijkhuizen, A.A. (1990) Economic losses due to bovine mastitis in Dutch dairy
herds. *Netherlands Journal of Agricultural Science* 38(1), 89–92.

Schepers, J.A. and Dijkhuizen, A.A. (1991) The economics of mastitis and mastitis control in dairy cattle: a
critical analysis of estimates published since 1970. *Preventive Veterinary Medicine* 10(3), 213–224.

Scholman, G.J. and Dijkhuizen, A.A. (1989) Determination and analysis of the economic optimum culling
strategy in swine breeding herds in Western Europe and the USA. *Netherlands Journal of Agricultural
Science* 57(1), 71–73.

Shah, S.N.H., Dijkhuizen, A.A., Willemse, A.H. and van de Wiel, D.F.M. (1991) Economic aspects of reproductive failure in dairy buffaloes of Pakistan. *Preventive Veterinary Medicine* 11(2), 147–155.

Sol, J., Stelwagen, J. and Dijkhuizen, A.A. (1984) A three year herd health and management program on
thirty Dutch dairy farms. 2. Culling strategy and losses caused by forced replacement of dairy cows.
Veterinary Quarterly 6(3), 149–157.

Stelwagen, J. and Dijkhuizen, A.A. (1998) An outbreak of bovine viral diarrhoea can be costly – a practical
example. [Dutch] BVD-uitbraak kan kostbaar zijn: een praktijkgeval. *Tijdschrift voor Diergeneeskunde*
123(9), 283–286.

van der Kamp, A., Dijkhuizen, A.A. and Peterse, D.J. (1990) A simulation of leptospirosis control in Dutch
dairy herds. *Preventive Veterinary Medicine* 9(1), 9–26.

van Schaik, G., Kalis, C.H.J., Benedictus, G., Dijkhuizen, A.A. and Huirne, R.B.M. (1996) Cost–benefit
analysis of vaccination against paratuberculosis in dairy cattle. *Veterinary Record* 139(25), 624–627.

van Schaik, G., Shoukri, M., Martin, S.W., Schukken, Y.H., Nielen, M., Hage, J.J. and Dijkhuizen, A.A.
(1999) Modeling the effect of an outbreak of bovine herpesvirus type 1 on herd-level milk production
of Dutch dairy farms. *Journal of Dairy Science* 82(5), 944–952.

Vos, C.J. de, Horst, H.S. and Dijkhuizen, A.A. (1999) Risk of animal movements for the introduction of contagious animal diseases to densely populated livestock areas of the European Union. In: Thrusfield,

M.V. and Goodall, E.A. (eds) *Society for Veterinary Epidemiology and Preventive Medicine. Proceedings of a Meeting Held at the University of Edinburgh on the 29th, 30th and 31st of March 2000*. Society for Veterinary Epidemiology and Preventive Medicine, Roslin, UK, pp. 124–136.

Wentink, G.H. and Dijkhuizen, A.A. (1990) Economic consequences of infection with bovine diarrhoea virus in 14 dairy herds. [Dutch] Economische gevolgen van een infectie met het Bovine Virus Diarree virus (BVD-virus) op 14 melkveebedrijven. *Tijdschrift voor Diergeneeskunde* 115(22), 1031–1040.

Tisdell, Ramsay and Harrison

Harrison, S.R. (1996) *Cost–Benefit Analysis with Applications to Animal Health Programmes*. Research Papers and Reports in Animal Health Economics, No. 18–23, The University of Queensland, Brisbane, Australia.

Harrison S.R. and Sharma P (1999) Interfacing GIS with economic models for managing livestock health. In: Sharma, P. and Baldock, C. (eds) *Understanding Animal Health in South-East Asia. Advances in the Collection, Management and Use of Animal Health Information*. ACIAR Monograph 58. ACIAR, Canberra, Australia, pp. 223–240.

Harrison, S.R. and Tisdell, C.A. (1997) Animal health programs in sustainable economic development: some observations from Thailand. In: Roy, K.C., Blomqvist, H.C. and Hossein, I. (eds) *Development that Lasts*. New Age International, New Delhi, pp. 201–214.

Harrison, S.R. and Tisdell, C.A. (1999) *Economic Analysis of Foot and Mouth Disease Control and Eradication in Thailand*. ACIAR, Canberra, Australia, 95 pp.

Harrison, S.R., Tisdell, C. and Ramsey, G. (1999) Economic issues in animal health programs. In: Sharma, P. and Baldock, C. (eds) *Understanding Animal Health in South-East Asia. Advances in the Collection, Management and Use of Animal Health Information*. ACIAR Monograph 58. ACIAR, Canberra, Australia, pp. 57–72.

Ramsay, G.C. (1997) Setting animal health priorities: a veterinary and economic analysis with special reference to the control of *Babesia bovis* in central Queensland. PhD thesis, Department of Economics, University of Queensland, Brisbane, Australia, 325 pp.

Ramsay, G.C., Tisdell, C.A. and Harrison, S.R. (1997a) *The Distribution of Benefits in Improved Animal Health Decision Making as a Result of the Collection of Additional Animal Health Information*. Research Papers and Reports in Animal Health Economics, No. 38, The University of Queensland, Brisbane, Australia.

Ramsay, G.C., Tisdell, C.A. and Harrison, S.R. (1997b) Distribution of benefits from improved animal health decision making. *Epidémiologie et Santé Animal* Special Issue 31–32, 10.01.1–10.01.3.

Ramsay, G.C., Tisdell, C.A. and Harrison, S.R. (1997c) *Private Decision in Livestock Disease Control and the Value of Additional Information in Animal Health*. Research Papers and Reports in Animal Health Economics, No. 37, The University of Queensland, Brisbane, Australia.

Ramsay, G.C., Tisdell, C.A. and Harrison, S.R. (1999a) Distribution of benefits from improved animal health. In: Sharma, P. and Baldock, C. (eds) *Understanding Animal Health in South-East Asia. Advances in the Collection, Management and Use of Animal Health Information*. ACIAR Monograph 58. ACIAR, Canberra, Australia, pp. 241–260.

Ramsay, G.C., Tisdell, C.A. and Harrison, S.R. (1999b) Assessing value of additional animal health information. In: Sharma, P. and Baldock, C. (eds) *Understanding Animal Health in South-East Asia. Advances in the Collection, Management and Use of Animal Health Information*. ACIAR Monograph 58. ACIAR, Canberra, Australia, pp. 261–282.

Tisdell, C.A. (1995) *Assessing the Approach of Cost–Benefit Analysis of Controlling Livestock Diseases of McInerney and Others*. Research Papers and Reports in Animal Health Economics, No. 3, Department of Economics, University of Queensland, Brisbane, Australia, 22 pp.

Tisdell, C.A., Harrison, S.R. and Ramsay, G.C. (1999) The economic impacts of endemic diseases and disease control programmes. *Revue Scientifique et Technique Office International des Epizooties* 18(2), 380–398.

Bennett

Anderson, J., Bennett, R. and Blaney, R. (1999) Moral importance, animal welfare and food policy. In: *Avhandlingar – Institutionen for Ekonomi, Sveriges Lantbruksuniversitet*, No. 29. Sveriges Lantbruksuniversitet, Institutionen for Ekonomi, Uppsala, Sweden, pp. 2–8.

Bennett, R. (1991) Dairy farmers, information and disease control. *Farm Management* 7(10), 485–493.

Bennett, R. (1993) Modelling to support decisions on leptospirosis control in dairy herds. In: Thrusfield, M.V. (ed.) *Society for Veterinary Epidemiology and Preventive Medicine: Proceedings of a Meeting Held at the University of Exeter, 31 March–2 April 1993.* Society for Veterinary Epidemiology and Preventive Medicine, Roslin, UK, pp. 6–19.

Bennett, R. (1995) The value of farm animal welfare. *Journal of Agricultural Economics* 46(1), 46–60.

Bennett, R. (1998) Measuring public support for animal welfare legislation: a case study of cage egg production. *Animal Welfare* 7(1), 1–10.

Bennett, R. (2000) Modelling the costs associated with BVD in dairy herds. *Cattle Practice* 8(1), 15–16.

Bennett, R. and Larson, D. (1996) Contingent valuation of the perceived benefits of farm animal welfare legislation: an exploratory survey. *Journal of Agricultural Economics* 47(2), 224–235.

Bennett, R., Christiansen, K. and Clifton-Hadley, R. (1997) An economic study of the importance of non-notifiable diseases of farm animals in Great Britain. *Epidémiologie et Santé Animale* 31/32, 10.19.1–10.19.3.

Bennett, R., Christiansen, K. and Clifton-Hadley, R. (1999a) Preliminary estimates of the direct costs associated with endemic diseases of livestock in Great Britain. In: Bennett, R.M. and Marshall, B.J. (eds) *Economic Assessment of Livestock Disease Problems. Proceedings of a Conference and Workshops Organised by the Department of Agricultural and Food Economics and the Centre for Agricultural Strategy, The University of Reading, Held at the Town Hall, Reading, UK, on 2 March 1999.* Department of Agricultural and Food Economics, University of Reading, Reading, UK, pp. 13–24.

Bennett, R., Christiansen, K. and Clifton-Hadley, R. (1999b) Preliminary estimates of the direct costs associated with endemic diseases of livestock in Great Britain. *Preventive Veterinary Medicine* 39(3), 155–171.

Blaney, R. and Bennett, R. (1997) Farm animal welfare: economics and epidemiology. *Epidémiologie et Santé Animale* 31/32, 10.C.04.

Perry and Mukhebi

Mukhebi, A.W., Wathanga, J., Perry, B.D., Irvin, A.D. and Morzaria, S.P. (1989) Financial analysis of East Coast fever control strategies on beef production under farm conditions. *The Veterinary Record* 125, 456–459.

Mukhebi, A.W., Morzaria, S.P., Perry, B.D., Dolan, T.T. and Norval, R.A.I. (1990) Cost analysis of immunization for East Coast fever by the infection treatment method. *Preventive Veterinary Medicine* 9, 207–219.

Mukhebi, A.W., Perry, B.D. and Kruska, R. (1992) Estimated economics of theileriosis control in Africa. *Preventive Veterinary Medicine* 12, 73–85.

Mukhebi, A.W., Chamboko, T., O'Callaghan, C.J., Peter, T.F., Kruska, R.L., Medley, G.F., Mahan, S.M. and Perry, B.D. (1999) An assessment of the economic impact of heartwater (*Cowdria ruminantium* infection) and its control in Zimbabwe. *Preventive Veterinary Medicine* 39, 173–189.

Perry, B.D. and Randolph, T.F. (1999) Improving the assessment of the economic impact of parasitic diseases and of their control in production animals. *Veterinary Parasitology* 84, 145–168.

Perry, B.D. and Young, A.S. (1995) The past and future roles of epidemiology and economics in the control of tick-borne diseases of livestock in Africa: the case of theileriosis. *Preventive Veterinary Medicine* 25, 107–120.

Perry, B.D., Mukhebi, A.W., Norval, R.A.I. and Barrett, J.C. (1990) *A Preliminary Assessment of Current and Alternative Tick and Tick-borne Disease Control Strategies in Zimbabwe.* ILRAD, Nairobi, Kenya.

Perry, B.D., Kalpravidh, W., Coleman, P.G., Mcdermott, J.J., Randolph, T.F. and Gleeson, L.J. (1999) The economic impact of foot and mouth disease and its control in South-East Asia: a preliminary assessment with special reference to Thailand. *Revue Scientifique et Technique Office International des Epizooties* 2, 478–497.

Perry, B.D., McDermott, J. and Randolph, T. (2001) Can epidemiology and economics make a meaningful contribution to national animal-disease control? *Preventive Veterinary Medicine* 48, 231–260.

Economic Assessment of Livestock Diseases

Delgado, C.L., Rosegrant, M.W. and Meijer, S. (2001) Livestock to 2020: the revolution continues. Paper presented at the annual meetings of the International Agricultural Trade Consortium (IATRC), Auckland, New Zealand, 18–19 January 2001.

Dufour, B. and Moutou, F. (1994) Economic analysis of the modification of the French system of foot and mouth disease control. [French] Etude économique de la modification de la lutte contre la fièvre aphteuse en France. *Annales de Médecine Vétérinaire* 138(2), 97–105.

James, A.D. and Carles, A. (1996) Measuring the productivity of grazing and foraging livestock. *Agricultural Systems* 52(2/3), 271–291.

PAN Livestock Services (1991) *LPEC The Livestock Production Efficiency Calculator User Guide*. PAN Livestock Services, Department of Agriculture, Earley Gate, PO Box 236, Reading RG6 6AT, UK, 113 pp.

Rushton, J., Thornton, P. and Otte, M.J. (1999) Methods of economic impact assessment. In: *The Economics of Animal Disease Control. OIE Revue Scientifique et Technique* 18(2), 315–338.

Shaw, A.P.M. (1989) *CLIPPER. Computerised Livestock Project Planning Exercise. User Notes*. AP Consultants, Andover, UK.

Yalcin, C., Cevger, Y., Turkyilmaz, K. and Uysal, G. (2000) Estimation of milk yield losses from subclinical mastitis in dairy cows. [Turkish] Sut ineklerinde subklinik mastitisten kaynaklanan sut verim kayiplarinin tahmini. *Turk Veterinerlik Ve Hayvancilik Dergisi* 24(6), 599–604.

Livestock Populations and Production Systems

Seré, S. and Steinfeld, H. (1995) *World Livestock Production Systems – Current Status, Issues and Trends*. FAO Animal Production and Health Paper No. 127. FAO, Rome, Italy.

Major Diseases

OIE (2001a) International Animal Health Code 2001. Available at: http://www.oie.int/eng/normes/mcode/A_summary.htm

OIE (2001b) A short history of the Office International des Epizooties. Available at: http://www.oie.int/eng/OIE/en_histoire.htm

OIE (2001c) Diseases of the OIE Classification. Available at: http://www.oie.int/eng/maladies/en_classification.htm

FMD

Amadori, M., Lodetti, E., Massirio, I. and Panina, G.F. (1991) Eradication of foot and mouth disease in Italy: cost benefit analysis of a change in strategy. [Italian] Eradicazione dell'afta epizootica in Italia: analisi so costo/beneficio nel cambio di strategia. *Selezione Veterinaria* 32(12), 1773–1780.

Astudillo, V.M. and Auge de Mello, P. (1980) Cost and effectiveness analysis of two foot-and-mouth disease vaccination procedures. *Boletin del Centro Panamericano de Fiebre Aftosa* 37/38, 49–63.

Berentsen, P.B.M., Dijkhuizen, A.A. and Oskam, A.J. (1990a) Cost–benefit analysis of foot and mouth disease control, with special attention to the effects of potential export bans. In: Noort, P.C. van den (ed.) *Costs and Benefits of Agricultural Policies and Projects. Proceedings of the 22nd Symposium of the European Association of Agricultural Economists (EAAE), 12–14 October 1989, Amsterdam, The Netherlands*. Wissenschaftsverlag Vauk Kiel KG, Kiel, Germany, pp. 173–191.

Berentsen, P.B.M., Dijkhuizen, A.A. and Oskam, A.J. (1990b) *Foot-and-mouth Disease and Export, an Economic Evaluation of Preventive and Control Strategies for The Netherlands*. Wageningse Economische Studies 20, Wageningen University, Wageningen, The Netherlands, 89 pp.

Berentsen, P.B.M., Dijkhuizen, A.A. and Oskam, A.J. (1992) A dynamic model for cost–benefit analyses of foot-and-mouth disease control strategy. *Preventive Veterinary Medicine* 12(3–4), 229–243.

Bulman, G. and Terrazas, M.I. (1976) Effect of foot-and-mouth disease on milk production at a model farm in Cochabamba, Bolivia. [Spanish] Consideraciones sobre el efecto de la fiebre aftosa en la produccion lactea de un tambo modelo en Cochabamba, Bolivia. *Revista de Medicina Veterinaria, Argentina* 57(1), 1–2, 5–6, 9–10.

Caporale, V.P., Battelli, G., Ghilardi, G. and Biancardi, V. (1980) Evaluation of the costs and benefits of the control campaigns against bovine tuberculosis, brucellosis, foot-and-mouth disease and swine fever in Italy. *Bulletin de l'Office International des Epizooties* 92(5/6), 291–304.

Cardona, A.G., Uribe, J.R., Arboleda, C.F. and Alzate, R.L. (1982) Economic evaluation of an outbreak of foot and mouth disease in a Colombian dairy herd. [Spanish] *Evaluacion economica de un brote de aftosa en una explotacion lechera*. Cenicafe No. 8, Seccion de Industria Animal, Chin, Caldas, Colombia, 40 pp.

Carpenter, T.E. and Thieme, A. (1980) A simulation approach to measuring the economic effects of foot-and-mouth disease in beef and dairy cattle. In: *Proceedings of the Second International Symposium on Veterinary Epidemiology and Economics, 7–11 May 1979*. ISVEE, Canberra, Australia, pp. 511–516.

Davies, G. (1988) An economic analysis of foot and mouth disease policy options – problems and opportunities. *Acta Veterinaria Scandinavica* 84(Supplement), 423–426.

Dijkhuizen, A.A. (1989b) Epidemiological and economic evaluation of foot-and-mouth disease control strategies in the Netherlands. *Netherlands Journal of Agricultural Science* 37(1), 1–12.

Dufour, B. and Moutou, F. (1994) Economic analysis of the modification of the French system of foot and mouth disease control. [French] Etude économique de la modification de la lutte contre la fièvre aphteuse en France. *Annales de Médecine Vétérinaire* 138(2), 97–105.

Ertan, H. and Nazlioglu, M. (1981) Animal health and economics in Turkey. *Bulletin de l'Office International des Epizooties* 93(5/6), 1045–1052.

Farag, M.A., Al-Sukayran, A., Mazloum, K.S. and Al-Bokmy, A.M. (1998) The role of small ruminants in the epizootiology of foot and mouth disease in Saudi Arabia with reference to the economic impact of the disease on sheep and goats. *Assiut Veterinary Medical Journal* 40(79), 23–41.

Farez, S. and Morley, R.S. (1997) Potential animal health hazards of pork and pork products. *Revue Scientifique et Technique Office International des Epizooties* 16(1), 65–78.

Garner, M.G. and Lack, M.B. (1995) Modelling the potential impact of exotic diseases on regional Australia. *Australian Veterinary Journal* 72(3), 81–87.

Ghilardi, G., Caporale, V.P., Battelli, G. and Cavrini, C. (1981) Updating of the economic evaluation of the control campaigns against bovine tuberculosis, brucellosis, foot-and-mouth disease and swine fever in Italy. *Bulletin de l'Office International des Epizooties* 93(5/6), 1015–1021.

Hafez, S.M., Farag, M.A. and Al-Sukayran, A.M. (1994) The impact of live animal importation on the epizootiology of foot-and-mouth disease in Saudi Arabia. *Deutsche Tierarztliche Wochenschrift* 101(10), 397–402.

James, A.D. and Ellis, P.R. (1978) Benefit–cost analysis in foot and mouth disease control programmes. *British Veterinary Journal* 134(1), 47–52.

Kazimi, S.E. and Shah, S.K. (1980) Effect on production performance in cattle due to foot-and-mouth disease. *Bulletin de l'Office International des Epizooties* 92(3/4), 159–166.

Kulkarni, M.D., Deshpande, P.D., Kale, K.M. and Narawade, V.S. (1990) Epidemiological investigation and economics on foot and mouth disease outbreak. *Livestock Adviser* 15(10), 29–33.

Leabad, A. (1981) The foot and mouth disease outbreak in Morocco in 1977. [French] L'épizootie de fièvre aphteuse au Maroc en 1977. Thèse, Ecole National Vétérinaire d'Alfort, 92 pp.

Lorenz, R.J. (1988) A cost effectiveness study on the vaccination against foot-and-mouth disease (FMD) in the Federal Republic of Germany. *Acta Veterinaria Scandinavica* 84(Supplement), 427–429.

Mahul, O. and Durand, B. (2000) Simulated economic consequences of foot-and-mouth disease epidemics and their public control in France. *Preventive Veterinary Medicine* 47(1/2), 23–38.

McCauley, H., Aulaqi, N., Sundquist, W.B. and New, J. (1978) Studies on economic impact of foot and mouth disease in the United States. Preliminary report of on-going research at the University of Minnesota. In: Ellis, P.R., Shaw, A.P.M and Stephens, A.J. (eds) *New Techniques in Veterinary Epidemiology and Economics*. Department of Agriculture, Reading University, Reading, UK, pp. 132–166.

Mendoza, J.W.M., Francis, D.G., Castro, L.M.B. and Machado Filho, F. (1978) Socio-economic factors involved in the programme to eradicate foot and mouth disease in two regions of Paraguay. [Portuguese] Fatores socio-economicos relacionados com o combate a febre aftosa em dois departamentos do Paraguai. *Revista Ceres* 25(139), 280–291.

Mersie, A., Tafesse, B., Getahun, F. and Teklu, W. (1992) Losses from foot-and-mouth disease in a mixed farming area of eastern Ethiopia. *Tropical Animal Health and Production* 24(3), 144.

Obiaga, J.A., Rosenberg, F.J., Astudillo, V. and Goic, M.R. (1979) Characteristics of livestock production as determinant of foot-and-mouth disease ecosystems. *Boletin del Centro Panamericano de Fiebre Aftosa* 33/34, 33–42, 43–52.

Oleksiewicz, M.B., Donaldson, A.I. and Alexandersen, S. (2001) Development of a novel real-time RT-PCR assay for quantitation of foot-and-mouth disease virus in diverse porcine tissues. *Journal of Virological Methods* 92(1), 23–35.

Perry, P.B., Kalpravidh, W., Coleman, P.G., Horst, H.S., McDermott, J.J., Randolph, T.F. and Gleeson, L.J. (1999) The economic impact of foot and mouth disease and its control in South-East Asia: a preliminary assessment with special reference to Thailand. *Revue Scientifique et Technique Office International des Epizooties* 18(2), 478–497.

Power, A.P. and Harris, S.A. (1973) A cost–benefit analysis of alternative control policies for foot-and-mouth disease in Great Britain. *Journal of Agricultural Economics* 24, 573–600.

Saini, S.S., Sharma, J.K. and Kwatra, M.S. (1992) Assessment of some factors affecting the prevalence of foot-and-mouth disease among traditionally managed animal population of Punjab State. Socio-economic and animal health related interests. *Indian Journal of Animal Sciences* 62(1), 1–4.

Saxena, R. (1994a) *Economic Value of Milk Loss Caused by Foot-and-mouth Disease (FMD) in India.* Working Paper No. 60 – Institute of Rural Management, Anand, 20 pp.

Saxena, R. (1994b) *Economic Value of Some Non-milk Losses Caused by Foot-and-mouth Disease (FMD) in India.* Working Paper No. 62 – Institute of Rural Management, Anand, 15 pp.

Stougaard, E. (1984) Fighting foot-and-mouth disease. The economic consequences of different methods of combating the disease. [Danish] Mund- og klovesygebekaempelse. Okonomiske konsekvenser ved forskellige bekaempelsesmetoder. *Tidsskrift for Landokonomi* 171(4), 173–176.

van Ham, M. and Zur, Y. (1994) Estimated damage to the Israeli dairy herd caused by foot and mouth disease outbreaks and a cost/benefit analysis of the present vaccination policy. *Israel Journal of Veterinary Medicine* 49(1), 13–16.

Anthrax

Akerejola, O.O., van Veen, T.W.S. and Njoku, C.O. (1979) Ovine and caprine diseases in Nigeria: a review of economic losses. *Bulletin of Animal Health and Production in Africa* 27(1), 65–70.

Barnes, H.J. (1997) Other bacterial diseases. In: Calnek, B.W. (ed.) *Diseases of Poultry*, 10th edn. Mosby Wolfe, London, pp. 289–302.

Department of Veterinary Services, Kenya (1972) *Annual Report 1969.* Government of Kenya, Kabete, Kenya, 41 pp.

Gill, I.J. (1982) Antibiotic therapy in the control of an outbreak of anthrax in dairy cows. *Australian Veterinary Journal* 58(5), 214–215.

Mattioli, A. and Gagliardi, G. (1980) Evaluation of the economic and social losses caused by contagious and infectious diseases notifiable under the Italian veterinary police regulations and not subject to disease control programmes. [French] Evaluation des dommages économiques et sociaux dus aux maladies infectieuses contagieuses déclarables aux termes du Réglement de Police Vétérinaire italien non sujettés à des plans de prophylaxie. *Bulletin de l'Office International des Epizooties* 92(5/6), 273–287.

Nurul Islam, F.A.M. (1984) *Livestock and Poultry in Rural Area: a Study of Four Villages in Comilla Kotwali Thana.* Bangladesh Academy for Rural Development, Kotbari, Bangladesh, 43 pp.

Ronohardjo, P., Wilson, A.J., Partoutomo, S. and Hirst, R.G. (1985) Some aspects of the epidemiology and economics of important diseases of large ruminants in Indonesia. In: *Proceedings of the 4th International Symposium on Veterinary Epidemiology and Economics, Singapore, 18–22 November 1985.* ISVEE, Singapore, pp. 303–305.

Rushton, J. (1995) An anthrax outbreak in a South India village. In: *The Society of Veterinary Epidemiology and Preventive Medicine Poster Display Booklet.* SVEPM, Reading, UK, pp. 160–163.

Tuberculosis

Alonge, D.O. and Ayanwale, F.O. (1984) Economic importance of bovine tuberculosis in Nigeria. *Journal of Animal Production Research* 4(2), 165–170.

Andrews, L.G., Johnston, J.H. and McNicholl, L.G. (1980) The economic impact of herd health programs in beef cattle lands within extensive areas of tropical Australia. In: *Proceedings of the Second International Symposium on Veterinary Epidemiology and Economics, 7–11 May 1979.* ISVEE, Canberra, Australia, pp. 426–436.

Awa, D.N., Njoya, A., Tama, A.C.N. and Ekue, F.N. (1999) The health status of pigs in North Cameroon. *Revue d'Elevage et de Médecine Vétérinaire des Pays Tropicaux* 52(2), 93–98.

Bernues, A., Manrique, E. and Maza, M.T. (1997) Economic evaluation of bovine brucellosis and tuberculosis eradication programmes in a mountain area of Spain. *Preventive Veterinary Medicine* 30(2), 137–149.

Berthelsen, J.D. (1974) Economics of the avian TB problem in swine. *Journal of the Veterinary Medical Association* 164(3), 307–308.

Bolitho, W.S. (1978) The economics of pig disease: the cost to the meat processor. In: Beynon, V.H. (ed.) *Pig Veterinary Society Proceedings,* Volume 2. Royal Veterinary College Field Station, Hatfield, UK, pp. 93–99.

Caporale, V.P., Battelli, G., Ghilardi, G. and Biancardi, V. (1980) Evaluation of the costs and benefits of the control campaigns against bovine tuberculosis, brucellosis, foot-and-mouth disease and swine fever in Italy. *Bulletin de l'Office International des Epizooties* 92(5/6), 291–304.

Denes, L. (1983) Tuberculosis in cattle in Hungary. IV. Statistics, conclusions, lessons. [Hungarian] A szarvasmarha-gumokor helyzete Magyarorszagon. IV. Statisztikak, kovetkeztetesek, tanulsagok. *Magyar Allatorvosok Lapja* 38(4), 195–201.

Dey, B.P. and Parham, G.L. (1993) Incidence and economics of tuberculosis in swine slaughtered from 1976 to 1988. *Journal of the American Veterinary Medical Association* 203(4), 516–519.

Eves, J.A. (1999) Impact of badger removal on bovine tuberculosis in east County Offaly. *Irish Veterinary Journal* 52(4), 199–203.

Ghilardi, G., Caporale, V.P., Battelli, G. and Cavrini, C. (1981) Updating of the economic evaluation of the control campaigns against bovine tuberculosis, brucellosis, foot-and-mouth disease and swine fever in Italy. *Bulletin de l'Office International des Epizooties* 93(5/6), 1015–1021.

Jaumally, M.R. and Sibartie, D. (1983) A survey of bovine tuberculosis in Mauritius. *Tropical Veterinary Journal* 1(1), 20–24.

Kao, R.R. and Roberts, M.G. (1999) A comparison of wildlife control and cattle vaccination as methods for the control of bovine tuberculosis. *Epidemiology and Infection* 122(3), 505–519.

McInerney, J.P. (1986) Bovine tuberculosis and badgers – technical, economic and political aspects of a disease control programme. *Journal of the Agricultural Society,* University College of Wales 67, 136–167.

Nfi, A.N. and Alonge, D.O. (1987) An economic survey of abattoir data in Fako division of the south west province, Cameroon (1978–1980). *Bulletin of Animal Health and Production in Africa* 35, 239–242.

Power, A.P. and Watts, B.G.A. (1987) *The Badger Control Policy: an Economic Assessment.* Ministry of Agriculture, Fisheries and Food, London.

Smolyaninov Yu, I. and Martynov, V.F. (1982) Economic effectiveness of control measures against bovine tuberculosis. [Russian] *Veterinariya, Moscow, USSR* 7, 35–36.

Stoneham, G. and Johnston, J. (1987) *The Australian Brucellosis and Tuberculosis Eradication Campaign. An Economic Evaluation of Options for Finalising the Campaign in Northern Australia.* Occasional Paper No. 97, Bureau of Agricultural Economics, Canberra, Australia, 112 pp.

Texdorf, I. (1981) Diseases that impair the quality of slaughter pigs. [German] Qualitatsmindernde Erkrankungen des Mastschweines. *Fleischwirtschaft* 61(7), 999–1003.

Thoen, C.O. (1997) Tuberculosis. In: Calnek, B.W. (ed.) *Diseases of Poultry.* Mosby Wolfe, London, pp. 167–178.

Tuyttens, F.A.M. and Macdonald, D.W. (1998) Sterilization as an alternative strategy to control wildlife diseases: bovine tuberculosis in European badgers as a case study. *Biodiversity and Conservation* 7(6), 705–723.

Valdespino Ortega, J.R. (1993) Losses from the premature culling of dairy cows in Mexico. [Spanish] Perdidas por desecho prematuro de vacas en un hato lechero en Mexico. *World Animal Review* 74–75, 64–67.

Vera, A., Cotrina, N., Botello, A., Riquelme, E. and Llorens, F. (1984) Experiences in the eradication of bovine tuberculosis in a district and its effect on milk production. [Spanish] Experiencias sobre la eliminacion de la tuberculosis bovina en un distrito ganadero y su efecto sobre la produccion lactea. *Revista Cubana de Ciencias Veterinarias* 15(1), 17–23.

Zhilinskii, A.G., Bashirov, R.G. and Zen'kov, A.V. (1986) Economic losses from bovine tuberculosis in the Belorussian Republic of the USSR. [Russian] *Veterinarnaya Nauka – Proizvodstvu* 24, 20–24.

Zorawski, C., Karpinski, T., Loda, M. and Szymanski, M. (1982) Tuberculin reactions and pathological changes in the lymph nodes of swine on an intensive farm of the 'Gi-Gi' type. [Polish] Odczyny tuberkulinowe i zmiany chlorobowe w wezlach chlonnych swin jednej z ferm typu Gi-Gi. *Medycyna Weterynaryjna* 37(11), 570–574.

Salmonellosis

Abdel-Ghani, M., Mohomed, A.H. and Yassein, S. (1987) Occurrence of salmonellae in sheep and goats in Egypt. *Journal of the Egyptian Veterinary Medical Association* 47(1/2), 161–170.

Ali, M.R., Borhanuddin, M., Rahman, M.M. and Choudhury, K.A. (1987) Incidence of microorganisms in market shell eggs and their impact on public health. *Bangladesh Veterinary Journal* 21(3–4), 9–13.

Ament, A.J.H.A., Jansen, J., van der Giessen, A. and Notermans, S. (1993) Cost–benefit analysis of a screening strategy for *Salmonella enteritidis* in poultry. *Veterinary Quarterly* 15(1), 33–37.

Anderson, D.A. (1992) The 1990–1991 *Salmonella pullorum* outbreak: overview and evaluation. *Animal Health Insight* Summer, 1–12.

Bender, F.E. and Ebel, E.D. (1992) Decision making when *Salmonella enteritidis* is present in laying flocks. *Journal of Applied Poultry Science* 1(2), 183–189.

Bernardo, F.M.A. and Machado, J.C.C. (1990) Prevalence of *Salmonella* in slaughter animals in Portugal. [Portuguese] Incidencia de *Salmonella* em animais de talho em Portugal. *Revista Portuguesa de Ciencias Veterinarias* 85(495), 94–102.

Bilbao, G.N. and Spath, E.J.A. (1997) Financial losses due to salmonellosis in dairy calves. [Spanish] Perdidas financieras causadas por la salmonelosis en terneros de tambo. *Revista de Medicina Veterinaria (Buenos Aires)* 78(3), 157–160.

Bisgaard, M., Folkersen, J.C.R. and Hoeg, C. (1981) Arthritis in ducks. II. Condemnation rate, economic significance and possible preventive measures. *Avian Pathology* 10(3), 321–327.

Blackburn, B.O., Sutch, K. and Harrington, R. Jr. (1980) The changing distribution of *Salmonella dublin* in the United States. *Proceedings of the United States Animal Health Association* 84, 445–451.

Borger, K. (1985) Aspects of salmonellosis control in agriculture, with reference to cost–benefit analysis. [German] Aspekte der Salmonellosebekampfung im Bereich der Landwirtschaft unter besonderer Berucksichtigung der Nutzen-Kosten-Analyse. *Zentralblatt fur Veterinarmedizin, A* 32(7), 505–525.

Branscheid, W. (1993) Consumer expectations on the quality of foods of animal origin. [German] Verbraucherwunsche an die Qualitat von Lebensmitteln tierischer Herkunft. In: *Kongressband 1993 Hamburg. Vortrage zum Generalthema des 105. VDLUFA-Kongresses vom 20.-25.9.1993 in Hamburg: Qualitat und Hygiene von Lebensmitteln in Produktion und Verarbeitung*. VDLUFA-Verlag, Darmstadt, Germany, pp. 23–32.

Brede, H.D. (1992) Salmonellosis on the increase. [German] Salmonellosen nehmen zu Munchener. *Medizinische Wochenschrift* 134(21), 355–356.

Bunte, F., Wolbrink, M., Rie, J.P. van and Burgers, S. (2001) As right as rain: a cost benefit analysis of a reduction in the contamination of poultry meat with salmonellosis and campylobacteriosis. [Dutch] *Kiplekker: een kosten-batenanalyse van een reductie in de besmetting van pluimveevlees met salmonella en campylobacter*. Rapport No. 3.01.03 – Landbouw-Economisch Instituut (LEI). Landbouw-Economisch Instituut (LEI), The Hague, Netherlands, 75 pp.

Buyukcoban, A.F. (1989) *Campylobacter* and *Salmonella* infections in sheep in Bursa province, Turkey. [Turkish] Bursa bolgesindeki koyunlarda Campylobacter ve Salmonella enfesiyonlari. *Pendik Hayvan Hastaliklari Merkez Avastirma Enstitusu Dergisi* 20(1), 17–24.

Buzby, J.C., Fox, J.A., Ready, R.C. and Crutchfield, S.R. (1998) Measuring consumer benefits of food safety risk reductions. *Journal of Agricultural and Applied Economics* 30(1), 69–82.

Caley, J.E. (1972) Salmonella in pigs in Papua New Guinea. *Australian Veterinary Journal* 48(11), 601–604.

Carraminana, J.J., Herrera, A., Agustin, A.I., Yanguela, J., Blanco, D. and Rota, C. (1994) Incidence of *Salmonella* on broiler carcasses and livers in a poultry slaughterhouse – impact of processing procedures on the contamination. [Spanish] Incidencia de *Salmonella* en canales e higados de pollos en un matadero de aves e influencia de los diferentes puntos del proceso de carnizacion obre la contaminacion. *Microbiologie, Aliments, Nutrition* 12(1), 75–85.

Caswell, J.A. (1991) An economic framework for assessing foodborne disease control strategies with an application to *Salmonella* control in poultry. In: Caswell, J.A. (ed.) *Economics of Food Safety*. Elsevier, New York, pp. 131–151.

Cohen, D.R., Porter, I.A., Reid, T.M.S., Sharp, J.C.M., Forbes, G.I. and Paterson, G.M. (1983) A cost benefit study of milk-borne salmonellosis. *Journal of Hygiene* 91(1), 17–23.

Cohen, M.L. and Tauxe, R.V. (1986) Drug-resistant *Salmonella* in the United States: an epidemiologic perspective. *Science, USA* 234(4779), 964–969.

Curtin, L. (1984) *Economic Study of Salmonella Poisoning and Control Measures in Canada*. Working Paper No. 11784, Marketing and Economics Branch, Agriculture Canada, Ottawa, Canada, vi + 96 pp.

Davies, R.H., McLaren, I.M. and Bedford, S. (1999) Observations on the distribution of *Salmonella* in a pig abattoir. *Veterinary Record* 145(23), 655–661.

Ding ChangChun and Li LiHu (1998) Causes of proctoptosis [rectal prolapse] in caged breeding chickens: prevention and treatment measures. *[Chinese] Poultry Husbandry and Disease Control* 10, 26.

Fontaine, M. and Fontaine, M.P. (1981) Epidemiological survey of brucellosis in the transhumant sheep population of Provence and Côte-d'Azur. [French] Etude épidémiologique de la brucellose dans le troupeau ovin transhumant de la région Provence – Côte-d'Azur. *Bulletin de la Société des Sciences Vétérinaires et de Médecine Comparée de Lyon* 83(1), 33–38.

Froyd, G. and McWilliam, N. (1975) Estimate of the economic implications of fascioliasis to the United Kingdom livestock industry. In: *Proceedings of the 20th World Veterinary Congress, 6–12 July 1975, Thessaloniki, Greece*, Volume 1. World Veterinary Congress, Thessaloniki, Greece, pp. 553–556.

Hemmatzadeh, F. and Sharifzadeh, A. (1999) A serological survey of *Salmonella abortus ovis* infection in sheep in Chaharmahal Bakhtiary province of Iran. [Persian] *Journal of the Faculty of Veterinary Medicine, University of Tehran* 54(1), 14–21.

Kane, D.W. (1979) The prevalence of salmonella infection in sheep at slaughter. *New Zealand Veterinary Journal* 27(6), 110–113.

Kiran, M.M., Baysal, T., Gozun, H., Guler, L., Gunduz, K., Kuyucuoglu, O. and Kucukayan, U. (1997) Pathological, bacteriological and serological studies on ovine abortion in Konya province. [Turkish] Konya yoresinde koyun abortuslari uzerinde patolojik, bakteriyolojik ve serolojik calismalar. *Etlik Veteriner Mikrobiyoloji Dergisi* 9(2), 109–128.

Laegaard, A. and Hedetoft, A. (1999) Salmonella and broiler chicken production. Economic evaluation of control measures. [Danish] *Salmonella i slagtekyllinge-produktionen – okonomisk vurdering af bekaempelsesstrategier*. Rapport No. 105 – Statens Jordbrugs- og Fiskeriokonomiske Institut. Statens Jordbrugs- og Fiskeriokonomiske Institut, Valby, Denmark, 111 pp.

Leslie, J. (1996) Simulation of the transmission of *Salmonella enteritidis* phage type 4 in a flock of laying hens. *Veterinary Record* 139(16), 388–391.

Lindgren, N.O., Sandstedt, K. and Nordblom, B. (1980) An evaluation of an avian salmonellosis control program in Sweden. In: *6. Europaische Geflugelkonferenz, Hamburg, 8–12 September 1980*, Volume I. World's Poultry Science Association, Hamburg, Germany, pp. 196–205.

Little, C.L. and de Louvois, J. (1999) Health risks associated with unpasteurized goats' and ewes' milk on retail sale in England and Wales. A PHLS Dairy Products Working Group Study. *Epidemiology and Infection* 122(3), 403–408.

Lowry, V.K., Tellez, G.I., Nisbet, D.J., Garcia, G., Urquiza, O., Stanker, L.H. and Kogut, M.H. (1999) Efficacy of *Salmonella enteritidis*-immune lymphokines on horizontal transmission of *S. arizonae* in turkeys and *S. gallinarum* in chickens. *International Journal of Food Microbiology* 48(2), 139–148.

Luthgen, W. (1979) *Salmonella pullorum* infection in a flock of laying hens. [German] *Salmonella pullorum – Ausbruch in einem Legehennenbestand*. *Deutsche Tierarztliche Wochenschrift* 86(2), 62–65.

Minev, M., Masalska, I. and Stoev, B. (1983) Veterinarna Stantsiya, Shumen, Bulgaria. Economic losses attributable to acute fowl typhoid. [Bulgarian] *Veterinarna Sbirka* 81(10), 30–33.

Nauta, M.J., van de Giessen, A.W. and Henken, A.M. (2000) A model for evaluating intervention strategies to control salmonella in the poultry meat production chain. *Epidemiology and Infection* 124(3), 365–373.

Noordhuizen, J.P. and Frankena, K. (1994) *Salmonella enteritidis*: clinical epidemiological approaches for prevention and control of *S. enteritidis* in poultry production. *International Journal of Food Microbiology* 21(1/2), 131–143.

Nursey, I. (1997) Control of *Salmonella*. [German] Salmonellen kontrollieren. *Kraftfutter* 10, 415–422.

Orr, M.B. (1989) Sheep abortions – Invermay [New Zealand] 1988. *Surveillance (Wellington)* 16(3), 24–25.

Ortenberg, E. (1998) Effective control of *Salmonella*. [Swedish] Effektiv kontroll av *Salmonella*. *Var Foda* 50(6), 6–8.

Otaru, M.M.M., Nsengwa, G.R.M. and Wagstaff, L. (1990) Animal salmonellosis in southern Tanzania. *Bulletin of Animal Health and Production in Africa* 38(2), 199–201.

Peters, A.R. (1985) An estimation of the economic impact of an outbreak of *Salmonella dublin* in a calf rearing unit. *Veterinary Record* 117(25/26), 667–668.

Radkowski, M. (2001) Occurrence of *Salmonella* spp. in consumption eggs in Poland. *International Journal of Food Microbiology* 64(1/2), 189–191.

Roberts, T. (1988) Salmonellosis control: estimated economic costs. *Poultry Science* 67(6), 936–943.

Saglam, Y.S., Turkutanit, S.S., Tastan, R., Bozoglu, H. and Otlu, S. (1998) Aetiological and pathological studies on bacterial abortion in sheep and cattle in the North-East Anatolian region. [Turkish] Kuzeydogu Anadolu Bolgesi'nde gorulen bakteriyel sigir ve koyun abortlarinin etiyolojik ve patolojik yonden incelenmesi. *Veteriner Bilimleri Dergisi* 14(1), 133–145.

Sander, J. (1993) Pathogenesis of salmonellosis in man. [German] Pathogenese der Salmonella-Infektionen des Menschen. *Deutsche Tierarztliche Wochenschrift* 100(7), 283–285.

Sawicka-Wrzosek, K. and Gosiewska, A. (1983) Causes of abortion in cows in central Poland in the years 1978–1982. [Polish] Przyczyny ronien u bydla w Polsce centralnej w latach 1978–1982. *Medycyna Weterynaryjna* 39(8), 494–496.

Sawicka-Wrzosek, K., Maciak, T. and Kubinski, T. (1997) Prevalence of *Salmonella* infections in animals in central Poland. [Polish] Czestotliwosc wystepowania drobnoustrojow z rodzaju *Salmonella* u zwierzat w Polsce Centralnej. *Zycie Weterynaryjne* 72(8), 322–325.

Schulz, W., Kiupel, H. and Gunther, H. (1975) Bovine salmonellosis: occurrence, economic implications, epidemiology. [German] Die Salmonellose des Rindes – Vorkommen, wirtschaftliche Bedeutung, Epizootiologie. *Monatshefte fur Veterinarmedizin* 30(14), 530–534.

Schweighardt, H. (1991) Specific causes of abortion in cattle and sheep with special reference to microbial agents (protozoa, bacteria, fungi). [German] Spezifische Abortursachen bei Rind und Schaf unter besonderer Berucksichtigung der mikrobiellen Erreger (Protozoen, Bakterien, Pilze). *Wiener Tierarztliche Monatsschrift* 78(1), 2–6.

Scottish Centre for Infection and Environmental Health (1997) Reports to SCIEH of isolates of salmonellas from animals and humans. *SCIEH Weekly Report* 32(9), 51.

Shahata, M.A., Ibrahim, A.A., Mousa, S. and Ahmed, S.H. (1983) A two-year study on duck salmonellosis in New-Valley, Egypt. I. Recovery of salmonellae from breeding duck flocks. II. Pathogenicity of isolated serotypes and their sensitivity to antimicrobial agents. *Assiut Veterinary Medical Journal* 11(21), 219–221.

Sharp, M.W. and Kay, R. (1988) The cost of *Salmonella typhimurium* phage type 204C infection in a group of purchased calves. *The State Veterinary Journal* 42(120), 61–67.

Steinbach, G. and Hartung, M. (1999) An attempt to estimate the share of human cases of salmonellosis attributable to *Salmonella* originating from pigs. [German] Versuch einer Schatzung des Anteils menschlicher Salmonellaerkrankungen, die auf vom schwein stammende Salmonellen zuruckzufuhren sind. *Berliner und Munchener Tierarztliche Wochenschrift* 112(8), 296–300.

Swanenburg, M., Urlings, H.A.P., Keuzenkamp, D.A. and Snijders, J.M.A. (2001) Salmonella in the lairage of pig slaughterhouses. *Journal of Food Protection* 64(1), 12–16.

Tadjbakhch, H., Baba-Ali, G.H. and Haghigat, M. (1992) Prevalence of *Salmonella* carriers among sheep and dromedaries in Iran. [French] Incidence des porteurs de *Salmonella* chez les moutons et les chameauz en Iran. *Revue de Médecine Vétérinaire* 143(4), 361–365.

Tenk, I., Gyorvary, I., Erdei, P., Szabo, Z., Kostyak, A. and Matray, D. (2000) Effects on *Salmonella* shedding in breeding turkey flocks of vaccine (Salenvac) against *Salmonella enteritidis*. [Hungarian] *Salmonella enteritidis* elleni vakcina (Salenvac) hatasa tenyeszpulyka-allomanyok *Salmonella*-uritesere. *Magyar Allatorvosok Lapja* 122(12), 737–741.

Todd, E.C.D. (1992) Foodborne disease in Canada – a 10-year summary from 1975 to 1984. *Journal of Food Protection* 55(2), 123–132.

Valheim, M. and Hofshagen, M. (1998) Occurrence of *Salmonella diarizonae* in rams in eastern and northern Norway. [Norwegian] Forekomst av *Salmonella diarizonae* hos vaerer pa Ostlandet og i Nord-Norge. *Norsk Veterinaertidsskrift* 110(1), 13–16.

Vodas, K., Elitsina, P. and Atanasov, Ch. (1986) Occurrence of *Salmonella* abortion among ewes in Bulgaria between 1970 and 1984. [Bulgarian] *Veterinarnomeditsinski Nauki* 23(5), 92–99.

Whiting, R.C. and Buchanan, R.L. (1997) Development of a quantitative risk assessment model for *Salmonella enteritidis* in pasteurized liquid eggs. *International Journal of Food Microbiology* 36(2/3), 111–125.

Wray, C. (1985) Is salmonellosis still a serious problem in veterinary practice? *Veterinary Record* 116(18), 485–489.

Yule, B.F., Sharp, J.C.M., Forbes, G.I. and MacLeod, A.F. (1988) Prevention of poultry-borne salmonellosis by irradiation: costs and benefits in Scotland. *Bulletin of the World Health Organization* 66(6), 753–758.

Brucellosis

Adesiyun, A.A. and Cazabon, E.P.I. (1996) Seroprevalences of brucellosis, Q-fever and toxoplasmosis in slaughter livestock in Trinidad. *Revue d'Elevage et de Médecine Vétérinaire des Pays Tropicaux* 49(1), 28–30.

Ajogi, I., Akinwumi, J.A., Esuruoso, G.O. and Lamorde, A.G. (1998) Settling the nomads in Wase and Wawa-Zange grazing reserves in the Sudan savannah zone of Nigeria III: estimated financial losses due to bovine brucellosis. *Nigerian Veterinary Journal* 19, 86–94.

Aller, B. (1975) Brucellosis in Spain. *International Journal of Zoonoses* 2(1), 10–15.

Amosson, S.H., Dietrich, R.A., Talpaz, H. and Hopkin, J.A. (1981) Economic and epidemiologic policy implications of alternative bovine brucellosis programs. *Western Journal of Agricultural Economics* 6(1), 43–56. 5 tables, 2 figs.

Amosson, S.H., Dietrich, R.A., Collins, G. and Hopkin, J.A. (1983) Economic implications for industry and society from US bovine brucellosis control/eradication programs. In: *Third International Symposium on Veterinary Epidemiology and Economics, Arlington, Virginia, United States of America, 6–10 September 1982*. Veterinary Medicine Publishing Company, Edwardsville, Kansas, pp. 535–542.

Atallah, S.T. and El-Kak, A.A. (1998) Economic loss due to infection of cattle and buffaloes with tuberculosis and brucellosis. *Alexandria Journal of Agricultural Research* 43(3), 367–376.

Bernues, A., Manrique, E. and Maza, M.T. (1997) Economic evaluation of bovine brucellosis and tuberculosis eradication programmes in a mountain area of Spain. *Preventive Veterinary Medicine* 30(2), 137–149.

Camus, E. and Landais, E. (1981) Methods of field evaluation of losses caused by two major diseases (trypanosomiasis and brucellosis) in cattle in the north of the Ivory Coast. [French] Méthodologie de l'évaluation sur le terrain des pertes provoquées par deux affections majeures (trypanosomose et brucellose) sur les bovins nord-ivoiriens. [XLIXe Session Generale du Comite de l'O.I.E., Paris, 25–29 mai 1981. Rapport No. 1.7] *Bulletin de l'Office International des Epizooties* 93(5/6), 839–847.

Caporale, V.P., Battelli, G., Ghilardi, G. and Biancardi, V. (1980) Evaluation of the costs and benefits of the control campaigns against bovine tuberculosis, brucellosis, foot-and-mouth disease and swine fever in Italy. *Bulletin de l'Office International des Epizooties* 92(5/6), 291–304.

Choudhary, S.P., Singh, S.N., Narayan, K.G. and Kalimuddin, M. (1983) Sero-prevalence of porcine brucellosis in Bihar. *Indian Veterinary Journal* 60(5), 336–338.

Domenech, J., Coulomb, J. and Lucet, P. (1982) Bovine brucellosis in central Africa. IV. Evaluation of its economic effect and cost benefit analysis of eradication campaigns. [French] La brucellose bovine en Afrique centrale. IV. Evaluation de son incidence économique et calcul du coût-bénéfice des opérations d'assainissement. *Revue d'Elevage et de Médecine Vétérinaire des Pays Tropicaux* 35(2), 113–124.

Ghilardi, G., Caporale, V.P., Battelli, G. and Cavrini, C. (1981) Updating of the economic evaluation of the control campaigns against bovine tuberculosis, brucellosis, foot-and-mouth disease and swine fever in Italy. *Bulletin de l'Office International des Epizooties* 93(5/6), 1015–1021.

Martinez, R., Vasquez, M.A. and Kourany, M. (1977) Epidemiological aspects of brucellosis in a high risk population in Panama. [Spanish] Aspectos epidemiologicos de la brucelosis en la poblacion de alto riesgo en Panama. *Boletin de la Oficina Sanitaria Panamericana* 83(2), 140–147.

Navarrete, S.M.G. (1979) Serological survey for swine brucellosis in the Cordoba region of Colombia. [Spanish] Evaluacion serologica de brucelosis en cerdos del corregimiento de Cacaotal departamento de Cordoba. *Revista – Instituto Colombiano Agropecuario* 14(1), 25–31.

Nordesjo, B. (1999) *A Survey of the Brucellosis Status of Dairy Cows in the Hanoi Peri-urban Area*. Minor Field Studies No. 84 – International Office, Swedish University of Agricultural Sciences. Sveriges Lantbruksuniversitet (Swedish University of Agricultural Sciences) International Office, Uppsala, Sweden, 18 pp.

O'Riordan, F. (1980) An economic evaluation of alternative programs to control brucellosis in Canadian cattle. *Canadian Farm Economics* 15(3), 1–26.

Pfeiffer, D. (1986) Epidemiology and economics of bovine brucellosis in Cordoba Province of Colombia. [German] *Untersuchungen uber die Epidemiologie und Okonomie der Rinderbrucellose in Departamento Cordoba*. Kolumbien Justus-Liebig Universitat, Giessen, 194 pp., 26 pp.

Priadi, A., Hirst, R.G., Chasanah, U., Nurhadi, A., Emmins, J.J., Darodjat, M. and Soeroso, M. (1985) Animal brucellosis in Indonesia – *Brucella suis* infection detected by an enzyme linked immunosorbent assay. Efficient animal production for Asian welfare. In: *Proceedings of the 3rd AAAP Animal Science Congress, 6–10 May 1985*, Volume 1. AAAP, Seoul, Korea, pp. 507–509.

Salman, M.D., Meyer, M.E. and Hird, D.W. (1984) Epidemiology of bovine brucellosis in the Mexicali Valley, Mexico: data gathering and survey results. *American Journal of Veterinary Research* 45(8), 1561–1566.

Shepherd, A.A., Simpson, B.H. and Davidson, R.M. (1980) An economic evaluation of the New Zealand bovine brucellosis eradication scheme. In: *Proceedings of the Second International Symposium on Veterinary Epidemiology and Economics, 7–11 May 1979*. ISVEE, Canberra, Australia, pp. 443–447.

Vito, E. de, Torre, G. la, Scarlini, G., D'Aguanno, G., Zampelli, A., Russo, S. di, Ricciardi, G. (1997) Health and economic impact of a human brucellosis epidemic in Central Italy. [Italian] Impatto sanitario ed economico di un focolaio epidemico di brucellosi umana in Italia Centrale. *Igiene Moderna* 107(5), 439–453.

Wyble, M.L. and Huffman, D.C. (1987) *Economics of Brucellosis Eradication and Prevention Programs for Louisiana Beef Cattle Herds*. DAE Research Report No. 672, Department of Agricultural Economics and Agribusiness, Louisiana Agricultural Experiment Station, Baton Rouge, Louisiana, ii + 38 pp.

Zhunushov, A.T. and Kim, V.I. (1991) Epidemiological and economic effectiveness of control measures for bovine brucellosis. [Russian] *Veterinariya (Moskva)* 2, 35–37.

Trypanosomiasis

Azungwe Suswam, E. (1997) Investigations on mechanisms of acquisition of drug resistance in trypanosomes. PhD thesis, University of Edinburgh, CTVM, Edinburgh, UK

Barrett, J.C. (1994) Economic issues in trypanosomiasis control: case studies from Southern Africa. PhD thesis, University of Reading, VEERU, Reading, UK.

Barrett, J.C. (1997) Economic issues in trypanosomiasis control. Bulletin No. 75 – Natural Resources Institute. Natural Resources Institute (NRI), Chatham, UK, xiii + 183 pp.

Barrett, J.C. (1998) Control strategies for African trypanosomiasis, their sustainability and effectiveness. In: Hide, G., Mottram, J.C., Coombes, G.H. and Holmes, P.H. (eds) *Trypanosomiasis and Leishmaniansis Biology and Control*. CAB International, Wallingford, UK, pp. 347–359.

Brandl, F.E. (1988) *Economics of Trypanosomiasis Control in Cattle*. Wissenschaftsverlag Vauk, Kiel, German Federal Republic, ix + 220 pp.

Budd, L.T. (1999) *DFID Funded Tsetse and Trypanosomiasis Research and Development Since 1980*, Vol. 2. *Economic Analysis*. DfID, London.

Cecere, M.C., Castanera, M.B., Canale, D.M., Chuit, R. and Gurtler, R.E. (1999) *Trypanosoma cruzi* infection in *Triatoma infestans* and other triatomines: long-term effects of a control program in rural northwestern Argentina. *Revista Panamericana de Salud Publica/Pan American Journal of Public Health* 5(6), 392–399.

Davison, H.C. (1997) Evaluation of diagnostic tests for *Trypanosoma evansi* and their application in epidemiological studies in Indonesia. PhD thesis, University of Edinburgh, CTVM, Edinburgh, UK.

Dwinger, R.H., Agyemang, K., Kaufmann, A.S., Grieve, A.S. and Bah, M.L. (1994) Effects of trypanosome and helminth infections on health and production parameters of village N'Dama cattle in the Gambia. *Veterinary Parasitology* 54, 353–365.

Fakae, B.B. and Chiejina, S.N. (1993) The prevalence of concurrent trypanosome and gastrointestinal nematode infections in West African Dwarf sheep and goats in Nsukka area of eastern Nigeria. *Veterinary Parasitology* 49, 313–318.

Finelle, P. (1974) African animal trypanosomiasis. Part IV. Economic problems. *World Animal Review* 10, 15–18.

Geerts, S. and Holmes, P.H. (1998) *Drug Management and Parasite Resistance in Bovine Trypanosomiasis in Africa*. PAAT Technical and Scientific Series 1, FAO, Rome.

Gurtler, R.E. (1999a) Epidemiology and ecology of Chagas disease in north-west Argentina. [Spanish] Epidemiologia y ecologia de la enfermedad de Chagas en el noroeste Argentino. In: Lanteri, A.A. (ed.) *Revista de la Sociedad Entomologica Argentina* 58(1/2), 259–268.

Gurtler, R.E. (1999b) Population monitoring of *Triatoma infestans* during the vigilance phase in a rural community in northwest Argentina. [Spanish] Monitoreo poblacional de *Triatoma infestans* durante la fase de vigilancia en una comunidad rural del noroeste argentino. *Medicina* 59(Supplement II), 47–54.

Gurtler, R.E., Chuit, R., Cecere, M.C., Castanera, M.B., Cohen, J.E. and Segura, E.L. (1988) Household prevalence of seropositivity for *Trypanosoma cruzi* in three rural villages in northwest Argentina: environmental, demographic, and entomologic associations. *American Journal of Tropical Medicine and Hygiene* 59(5), 741–749.

Habtemariam, T., Ruppanner, R., Riemann, H.P. and Theis, J.H. (1983) [I] An epidemiologic systems analysis model for African trypanosomiasis. [II] Epidemic and endemic characteristics of trypanosomiasis in cattle: a simulation model. [III] Evaluation of trypanosomiasis control alternative using an epidemiologic simulation model. [IV] The benefit–cost analysis of alternative strategies for the control of bovine trypanosomiasis in Ethiopia. *Preventive Veterinary Medicine* 1(2), 125–136, 137–145, 147–156, 157–168.

Ibrahim, H.A. (1996) A study of the camel and the importance of *Trypansoma evansi* in Somali region of Ethiopia. MSc dissertation, University of Reading, VEERU, Reading, UK.

Itty, P. (1992) *Economics of Village Cattle Production in Tsetse Affected Areas of Africa: a Study of Trypanosomiasis Control Using Trypanotolerant Cattle and Chemotherapy in Ethiopia, Kenya, Cote d'Ivoire, The Gambia, Zaire and Togo*. Hartung-Gorre Verlag, Konstanz, Germany, xix + 316 [+ 43] pp.

Itty, P. (1993) Economics of trypanosomiasis control: research implications. In: Kategile, J.A. and Mubi, S. (eds) *Future of Livestock Industries in East and Southern Africa: Proceedings of the Workshop Held at Kadoma Ranch Hotel, Zimbabwe, 20–23 July 1992.* Publications Section, International Livestock Centre for Africa (ILCA), Addis Ababa, Ethiopia, pp. 127–134.

Jahnke, H.E. (1976) *Tsetse Flies and Livestock Development in East Africa.* Afrika-Studien Weltforum Verlag, Munich.

Jordan, A.M. (1986) The economics of trypanosomiasis control. In: *Trypanosomiasis Control and African Rural Development.* Longman Group Limited, Chelmsford, UK, pp. 223–242.

Kamara Mwanga, D. (1996) Socio-economic factors affecting implementation of community-managed tsetse control in Busia District, Kenya. PhD thesis, University of Reading, VEERU, Reading, UK.

Kanyari, P.W.N., Allonby, E.W., Wilson, A.J. and Munyua, W.K. (1983) Some economic effects of trypanosomiasis in goats. *Tropical Animal Health and Production* 15(3), 153–160.

Kaufman, J., Dwinger, R.H., Hallebeek, A., van Dijk, B. and Pfister, K. (1992) The interaction of *Trypanosoma congolense* and *Haemonchus contortus* infection in trypanotolerant N'Dama cattle. *Veterinary Parasitology* 43, 157–170.

Kristjanson, P.M., Swallow, B.M., Rowlands, G.J., Kruska, R.L. and de Leeuw, P.N. (1999) Measuring the costs of African animal trypanosomiasis, the potential benefits of control and returns to research. *Agricultural Systems* 59, 79–98.

Leak, G.A. (1998) *Tsetse Biology and Ecology. Their Role in the Epidemiology and Control of Trypanosomiasis.* CAB International, Wallingford, UK.

Lemecha, H. (1984) Prospects for exploitation of lowered susceptibility to trypanosomiasis by young cattle. MSc dissertation, University of Edinburgh, CTVM, Edinburgh, UK.

Marumben Lemunyete, R. (1994) An evaluation of the benefits of the control of camel trypanosomiasis among the camel keeping pastoralists of Northern Kenya. MSc dissertation, University of Edinburgh, CTVM, Edinburgh, UK.

Mattioli, R.C., Zinsstag, J. and Pfister, K. (1994) Frequency of trypanosomosis and gastrointestinal parasites in draught donkeys in the Gambia in relation to animal husbandry. *Tropical Animal Health and Production* 26, 102–108.

Minter-Goedbloed, E. and Croon, J.J.A.B. (1981) The insusceptibility of chickens to *Trypanosoma (Schizotrypanum) cruzi. Transactions of the Royal Society of Tropical Medicine and Hygiene* 75(3), 350–353.

Mortelmans, J. (1984) Socio-economic problems related to animal trypanosomiasis in Africa. *Social Science and Medicine* 19(10), 1105–1107.

Muthui Mwangi, D. (1991) *Trypanosoma (Nannomonas) congolense*: pathogenesis and cellular responses during the early stages of infection in sheep. PhD thesis, University of Edinburgh, CTVM, Edinburgh, UK.

Otte, M.J., Abuabara, J.Y. and Wells, E.A. (1994) *Trypanosoma vivax* in Colombia: epidemiology and production losses. *Tropical Animal Health and Production* 26(3), 146–156.

Pires, H.H.R., Borges, E.C., Andrade, R.E. de, Lorosa, E.S. and Diotaiuti, L. (1999) Peridomiciliary infestation with *Triatoma sordida* Stal, 1859 in the county of Serra do Ramalho, Bahia, Brazil. *Memorias do Instituto Oswaldo Cruz* 94(2), 147–149.

Prastyawati Sukanto, I. (1998) Molecular characterisation of *Trypanosoma evansi* stocks from Indonesia. PhD thesis, University of Edinburgh, CTVM, Edinburgh, UK.

Putt, S.N.H. and Shaw, A.P.M. (1983) The socio-economic effects of the control of tsetse transmitted trypanosomiasis in Nigeria. In: *Third International Symposium on Veterinary Epidemiology and Economics. Arlington, Virginia, United States of America, 6–10 September 1982.* Veterinary Medicine Publishing Co., Edwardsville, Kansas, pp. 515–523.

Putt, S.N.H., Shaw, A.P.M., Mathewman, R.W., Bourn, D.M., Underwood, M., James, A.D., Hallam, M.J. and Ellis, P.R. (1980) *The Social and Economic Implications of Trypanosomiasis Control. A Study of its Impact on Livestock Production and Rural Development in Northern Nigeria.* University of Reading, VEERU study No. 25, Reading, UK.

Roderick, S. (1995) Pastoralist cattle productivity in tsetse infested area, South West Kenya. PhD thesis, The University of Reading, VEERU, Reading, UK.

Rushton, J., Pilling, P and Heffernan, C. (2001) *Review of Livestock Diseases and their Importance in the Lives of Poor People.* A study commissioned by ILRI. ILRI, Nairobi, Kenya.

Shaw, A.P.M. (1986) The economics of trypanosomiasis control in the Sudan and northern Guinea zones of West Africa. A study based on examples from Nigeria and Mali. PhD thesis, University of Reading, VEERU, Reading, UK.

Shaw, A.P.M. and Kamate, C. (1982) An economic evaluation of the trypanosomiasis problem in Zone 1. *AIDS Research and Development Abstracts* 10, 1–2.

Springer, W.T. (1997) Other blood and tissue protozoa. In: Calnek, B.W. (ed.) *Diseases of Poultry 10th Edition*. Mosby Wolfe, London, pp. 900–912.

Stephen, L.E. (1966) *Pig Trypanosomiasis in Tropical Africa*. Commonwealth Agricultural Bureaux, Farnham Royal, UK.

Swallow, B. (2000) *Impacts of Trypanosomiasis on African Agriculture*. Programme Against African Trypanosomiasis (PAAT) technical and scientific series No. 2. ILRI, Nairobi, Kenya.

Tacher, G., Jahnke, H.E., Rojat, D. and Kell, P. (1988) Livestock development and economic production in tsetse-infested Africa. In: *Livestock Production in Tsetse Affected Areas of Africa*. Proceedings of a meeting, November 1987, Nairobi, Kenya. ILRI, Nairobi, Kenya.

Wilson, A.J., Njogu, A.R., Gatuta, G., Mgutu, S.P., Alushula, H. and Dolau, R. (1983) An economic study on the use of chemotherapy to control trypanosomiasis in cattle on Galana Ranch, Kenya. In: *Seventeenth Meeting of the International Scientific Council for Trypanosomiasis Research and Control, Arusha, Tanzania, 19–24 October 1981*. Organization of African Unity/Scientific, Technical and Research Commission, Nairobi, Kenya, pp. 306–317.

Bluetongue

Alexander, G.I., Alexander, M.P., St. George, T.D. (1996) Bluetongue – its impact on international trade in meat and livestock. In: St. George, T.D. and Kegao, P. (eds) *Bluetongue Disease in Southeast Asia and the Pacific. Proceedings of the First Southeast Asia and Pacific Regional Bluetongue Symposium, Greenlake Hotel, Kunming, P.R. China, 22–24 August 1995*. Australian Centre for International Agricultural Research (ACIAR), Canberra, Australia, pp. 254–258.

Barnard, B.J.H., Gerdes, G.H. and Meiswinkel, R. (1998) Some epidemiological and economic aspects of a bluetongue-like disease in cattle in South Africa – 1995/96 and 1997. *Onderstepoort Journal of Veterinary Research* 65(3), 145–151.

Ertan, H.N. and Nazlioglu, M. (1981) Animal health and economics in Turkey. *Bulletin de l'Office International des Epizooties* 93(5/6), 1045–1052.

Geering, W.A. (1985) Australia. In: Della-Porta, A.J. (ed.) *Veterinary Viral Diseases, Their Significance in South-East Asia and the Western Pacific*. Academic Press, Sydney, Australia, pp. 161–167.

Metcalf, H.E., Lomme, J. and Beal, V.C. Jr. (1980) Estimate of incidence and direct economic losses due to bluetongue in Mississippi cattle during 1979. *Proceedings of the United States Animal Health Association* 84, 186–202.

Osburn, B.I., Huffman, E.M., Sawyer, M. and Hird, D. (1986) Economics of bluetongue in the United States. In: St. George, T.D., Kay, B.H. and Blok, J. (eds) *Arbovirus Research in Australia. Proceedings Fourth Symposium 6–9 May 1986, Brisbane, Australia*. CSIRO, Melbourne, Australia, pp. 245–247.

Oviedo, M.T., Mo, C.L., Homan, E.J. and Thompson, L.H. (1992) Analysis of evidence of clinical bluetongue disease in Central America and the Caribbean. Bluetongue, African horse sickness, and related orbiviruses. In: Walton, T.E. and Osburn, B.I. (eds) *Proceedings of the Second International Symposium*. CRC Press, Boca Raton, Florida, pp. 114–119.

Taylor, W.P. (1987) What harm could bluetongue do in Europe. In: Taylor, W.P. (ed.) *Blue Tongue in the Mediterranean Region. Proceedings of a Meeting in the Community Programme for Coordination of Agricultural Research, Istituto Zooprofilatico Sperimentale dell' Abruzzo e del Molise, Teramo, Italy, 3–4 October 1985*. Commission of the European Communities, Luxembourg, pp. 103–105.

Paratuberculosis

Benedictus, G., Dijkhuizen, A.A.and Stelwagen, J. (1985) Economic losses due to paratuberculosis in cattle. [Dutch] Bedrijfseconomische schade van paratuberculose bij het rund. *Tijdschrift voor Diergeneeskunde* 110(8), 310–319.

Bennett, R.M., Christiansen, K. and Clifton-Hadley, R.S. (1999) *An economic study of the importance of non-notifiable diseases of farm animals in Great Britain*. Available at: http://www.rdg.ac.uk/AcaDepts/ae/AEM/livestockdisea

Chiodini, R.J. and van Kruiningen, H.J. (1986) The prevalence of paratuberculosis in culled New England cattle. *Cornell Veterinarian* 76(1), 91–104.

Collins, M.T. and Morgan, I.R. (1991) Economic decision analysis model of a paratuberculosis test and cull program. *Journal of the American Veterinary Medical Association* 199(12), 1724–1729.

Everett, R.E., North, R.N., Ottaway, S.J. and Scott-Orr, H. (1989) The status of Johne's disease in New South Wales. In: Milner, A.R. and Wood, P.R. (eds) *Johne's Disease: Current Trends in Research, Diagnosis and Management*. CSIRO Publications, East Melbourne, Australia, pp. 14–18.

Gill, I.J. (1989) The economic impact of Johne's disease in cattle in Australia. In: Milner, A.R. and Wood, P.R. (eds) *Johne's Disease: Current Trends in Research, Diagnosis and Management*. CSIRO Publications, East Melbourne, Australia, pp. 36–40.

Hillion, E. and Argente, G. (1987) Control of bovine paratuberculosis in the Côtes-du-Nord region of France: health and economic aspects. [French] Plan de lutte contre la paratuberculose dans les Côtes-du-Nord: aspects sanitaires et économiques. *Le Point Vétérinaire* 19(104), 123–130.

Johnson-Ifearulundu, Y., Kaneene, J.B. and Lloyd, J.W. (1999) Herd-level economic analysis of the impact of paratuberculosis on dairy herds. *Journal of the American Veterinary Medical Association* 214(6), 822–825.

Juste, R.A. and Casal, J. (1993) An economic and epidemiologic simulation of different control strategies for ovine paratuberculosis. *Preventive Veterinary Medicine* 15(2–3), 101–115.

Lisle, G.W. de and Milestone, B.A. (1989) The economic impact of Johne's disease in New Zealand. In: Milner, A.R. and Wood, P.R. (eds) *Johne's Disease: Current Trends in Research, Diagnosis and Management*. CSIRO Publications, East Melbourne, Australia, pp. 41–45.

Ott, S.L., Wells, S.J. and Wagner, B.A. (1999) Herd-level economic losses associated with Johne's disease on US dairy operations. *Preventive Veterinary Medicine* 40(3/4), 179–192.

Stabel, J.R. (1998) Johne's disease: a hidden threat. *Journal of Dairy Science* 81(1), 283–288.

Thurtell, D., Davenport, S., Roth, I., Jane, D., Scott-Orr, H. and Everett, R. (1994) *Controlling Bovine Johne's Disease in New South Wales*. Economic Policy Report No. 7 – Economic Services Unit, NSW Agriculture, Orange, Australia, vi + 26 pp.

van Schaik, G., Kalis, C.H.J., Benedictus, G., Dijkhuizen, A.A. and Huirne, R.B.M. (1996) Cost–benefit analysis of vaccination against paratuberculosis in dairy cattle. *Veterinary Record* 139(25), 624–627.

Echinococcosis/Hydatidosis

Majorowski, M.M., Carabin, H., Kilani, M. and Bensalah, A. (2001) Echinococcosis in Tunisia: an economic analysis. In: Menzies, F.D. and Reid, S.W.J. (eds) *Proceedings of a Meeting Held at the Golden Tulip Conference Centre, Leeuwenhorst, Noordwijkerhout, The Netherlands, 28–30 March 2001*. Society for Veterinary Epidemiology and Preventive Medicine, Wageningen, The Netherlands, pp. 187–201.

Bovine diarrhoea virus and border disease virus

Burgu, I., Ozturk, F., Akzca, Y., Toker, A., Frey, H.R. and Liess, B. (1987) Investigations on the occurrence and impact of bovine viral diarrhea (BVD) virus infections in sheep in Turkey. *Deutsche Tierarztliche Wochenschrift* 94(5), 292–294.

Sharp, M.W. and Rawson, B.C. (1986) The cost of border disease infection in a commercial flock. *Veterinary Record* 119(6), 128–130.

Sweasey, D., Patterson, D.S.P., Richardson, C., Harkness, J.W., Shaw, I.G. and Williams, W.W. (1979) Border disease: a sequential study of surviving lambs and an assessment of its effect on profitability. *Veterinary Record* 104(20), 447–450.

Minor Diseases

Campylobacter

Anderson, S.A., Woo, R.W.Y. and Crawford, L.M. (2001) Risk assessment of the impact on human health of resistant *Campylobacter jejuni* from fluoroquinolone use in beef cattle. *Food Control* 12(1), 13–25.

Shane, S.M. (1997) Campylobacteriosis. In: Calnek, B.W. (ed.) *Diseases of Poultry*. Mosby Wolfe, London, pp. 235–246.

Chlamydia/Chlamydophila

Ansell, D.J. and Done, J.T. (1988) *Veterinary Research and Development: Cost–Benefit Studies on Products for the Control of Animal Diseases*. Centre for Agricultural Strategy, University of Reading, Reading, UK, vii + 69 pp.

Yersinia

Adesiyun, A.A. and Kaminjolo, J.S. (1994) Prevalence and epidemiology of selected enteric infections of livestock in Trinidad. *Preventive Veterinary Medicine* 19(3/4), 151–165.

Adesiyun, A.A., Lombin, L.H. and Agbonlahor, D.E. (1986) Prevalence of antibodies to *Yersinia enterocolitica* serogroups 0:3, 0:8 and 0:12,26 in domestic animals in Nigeria. *British Veterinary Journal* 142(4), 381–388.

Akkermans, J.P.W.M. (1975) [Fertility problems caused by infectious agents in pigs in the Netherlands]. [Dutch] Fertiliteitsstoringen bij het varken in Nederland door infectieuze agentia. *Tijdschrift voor Diergeneeskunde* 100(15), 809–820.

Czernomysy-Furowicz, D., Furowicz, A.J., Karakulska, J., Nawrotek, P., Peruzynska, A. and Kalisinska, E. (1999) A case of isolation of *Yersinia enterocolitica* from duck muscles. *Advances in Agricultural Sciences* 6(1), 19–24.

Gad El-Said, W.A., El-Danaf, N.A., Tanios, A.I., Shaaban, A.I. and Rashed, M.E. (1996) Seroprevalence of *Yersinia enterocolitica* 'O:3 and/or O:9'2 in animals in Egypt with reference to its serological cross-reactions with *Brucella abortus*. *Veterinary Medical Journal Giza* 44(3), 629–635.

Hodges, R.T., Carman, M.G. and Mortimer, W.J. (1984) Serotypes of *Yersinia pseudotuberculosis* recovered from domestic livestock. *New Zealand Veterinary Journal* 32(1/2), 11–13.

Hu, J.Y. (1988) A survey of *Yersinia enterocolitica* infection in Pingxiang, Jiangxi, China. [Chinese] *Chinese Journal of Veterinary Medicine* 14(9), 31–33.

Jensen, N. and Hughes, D. (1980) Public health aspects of raw goats' milk produced throughout New South Wales. *Food Technology in Australia* 32(7), 336–338, 340–341.

Lautner, B. and Friendship, R.M. (1992) Human health in swine veterinary practice. *Compendium on Continuing Education for the Practicing Veterinarian* 14(1), 99–101, 110.

Nattermann, H., Horsch, F. and Zimmermann, H. (1980) Reproduction of *Brucella* titres in pigs by means of experimental infection with *Yersinia enterocolitica* serotypes 0:9 and 0:6. [German] Reproduktion von Brucellatitern beim Schwein mittels experimenteller Infektion mit den *Yersinia-enterocolitica*-Serotypen 0:9 und 0:6. *Archiv fur Experimentelle Veterinarmedizin* 34(5), 741–752. 11 refs.

Roberts, D. (1990) Sources of infection: food. *Lancet* (British edition) 336(8719), 859–861.

Schiemann, D.A. and Fleming, C.A. (1981) *Yersinia enterocolitica* isolated from throats of swine in eastern and western Canada. *Canadian Journal of Microbiology* 27(12), 1326–1333.

Shiozawa, K., Hayashi, M., Akiyama, M., Nishina, T., Nakatsugawa, S., Fukushima, H. and Asakawa, Y. (1988) Virulence of *Yersinia pseudotuberculosis* isolated from pork and from the throats of swine. *Applied and Environmental Microbiology* 54(3), 818–821.

Slee, K.J. and Skilbeck, N.W. (1992) Epidemiology of *Yersinia pseudotuberculosis* and *Y. enterocolitica* infections in sheep in Australia. *Journal of Clinical Microbiology* 30(3), 712–715.

Staroniewicz, Z. (1986) *Yersinia enterocolitica* antibodies in animals. [Polish] Badania nad wystepowaniem przeciwcial anty-*Yersinia enterocolitica* u zwierzat. *Medycyna Weterynaryjna* 42(2), 97–99.

Neospora caninum

Agerholm, J.S., Willadsen, C.M., Nielsen, T.K., Giese, S.B., Holm, E., Jensen, L. and Agger, J.F. (1997) Diagnostic studies of abortion in Danish dairy herds. *Journal of Veterinary Medicine – Series A* 44(9/10), 551–558. 16 refs.

Antony, A. and Williamson, N.B. (2001) Recent advances in understanding the epidemiology of *Neospora caninum* in cattle. *New Zealand Veterinary Journal* 49(2), 42–47.

Bartels, C.J.M., Wouda, W. and Schukken, Y.H. (1999) Risk factors for *Neospora caninum*-associated abortion storms in dairy herds in the Netherlands (1995–1997). *Theriogenology* 52(2), 247–257. 37 refs.

French, N.P., Davison, H.C., Clancy, D., Begon, M. and Trees, A.J. (1998) Modelling of *Neospora* infection in dairy cattle: the importance of horizontal and vertical transmission and differential culling. In: Thrusfield, M.V. and Goodall, E.A. (eds) *Proceedings of the Society for Veterinary Epidemiology and Preventive Medicine Annual Meeting Held on 25–27 March 1998*. SVEPM, Reading, UK, pp. 113–122. 17 refs.

French, N.P., Clancy, D., Davison, H.C. and Trees, A.J. (1999) Mathematical models of *Neospora caninum* infection in dairy cattle: transmission and options for control. *International Journal for Parasitology* 29(10), 1691–1704. 20 refs.

Kasari, T.R., Barling, K. and McGrann, J.M. (1999) Estimated production and economic losses from *Neospora caninum* infection in Texas beef herds. *Bovine Practitioner* 33(2), 113–120. 16 refs.

Otter, A. (1996) Bovine neosporosis – a new and emerging condition. *The State Veterinary Journal* 6(1), 13–15. 15 refs.

Otter, A. (1997) Neospora and bovine abortion. *Veterinary Record* 140(9), 239. 4 refs.

Thurmond, M.C. and Hietala, S.K. (1996) Culling associated with *Neospora caninum* infection in dairy cows. *American Journal of Veterinary Research* 57(11), 1559–1562. 14 refs.

Yamane, I., Koiwai, M., Haritani, M. and Hamaoka, T. (2000) Economic losses from *Neospora caninum* infection in dairy cattle in Japan. [Japanese] *Journal of the Japan Veterinary Medical Association* 53(2), 67–69.

Cryptosporidiosis

de Graaf, D.C., Vanopdenbosch, E., Ortega-Mora, L.M., Abbassi, H. and Peeters, J.E. (1999) A review of the importance of cryptosporidiosis in farm animals. *International Journal for Parasitology* 29(8), 1269–1287.

Diseases of Large Ruminants

Adlakha, S.C. (1985) India. In: Della-Porta, A.J. (ed.) *Veterinary Viral Diseases. Their Significance in South-East Asia and the Western Pacific*. Proceedings of an international symposium held at Australian Animal Health Laboratory, CSIRO, Geelong, Australia, 27–30 August 1984. CSIRO, Geelong, Australia, pp. 178–183.

Bennett, R.M., Christiansen, K. and Clifton-Hadley, R.S. (1999) *An economic study of the importance of non-notifiable diseases of farm animals in Great Britain*. Available at: http://www.rdg.ac.uk/AcaDepts/ae/AEM/livestockdisea

Bölske, G., Msami, G., Gunnarson, A., Kapaga, A.M. and Loomu, P.M. (1995) Contagious bovine pleuropneumonia in northern Tanzania, culture, confirmation and seriological studies. *Tropical Animal Health and Production* 27, 193–201.

Cheneau, Y. (1993) Les nouvelles stratégies d'intervention zoosanitaire dans les pays en développement. *World Animal Review* 74/75, 12–16.

Da, Y., Shanks, R.D., Stewart, J.A. and Lewin, H.A. (1993) Milk and fat yields decline in bovine leukemia virus-infected Holstein cattle with persistent lymphocytosis. *Proceedings of the National Academy of Sciences of the USA* 90(14), 6538–6541.

Davies, G., Edwards, W.A. and Irving, R. (1980) Enzootic bovine leukosis in Great Britain: its prevalence and its potential cost. In: Markson, L.M. (ed.) *CEC Scientific Workshop on Bovine Leucosis*. Commission of the European Communities, Luxembourg, pp. 21–25.

Davis, S.S., Gibson, D.S. and Clark, R. (1984) The effect of bovine ephemeral fever on milk production. *Australian Veterinary Journal* 61(4), 128–130.

De Alwis, M.C.L. (1993a) Pasteurellosis in production animals: a review. In: Patten, B.E., Spencer, T.L., Johnson, R.B., Hoffmann, D. and Lehane, L. (eds) *Pasteurellosis in Production Animals*. An international workshop sponsored by ACIAR held at Bali, Indonesia, 10–13 August 1992. ACIAR Proceedings, No. 43. Australian Centre for International Agricultural Research, Canberra, Australia, pp. 11–22.

De Alwis, M.C.L. (1993b) The epidemiology of haemorrhagic septicaemia in Sri Lanka. In: Patten, B.E., Spencer, T.L., Johnson, R.B., Hoffmann, D. and Lehane, L. (eds) *Pasteurellosis in Production Animals*. An international workshop sponsored by ACIAR held at Bali, Indonesia, 10–13 August 1992. ACIAR Proceedings, No. 43. Australian Centre for International Agricultural Research, Canberra, Australia, pp. 98–102.

Debnath, N.C., McGrane, J., Sil, B.K., Selim, S.A., Selim, S.A., Taimur, M.J.F.D.A., Mia, M.F., Chowdhury, S.M.Z.H., Prodhan, M.A.M., Howlader, M.M.R. and Rahman, M.F. (1994) Point seroprevalence of rinderpest antibody in cattle in Bangladesh. *Preventive Veterinary Medicine* 19, 145–149.

Dufour, B., Repiquet, D. and Touratier, A. (1999) Economic studies in animal health decision-making: the cost–benefit ratio of eradicating bovine virus diarrhoea in France. [French] Place des études économiques dans les décisions de santé animale: exemple du rapport coût/bénéfice de l'éradication de la diarrhée virale bovine en France. *Revue Scientifique et Technique Office International des Epizooties* 18(2), 520–532.

Durrani, N.U., Athar, S.M., Asif, M. and Hussain, Z. (1988) Rinderpest in the Landhi Dairy Colony. *Tropical Animal Health and Production* 20, 177–180.

Edelsten, R.M., Gourlay, R.N., Lawson, G.K.H., Morrow, A.N. and Ramachandran, S. (1990) Diseases caused by bacteria. In: Sewell, M.M.H. and Brocklesby, D.W. (eds) *Handbook on Animal Diseases in the Tropics*. Baillière Tindall, London, pp. 216–245.

Empres (1997) SADC declares war on CBPP. *Empres Transboundary Animal Diseases Bulletin* 4. Available at: www.fao.org

Empres (1998a) Contagious bovine pleuropneumonia control in Botswana, February 1995 to July 1997. *Empres Transboundary Animal Diseases Bulletin* 6. Available at: www.fao.org

Empres (1998b) Epidemiological considerations for CBPP vaccination. *Empres Transboundary Animal Diseases Bulletin* 5. Available at: www.fao.org

Empres (1998c) New introduction of CBPP into Burundi January 1997. *Empres Transboundary Animal Diseases Bulletin* 4. Available at: www.fao.org

Empres (1999a) Rinderpest in Kenya. *Empres Transboundary Animal Diseases Bulletin*, 10. Available at: www.fao.org

Empres (1999b). Suspected rinderpest in Somalia. *Empres Transboundary Animal Diseases Bulletin*, 10. Available at: www.fao.org

Empres (2000) Contagious bovine pleuropneumonia. *Empres Transboundary Animal Diseases Bulletin* 14. Available at: www.fao.org

Esslemont, R.J. and Peeler, E.J. (1993) The scope for raising margins in dairy herds by improving fertility and health. *British Veterinary Journal* 149(6), 537–547.

Fourichon, C., Seegers, H., Bareille, N. and Beaudeau, F. (1999) Effects of disease on milk production in the dairy cow: a review. *Preventive Veterinary Medicine* 41(1), 1–35.

GREP (2001) Rinderpest detected in Pakistan. Global Rinderpest Eradication Campaign – News. Available at: www.fao.org

GREP (undated) Global Rinderpest Eradication Campaign. Available at: www.fao.org

Heffernan, C. and Misturelli, F. (2000) The delivery of veterinary services to the rural poor: preliminary findings from Kenya. Report for the DFID funded study R7359. Available at: www.livestockdevelopment.org

Hiramune, T. and De Alwis, M.C.L. (1982) Haemorrhagic septicaemia carrier status and buffalo in Sri Lanka. *Tropical Animal Health and Production* 14, 91–92.

Hird, D.W., Weigler, B.J., Salman, M.D., Danaye-Elmi, C., Palmer, C.W., Holmes, J.C., Utterback, W.W. and Sischo, W.M. (1991) Expenditures for veterinary services and other costs of disease and disease prevention in 57 California beef herds in the National Animal Health Monitoring System (1988–1989). *Journal of the American Veterinary Medical Association* 198(4), 554–558.

Houe, H., Pedersen, K.M. and Meyling, A. (1993) A computerized spread sheet model for calculating total annual national losses due to bovine viral diarrhoea virus infection in dairy herds and sensitivity analysis of selected parameters. In: Edwards, S. (ed.) *Proceedings of the Second Symposium on Pestiviruses, 1–3 October 1992*. Fondation Marcel Mérieux, Lyon, France, pp. 179–184.

House, J.A. (1978) Economic impact of rotavirus and other neonatal disease agents of animals. *Journal of the American Veterinary Medical Association* 173(5), II, 573–576.

Hugoson, G. and Wold-Troell, M. (1983) Benefit/cost aspects on voluntary control of bovine leukosis. *Nordisk Veterinaermedicin* 35(1), 1–17.

Interior, M.M. (1993) Philippines. In: Patten, B.E., Spencer, T.L., Johnson, R.B., Hoffmann, D. and Lehane, L. (eds) *Pasteurellosis in Production Animals*. An international workshop sponsored by ACIAR held at

Bali, Indonesia, 10–13 August 1992. ACIAR Proceedings, No. 43. Australian Centre for International Agricultural Research, Canberra, Australia, pp. 254–255.

Jamaludin, R. (1993) Malaysia. In: Patten, B.E., Spencer, T.L., Johnson, R.B., Hoffmann, D. and Lehane, L. (eds) *Pasteurellosis in Production Animals*. An international workshop sponsored by ACIAR held at Bali, Indonesia, 10–13 August 1992. ACIAR Proceedings, No. 43. Australian Centre for International Agricultural Research, Canberra, Australia, pp. 238–239.

Johnson, R. and Kaneene, J.B. (1991) Bovine leukemia virus. Part IV. Economic impact and control measures. *Compendium on Continuing Education for the Practicing Veterinarian* 13(11), 1727–1734, 1736–1737.

Kaneene, J.B. and Hurd, H.S. (1990a) The National Animal Health Monitoring System in Michigan. III. Cost estimates of selected dairy cattle diseases. *Preventive Veterinary Medicine* 8(2–3), 127–140.

Kaneene, J.B. and Hurd, H.S. (1990b) The National Animal Health Monitoring System in Michigan. I. Design, data and frequencies of selected dairy cattle diseases. *Preventive Veterinary Medicine* 8(2–3), 103–114.

Kautzsch, S. and Schluter, H. (1990) Prospects for and economic aspects of the control of enzootic bovine leukosis in the German Democratic Republic. [German] Prognose und okonomische Aspekte der Bekampfung der enzootischen Rinderleukose. *Monatshefte für Veterinarmedizin* 45(2), 41–45.

Kellar, J.A. (1981) The economic impact of enzootic bovine leucosis in Canada. *Bulletin de l'Office International des Epizooties* 93(5/6), 879–891.

Khan, M.A., Yamin, M., Khan, M.S. and Khan, A.G. (1994) Epidemiological and economical based ranking order of buffalo and cattle diseases through active disease surveillance system. In: *Proceedings of the 8th International Congress on Animal Hygiene, St Paul, Minnesota*. Available at: http://www.isah_sac.org/

Kim JongShu, Kim YongHwan, Lee HyoJong, Kim GonSup, Kim ChungHui, Park JeongHee, Hah DaeSik and Choi MinCheol (1999) Development of a model for a National Animal Health Monitoring System in Gyeongnam. III. Cost estimates of selected dairy cattle diseases. [Korean] *Korean Journal of Veterinary Clinical Medicine* 16(2), 428–438.

Kundu, P.B. (1993) India. In: Patten, B.E., Spencer, T.L., Johnson, R.B., Hoffmann, D. and Lehane, L. (eds) *Pasteurellosis in Production Animals*. An international workshop sponsored by ACIAR held at Bali, Indonesia, 10–13 August 1992. ACIAR Proceedings, No. 43, Australian Centre for International Agricultural Research, Canberra, Australia, pp. 232–233.

Lamichang, C.M. (1985) Nepal. In: Della-Porta, A.J. (ed.) *Veterinary Viral Diseases. Their Significance in South East Asia and the Western Pacific*. Proceedings of an international symposium held at the Australian Animal Health Laboratory, Geelong, Australia, 27–30 August 1984. Academic Press, Sydney, Australia, pp. 204–209.

Langston, A., Ferdinand, G.A.A., Ruppanner, R., Theilen, G.H., Drlica, S. and Behymer, D. (1978) Comparison of production variables of bovine leukemia virus antibody-negative and antibody-positive cows in two California dairy herds. *American Journal of Veterinary Research* 39(7), 1093–1098.

McCosker, P.J. (1979) Global aspects of the management and control of ticks of veterinary importance. *Recent Advances in Acarology* 11, 45–53.

Meszaros, J., Antal, T., Polner, A., Szabo, I., Szentmiklossy, C. and Tekes, L. (1986) Experiences of the eradication of bovine leukosis in Hungary. [Hungarian] A szarvasmarha-leucosistol valo mentesites eddigi tapasztalatai. *Magyar Allatorvosok Lapja* 41(5), 277–285.

Miller, G.Y. and Dorn, C.R. (1990) Costs of dairy cattle diseases to producers in Ohio. *Preventive Veterinary Medicine* 8(2–3), 171–182.

Minjauw, B. and McLeod, A. (2001) *Epidemiology and Economics of Tick-Borne Diseases and Its Effects on the Livelihoods of the Poor in East, Southern Africa and India*. DfID, London.

Minjauw, B., Rushton, J., James, A.D. and Upton, M. (1999) Financial analysis of East Coast fever control strategies in traditionally managed Sanga cattle in Central Province of Zambia. *Preventive Veterinary Medicine* 38, 35–45.

Mouchet, C., Denis, B. and Drouin, B. (1986) Veterinary expenses in dairy farming. A study in Ille-et-Vilaine (1982–1984). [French] Les frais vétérinaires en élevage bovin laitier. Etude en Ille-et-Vilaine (1982–1984). *Recueil de Médecine Vétérinaire* 162(4), 485–494.

Mukhebi, A.W., Perry, B.D. and Kruska, R. (1992) Estimated economics of theileriosis control in Africa. *Preventive Veterinary Medicine* 12, 73–85.

Muller, M. and Wittmann, W. (1990) Cost–benefit analysis of the control and eradication of bovine leukosis in a selected region. [German] Kosten-Nutzen-Analyse zur Bekampfung und Sanierung der enzootischen Rinderleukose, dargestellt am Beispiel eines ausgewahlten Territoriums. *Archiv für Experimentelle Veterinarmedizin* 44(2), 213–222.

Mustafa, A.A., Ghalib, H.W. and Shigidi, M.T. (1978) Carrier rate of *Pasteurella multocida* in a cattle herd associated with an outbreak of haemorrhagic septicaemia in the Sudan. *British Veterinary Journal* 134, 375–378.

Neramitmansook, P. (1993) Thailand. In: Patten, B.E., Spencer, T.L., Johnson, R.B., Hoffmann, D. and Lehane, L. (eds) *Pasteurellosis in Production Animals*. An international workshop sponsored by ACIAR held at Bali, Indonesia, 10–13 August 1992. ACIAR Proceedings, No. 43. Australian Centre for International Agricultural Research, Canberra, Australia, pp. 234–237.

Noordegraaf, A.V., Buijtels, J.A.A.M., Dijkhuizen, A.A., Franken, P., Stegeman, J.A. and Verhoeff, J. (1998) An epidemiological and economic simulation model to evaluate the spread and control of infectious bovine rhinotracheitis in the Netherlands. *Preventive Veterinary Medicine* 36(3), 219–238.

OIE (2001) Handistatus II. Office International des Epizooties. Available at: www.OIE.int

Otesile, E.B., Kasali, O.B., Oyejide, A. and Trimnell, M.T. (1983) Calf losses on the University of Ibadan farm, Nigeria, 1968–1977. *Tropical Veterinarian* 1(3), 164–171.

Paramatma, S., Sissdia, B.V.S. and Kunzru, O.N. (1987) An economic analysis of livestock disease losses. *Indian Veterinary Journal* 64(3), 227–230.

Partoutomo, S., Ronohardjo, P., Wilson, A.J. and Stevenson, P. (1985) Review of diseases in Indonesia affecting draught power in domestic animals. In: *ACIAR Proceedings Series* No. 10, Australian Centre for International Agricultural Research, pp. 140–146.

Pasman, E.J., Dijkhuizen, A.A. and Wentink, G.H. (1994) A state-transition model to simulate the economics of bovine virus diarrhoea control. *Preventive Veterinary Medicine* 20(4), 269–277.

Perry, B.D. and Young, A.S. (1995) The past and future roles of epidemiology and economics in the control of tick-borne diseases of livestock in Africa: the case of theileriosis. *Preventive Veterinary Medicine* 25, 107–120.

Phoung, P.T. (1993) Vietnam. In: Patten, B.E., Spencer, T.L., Johnson, R.B., Hoffmann, D. and Lehane, L. (eds) *Pasteurellosis in Production Animals*. An international workshop sponsored by ACIAR held at Bali, Indonesia, 10–13 August 1992. ACIAR Proceedings, No. 43. Australian Centre for International Agricultural Research, Canberra, Australia, pp. 240–242.

Putra, A.A.G. (1993) Indonesia. In: Patten, B.E., Spencer, T.L., Johnson, R.B., Hoffmann, D. and Lehane, L. (eds) *Pasteurellosis in Production Animals*. An international workshop sponsored by ACIAR held at Bali, Indonesia, 10–13 August 1992. ACIAR Proceedings, No. 43. Australian Centre for International Agricultural Research, Canberra, Australia, pp. 229–231.

Raja, R.H. (1985) Pakistan. In: Della-Porta, A.J. (ed.) *Veterinary Viral Diseases. Their Significance in South East Asia and the Western Pacific*. Proceedings of an International symposium held at the Australian Animal Health Laboratory, Geelong, Australia, 27–30 August 1984. Academic Press, Sydney, Australia, pp. 216–222.

Rajala-Schultz, P.J. and Grohn, Y.T. (1999) Epidemiology of production diseases in Finnish Ayrshire cows. II Effect of disease on milk yield. [Finnish] Tuotantosairauksien epidemiologiaa suomalaisilla ayrshire-lehmilla II sairauksien vaikutus maidontuotantoon. *Suomen Elainlaakarilehti* 105(12), 655–660.

Reinhardt, G., Hochstein-Mintzel, V., Riedemann, S., Leal, H. and Niedda, M. (1988) Serological study of enzootic bovine leukosis on a farm in the province of Valdivia in relation to production and reproduction values. [Spanish] Estudio serologico de leucosis enzootica bovina en un predio de la provincia de Valdivia y su relacion a parametros productivos y reproductivos. *Journal of Veterinary Medicine, B (Infectious Diseases, Immunology, Food Hygiene, Veterinary Public Health)* 35(3), 178–185.

Roeder, P. (2000a) Emergency strengthening of rinderpest surveillance and control in Western Sudan. A workshop on rinderpest disease surveillance and epdemiology. Khartoum 17–22 January 2000. Available at: www.fao.org

Roeder, P. (2000b) Strengthening disease surveillance for rinderpest and development of and eradication strategy. A preliminary appraisal of current rinderpest epidemiology in Pakistan and implications for rinderpest control. Available at: www.fao.org

Ronohardjo, P. and Rastiko, P. (1982) Some epidemiological aspects and economic loss of bovine ephemeral fever outbreak in Tuban and surrounding areas, East Java, Indonesia. *Penyakit Hewan* 14(24), 25–29.

Ronohardjo, P., Wilson, A.J., Partoutomo, S. and Hirst, R.G. (1986) Some aspects of the epidemiology and economics of important diseases of large ruminants in Indonesia. In: *Proceedings of the 4th International Symposium on Veterinary Epidemiology and Economics, Singapore, 18–22 November 1985*. ISVEE, Singapore, pp. 303–305.

Rossiter, P.B. and James, A.D. (1989) An epidemiological model of rinderpest. II Simulations of the behaviour of rinderpest virus in populations. *Tropical Animal Health and Production* 21, 69–84.

Rossiter, P.B., Karstad, L., Jesset, D.M., Yamamoto, T., Dardiri, A.H. and Mushi, E.Z. (1983) Neutralizing antibodies to rinderpest virus in wild animal sera collected in Kenya between 1970 and 1981. *Preventive Veterinary Medicine* 1, 257–264.

Rushton, J., Pilling, P. and Heffernan, C. (2001) *Review of Livestock Diseases and their Importance in the Lives of Poor People*. A study commissioned by ILRI. ILRI, Nairobi, Kenya.

Schramm, G. and Aragon, A. (1994) Effects of enzootic bovine leukosis and its control on bovine production and reproduction performance on a dairy farm in Costa Rica. [German] Fallstudie uber den Einfluss von Leukose und Leukosebekampfungsmassnahmen auf die Produktions- und Reproduktionsleistung einer Milchviehherde in Costa Rica. *Tierarztliche Umschau* 49(1), 26–31.

Scott, G.R. (1990) Diseases caused by viruses. In: Sewell, M.M.H. and Brocklesby, D.W. (eds) *Handbook on Animal Diseases in the Tropics*. Baillière Tindall, London, pp. 257–362.

Seegers, H., Beaudeau, F., Fourichon, C. and Bareille, N. (1998) Reasons for culling in French Holstein cows. *Preventive Veterinary Medicine* 36(4), 257–271.

Seré, S. and Steinfeld, H. (1995) *World Livestock Production Systems – Current Status, Issues and Trends*. FAO Animal Production and Health Paper No. 127. FAO, Rome, Italy.

Siddique, M.R. (1985) Status of rinderpest. Its control and eradication programme in Bangladesh. In: Della-Porta, A.J. (ed.) *Veterinary Viral Diseases. Their Significance in South East Asia and the Western Pacific*. Proceedings of an International Symposium held at the Australian Animal Health Laboratory, Geelong, Australia, 27–30 August 1984. Academic Press, Sydney, Australia, pp. 497–501.

Sorensen, J.T., Enevoldsen, C. and Houe, H. (1995) A stochastic model for simulation of the economic consequences of bovine virus diarrhoea virus infection in a dairy herd. *Preventive Veterinary Medicine* 23(3/4), 215–227.

Stark, K.D.C., Frei-Staheli, C., Frei, P.P., Pfeiffer, D.U., Danuser, J., Audige, L., Nicolet, J., Strasser, M., Gottstein, B. and Kihm, U. (1997) Incidence and costs of health problems in Swiss dairy cattle and their calves (1993–1994) [German] Haufigkeit und Kosten von Gesundheits-problemen bei Schweizer Milchkuhen und deren Kalbern (1993–1994). *Schweizer Archiv für Tierheilkunde* 139(8), 343–353.

Tambi, E.N., Maina, O.W., Mukhebi, A.W. and Randolph, T.F. (1999) Economic impact assessment of rinderpest control in Africa. *Revue Scientifique et Technique Office International des Epizooties* 2, 458–477.

Theodoridis, A., Giesecke, W.H. and du Toit, I.J. (1973) Effects of ephemeral fever on milk production and reproduction of dairy cattle. *Onderstepoort Journal of Veterinary Research* 40(3), 83–91.

Thompson, K.G., Johnstone, A.C. and Hilbink, F. (1993) Enzootic bovine leukosis in New Zealand – a case report and update. *New Zealand Veterinary Journal* 41(4), 190–194.

Vagsholm, I., Carpenter, T.E. and Howitt, R.E. (1991) Shadow costs of disease and its impact on output supply and input demand: the dual estimation approach. *Preventive Veterinary Medicine* 10(3), 195–212.

Valdespino, J.R.O. (1993) Losses from the premature culling of dairy cows in Mexico. [Spanish] Perdidas por desecho prematuro de vacas en un hato lechero en Mexico. *World Animal Review* 74–75, 64–67.

Van Khar, U.R. and Myint, A. (1993) Myanmar. In: Patten, B.E., Spencer, T.L., Johnson, R.B., Hoffmann, D. and Lehane, L. (eds) *Pasteurellosis in Production Animals*. An international workshop sponsored by ACIAR held at Bali, Indonesia, 10–13 August 1992. ACIAR Proceedings, No. 43. Australian Centre for International Agricultural Research, Canberra, Australia, pp. 249–251.

Voigts, A.A., Ngaisure, G., Henton, M.M. and Hubschle, O.B.J. (1997) Haemorrhagic septicaemia due to *Pasteurella multocida* type B2 in Namibia. *Tropical Animal Health and Production* 29, 247–248.

Wafula, J.S. and Kariuki, D.P. (1987) A recent outbreak of rinderpest in East Africa. *Tropical Animal Health and Production* 19, 173–176.

Walsh, J. (1987) War on cattle disease divides the troops. *Science* 137, 1289–1291.

Wells, S.J., Ott, S.L. and Seitzinger, A.H. (1998) Key health issues for dairy cattle – new and old. *Journal of Dairy Science* 81(11), 3029–3035.

Wentink, G.H. and Dijkhuizen, A.A. (1990) Economic consequences of infection with bovine diarrhoea virus in 14 dairy herds. [Dutch] Economische gevolgen van een infectie met het Bovine Virus Diarree virus (BVD-virus) op 14 melkveebedrijven. *Tijdschrift voor Diergeneeskunde* 115(22), 1031–1040.

Wittkowski, G. and Orban, S. (1984) Increased prevalence of abortions, premature birth and neonatal calf losses in a dairy herd – a consequence of bovine diarrhoea virus infection. [German] Gehauftes Auftreten von Aborten, Fruhgeburten und neonatalen Kalberverlusten in einem Rinderbestand-Folge einer BVD-Virusinfektion. *Berliner und Munchener Tierarztliche Wochenschrift* 97(9), 305–310.

Yeo, B.K. and Mokhtar, I. (1993) Haemorrhagic septicaemia in Sabah, Malaysia. In: Patten, B.E., Spencer, T.L., Johnson, R.B., Hoffmann, D. and Lehane, L. (eds) *Pasteurellosis in Production Animals*. An international workshop sponsored by ACIAR held at Bali, Indonesia, 10–13 August 1992. ACIAR Proceedings, No. 43. Australian Centre for International Agricultural Research, Canberra, Australia, pp. 112–115.

Diseases of Small Ruminants

Adu, F.D. and Joannis, T.E. (1984) Serum-virus simultaneous method of immunisation against peste des petits ruminants. *Tropical Animal Health and Production* 16, 115–118.

Akerejola, O.O., Veen, T.W.S. van and Njoku, C.O. (1979) Ovine and caprine diseases in Nigeria: a review of economic losses. *Bulletin of Animal Health and Production in Africa* 27(1), 65–70.

Awa, D.N., Njoya, A. and Ngo Tama, A.C. (2000) Economics of prophylaxis against peste des petits ruminants and gastrointestinal helminthosis in small ruminants in north Cameroon. *Tropical Animal Health and Production* 32(6), 391–403.

Ba, S.B., Udo, H.M.J. and Zwart, D. (1996) Impact of veterinary treatments on goat mortality and offtake in semi-arid area of Mali. *Small Ruminant Research* 19, 1–8.

Bennett, R.M., Christiansen, K. and Clifton-Hadley, R.S. (1999) *An economic study of the importance of non-notifiable diseases of farm animals in Great Britain*. Available at: http://www.rdg.ac.uk/AcaDepts/ae/AEM/livestockdisea

Cole, D.J.W. and Heath, A.C.G. (1999) Progress towards development and adoption of integrated management systems against flystrike and lice in sheep. *Proceedings of the New Zealand Grassland Association* 61, 37–42.

Empres (1998) Assessment of PPR in the Middle East and the Horn of Africa. *Empres Transboundary Animal Diseases Bulletin* 6. Available at: www.fao.org

Kanyari, P.W.N., Allonby, E.W., Wilson, A.J. and Munyua, W.K. (1983) Some economic effects of trypanosomiasis in goats. *Tropical Animal Health and Production* 15(3), 153–160.

Martrenchar, A., Boucher, D., Zoyem, N., Thiacourt, F. and Lambert, M. (1997) Risk factors responsible for the appearance of individual clinical signs in small ruminants in North Cameroon. *Small Ruminant Research* 26, 45–52.

Martrenchar, A., Zoyem, N., Njoya, A., Ngo Tama, A.C., Bouchel, D. and Diallo, A. (1999) Field study of a homologous vaccine against peste des petits ruminants in northern Cameroon. *Small Ruminant Research* 31, 277–280.

Mukasa-Mugerwa, E., Lahlou-Kassi, A., Anindo, D., Rege, J.E.O., Tembely, S., Tibbo, M. and Baker, R.L. (2000) Between and within breed variation in lamb survival and the risk factors associated with major causes of mortality in indigenous Horro and Menz sheep in Ethiopia. *Small Ruminant Research* 37(1/2), 1–12.

Nawathe, D.R. (1984) Control of peste des petits ruminants in Nigeria. *Preventive Veterinary Medicine* 2, 147–155.

New Agriculturalist (2000) Peste des petits ruminants – an emerging plague? *New Agriculturalist on line*. Available at: www.newagri.co.uk/00–6

OIE (2001) Handistatus II. Office International des Epizooties. Available at: www.OIE.int

Reynolds, L. and Francis, P.A. (1988) The effect of PPR control and dipping on village goat populations in southwest Nigeria. *ILCA Bulletin* 32, 22–27.

Roeder, P.L., Abraham, G., Kenfe, G. and Barret, T. (1994) Peste des petits ruminants in Ethiopian goats. *Tropical Animal Health and Production* 26, 69–73.

Seré, S. and Steinfeld, H. (1995) *World Livestock Production Systems – Current Status, Issues and Trends*. FAO Animal Production and Health Paper No. 127. FAO, Rome, Italy.

Stem, C. (1993) An economic analysis of the prevention of peste des petits ruminants in Nigerian goats. *Preventive Veterinary Medicine* 16, 141–150.

Sweasey, D., Patterson, D.S.P., Richardson, C., Harkness, J.W., Shaw, I.G. and Williams, W.W. (1979) Border disease: a sequential study of surviving lambs and an assessment of its effect on profitability. *Veterinary Record* 104(20), 447–450.

Taylor, W.P. (1984) The distribution and prevalence of peste des petits ruminants. *Preventive Veterinary Medicine* 2, 157–166.

Diseases of Pigs

Awa, D.N., Njoya, A., Tama, A.C.N. and Ekue, F.N. (1999) The health status of pigs in North Cameroon. *Revue d'Elevage et de Médesine Vétérinaire des Pays Tropicaux* 52(2), 93–98.

Bennett, R.M., Christiansen, K. and Clifton-Hadley, R.S. (1999). *An economic study of the importance of non-notifiable diseases of farm animals in Great Britain*. Available at: http://www.rdg.ac.uk/AcaDepts/ae/AEM/livestockdisea

Blanquefort, P. (1995) Overall evaluation of control programme of PRRS in the Loire region. [French] Evaluation globale du programme de lutte contre le syndrome dysgénésique et respiratoire porcin dans les Pays de la Loire. *Epidémiologie et Santé Animale* 28, 47–60.

Braco-Forte Junior, M. da C. (1970) African swine fever in Portugal. Peste suina Africana em Portugal. *Anais da Escola Superior de Medicina Veterinaria, Lisboa* 12, 37–69.

Brouwer, J., Frankena, K., de Jong, M.F., Voets, R., Dijkhuizen, A., Verheijden, J. and Komijn, R.E. (1994) PRRS: effect on herd performance after initial infection and risk analysis. *Veterinary Quarterly* 16(2), 95–100.

Buijtels, J., Huirne, R., Dijkhuizen, A., Jong, M. de and Nes, A. van (1997) Computer simulation to support policy making in the control of pseudorabies. *Veterinary Microbiology* 55(1/4), 181–185.

Chae ChanHee, Kim OkJin, Min KyoungSub, Choi ChangSun, Kim JungHyun and Cho WanSeob (2000) Seroprevalence of porcine respiratory coronavirus in selected Korean pigs. *Preventive Veterinary Medicine* 46(4), 293–296.

Christensen, J., Ellegaard, B., Petersen, B.K., Willeberg, P. and Mousing, J. (1994) Pig health and production surveillance in Denmark: sampling design, data recording and measures of disease frequency. *Preventive Veterinary Medicine* 20(1/2), 47–61.

Dee, S.A., Joo, H.S., Polson, D.D. and Marsh, W.E. (1997) Evaluation of the effects of nursery depopulation on the profitability of 34 pig farms. *Veterinary Record* 140(19), 498–500.

Dee, S.A., Bierk, M.D., Deen, J. and Molitor, T.W. (2001) An evaluation of test and removal for the elimination of porcine reproductive and respiratory syndrome virus from 5 swine farms. *Canadian Journal of Veterinary Research* 65(1), 22–27.

Dijkhuizen, A.A., Jalvingh, A.W., Bolder, F.W.M.M., Stelwagen, J. and Schukken, Y.H. (1991) Determining the economic impact of the 'new' pig disease. In: *Porcine Reproductive and Respiratory Syndrome (the New Pig Disease)*. A report on the seminar held in Brussels on 4–5 November 1991 and organized by the European Commission (Directorate-General for Agriculture). European Commission, Brussels, Belgium, pp. 53–60.

Done, J.T. and Ellis, P.R. (1988) Aujeszky's disease: need for economic review. *Veterinary Record* 122(25), 615–616.

Ellis, P.R. (1972) *An Economic Evaluation of the Swine Fever Eradication Programme in Great Britain Using Cost–Benefit Analysis Techniques*. University of Reading, Department of Agriculture, Study No. 11, 76 pp.

Ellis, P.R., James, A.D. and Shaw, A.P.M. (1977) *Studies on the Epidemiology and Economics of Swine Fever Eradication in the EEC*. Commission of the European Communities, Luxembourg.

Empres (1998) Update on ASF. Situation in West Africa. *Empres Transboundary Animal Diseases Bulletin* 8. Available at: www.fao.org

Empres (1999) African Swine Fever (ASF). ASF in Botswana. *Empres Transboundary Animal Diseases Bulletin* 11. Available at: www.fao.org

Empres (2000) African Swine Fever, Epidemiosurveillance with TADINFO in Ghana. *Empres Transboundary Animal Diseases Bulletin* 14. Available at: www.fao.org

FAO (1998) News and highlights. Food and Agriculture Organisation of the United Nations. Available at: www.fao.org/news/1998

Farez, S. and Morley, R.S. (1997) Potential animal health hazards of pork and pork products. *Revue Scientifique et Technique Office International des Epizooties* 16(1), 65–78.

Griglio, B., Stannino, G, Grivetto, V., Filippi, E., Rossignoli, M. and Guarda, F. (1992) Monitoring of swine diseases at slaughter as a basis for epidemiological studies. [Italian] Il monitoraggio delle patologie del suino al macello come base per gli studi epidemiologici. *Nuovo Progresso Veterinario* 47(19), 597–602.

Hall, R.E. (1984) A 1984 swine health survey conducted by the American Association of Swine Practitioners (AASP). *Proceedings of the United States Animal Health Association* 88, 40–57.

Haresnape, J.M. (1984) African swine fever in Malawi. *Tropical Animal Health and Production* 16, 123–125.

Haresnape, J.M. (1988) Isolation of African swine fever from ticks of the *Ornithodoros moubata* complex (Ixodoidea: Argasidae) collected within the African Swine Fever enzootic area of Malawi. *Epidemiology and Infection* 101, 173–185.

Haresnape, J.M., Lungu, S.A.M. and Mamu, F.D. (1987) An updated survey of African Swine Fever in Malawi. *Epidemiology and Infection* 99, 723–732.

Lai Thi Kim Lan (2000) Epidemiology and economics of classical swine fever at smallholder level in Vietnam. MSc dissertation, University of Reading, VEERU, Reading, UK.

Madec, F., Eveno, E., Morvan, P., Hamon, L., Blanchard, P., Cariolet, R., Amenna, N., Morvan, H., Truong, C., Mahe, D., Albina, E. and Jestin, A. (2000) Post-weaning multisystemic wasting syndrome (PMWS)

in pigs in France: clinical observations from follow-up studies on affected farms. *Livestock Production Science* 63(3), 223–233.

Mangen, M.J.J., Jalvingh, A.W., Nielen, M., Mourits, M.C.M., Klinkenberg, D. and Dijkhuizen, A.A. (2001) Spatial and stochastic simulation to compare two emergency-vaccination strategies with a marker vaccine in the 1997/1998 Dutch Classical Swine Fever epidemic. *Preventive Veterinary Medicine* 48(3), 177–200.

Nana-Nukechap, M.F. and Gibbs, E.P.F. (1985) Socioeconomic effects of African swine fever in Cameroon. *Tropical Animal Health and Production* 17, 183–184.

New Agriculturalist (2000) CSF a communication crisis? *New Agriculturalist on line.* Available at: www. newagri.co.uk/00–6

Nielen, M., Jalvingh, A.W., Meuwissen, M.P.M., Horst, S.H. and Dijkhuizen, A.A. (1999) Spatial and stochastic simulation to evaluate the impact of events and control measures on the 1997–1998 classical swine fever epidemic in The Netherlands. II. Comparison of control strategies. In: Dijkhuizen, A.A. (ed.) *Preventive Veterinary Medicine* 39(4), 297–317.

Nodelijk, G., Jong, M.C.M. de, Nes, A. van, Vernooy, J.C.M., Leengoed, L.A.M.G. van, Pol, J.M.A. and Verheijden, J.H.M. (2000) Introduction, persistence and fade-out of porcine reproductive and respiratory syndrome virus in a Dutch breeding herd: a mathematical analysis. *Epidemiology and Infection* 124(1), 173–182.

OIE (2001) Handistatus II. Office International des Epizooties. Available at: www.OIE.int

Pejsak, Z., Stadejek, T. and Markowska-Daniel, I. (1997) Clinical signs and economic losses caused by porcine reproductive and respiratory syndrome virus in a large breeding farm. *Veterinary Microbiology* 55(1/4), 317–322.

Pejsak, Z., Lipowski, A. and Stadejek, T. (2000) Outbreak of PRRS in pig herd – epidemiological and economic analysis. [Polish] Analiza epizootyczna i ekonomiczna wystapienia zespolu rozrodczo-oddechowego w stadzie swin. *Medycyna Weterynaryjna* 56(4), 226–228.

Penny, R.H.C. and Penny, J.C. (1978) Priorities for pig research: the results of the second pig veterinary society questionnaire. *Pig Veterinary Society Proceedings* 3, 119–124.

Regula, G., Lichtensteiger, C.A., Mateus-Pinilla, N.E., Scherba, G., Miller, G.Y. and Weigel, R.M. (2000) Comparison of serologic testing and slaughter evaluation for assessing the effects of subclinical infection on growth in pigs. *Journal of the American Veterinary Medical Association* 217(6), 888–895.

Rodrigues, C.A., Gardner, I.A. and Carpenter, T.E. (1990) Financial analysis of pseudorabies control and eradication in swine. *Journal of the American Veterinary Medical Association* 197(10), 1316–1323.

Saatkamp, H.W., Dijkhuizen, A.A., Geers, R., Huirne, R.B.M., Noordhuizen, J.P.T.M. and Goedseels, V. (1997) Economic evaluation of national identification and recording systems for pigs in Belgium. *Preventive Veterinary Medicine* 30(2), 121–135.

Seré, S. and Steinfeld, H. (1995) *World Livestock Production Systems – Current Status, Issues and Trends.* FAO Animal Production and Health Paper No. 127. FAO, Rome, Italy.

Smits, J.M. and Merks, J.W.M. (2001) The importance of different pig diseases in the Netherlands. [Dutch] Het belang van de verschillende varkensziekten in Nederland. *Tijdschrift voor Diergeneeskunde* 126(1), 2–8.

Sumption, K.J. (1992) Genotypic comparison of African swine fever virus isolated from Zambia and Malawi. PhD thesis, University of Reading, Reading, UK.

Teuffert, J., Ohlinger, V.F., Wohlfarth, E., Schopeck, W. and Haas, B. (1993) Investigations on the occurrence of porcine reproductive and respiratory syndrome in Sachsen-Anhalt. I. Its course and economic effects in a large sow breeding unit during the 20 months after the disease outbreak. [German] Untersuchungen zum Auftreten des 'Porcine Reproductive and Respiratory Syndrome (PRRS)' in Sachsen-Anhalt. I. Verlauf und betriebswirtschaftliche Auswirkungen in einer geschlossenen Sauengrossanlage innerhalb 20 Monaten nach Seuchenausbruch. *Tierarztliche Umschau* 48(9), 539–549.

Texdorf, I. (1981) Diseases that impair the quality of slaughter pigs. [German] Qualitatsmindernde Erkrankungen des Mastschweines. *Fleischwirtschaft* 61(7), 999–1003.

Wesley, R.D., Woods, R.D., McKean, J.D., Senn, M.K. and Elazhary, Y. (1997) Prevalence of coronavirus antibodies in Iowa swine. *Canadian Journal of Veterinary Research* 61(4), 305–308.

Wilkinson, P.J. (1993) Special features of African swine fever. In: Galo, A. (ed.) *Agriculture. Coordination of Agricultural Research. African Swine Fever.* Proceedings of a workshop with the community programme for coordination of agricultural research, held in Lisbon on 7–9 October 1991. Commission of the European Communities, Luxembourg, 275 pp.

Wilkinson, P.J., Wardley, R.C. and Williams, S.M. (1981) African swine fever virus (Malta/78) in pigs. *Journal of Comparative Pathology* 91(2), 277–284.

Wilkinson, P.J., Pegram, R.G., Perry, B.D., Lemche, J. and Schells, H.F. (1988) The distribution of African swine fever virus isolated from *Ornithodoros moubata* in Zambia. *Epidemiology and Infection* 101, 547–564.

Willeberg, P., Leontides, L., Ewald, C., Mortensen, S., McInerney, J.P., Howe, K.S. and Kooij, D. (1996) Effect of vaccination against Aujeszky's disease compared with test and slaughter programme: epidemiological and economical evaluations. *Acta Veterinaria Scandinavica Supplementum* 90, 25–51.

Diseases of Poultry

Aichberger, L. (1986) Health status of flocks of broiler fowl. [German] Gesundheitsstatus in Geflugelmastbetrieben. *Wiener Tierarztliche Monatsschrift* 73(7), 253–254.

Ansell, D.J. (1988) Marek's disease an economic appraisal. In: Ansell, D.J and Done, J.T. (eds) *Veterinary Research and Development: Cost–Benefit Studies on Products for the Control of Animal Diseases*. Centre for Agricultural Strategy, University of Reading, Reading, UK, pp. 1–26.

Awan, A.W., Otte, M.J. and James, A.D. (1994) The epidemiology of Newcastle disease in rural poultry: a review. *Avian Pathology* 23, 405–423.

Bennett, R.M., Christiansen, K. and Clifton-Hadley, R.S. (1999) *An economic study of the importance of non-notifiable diseases of farm animals in Great Britain*. Available at: http://www.rdg.ac.uk/AcaDepts/ae/AEM/livestockdisea

Binta, M.G., Mushi, E.Z. and Adom, E.K. (1995) The impact of infectious bursal disease in Botswana. *Zimbabwe Veterinary Journal* 26(3/4), 110–115.

Bisgaard, M., Folkersen, J.C.R. and Hoeg, C. (1981) Arthritis in ducks. II. Condemnation rate, economic significance and possible preventive measures. *Avian Pathology* 10(3), 321–327.

Branton, S.L., Lott, B.D., May, J.D., Maslin, W.R., Boyle, C.R. and Pharr, G.T. (1997) The effects of F strain *Mycoplasma gallisepticum*, *Mycoplasma synoviae*, and the dual infection in commercial layer hens over a 44-week laying cycle when challenged before beginning of lay. I. Egg production and selected egg quality parameters. *Avian Diseases* 41(4), 832–837.

Calnek, B.W. and Witter, R.L. (1997) Marek's disease. In: Calnek, B.W. (ed.) *Diseases of Poultry*, 10th edn. Mosby Wolfe, London, pp. 369–413.

Carpenter, T.E. (1980) Economic evaluation of *Mycoplasma meleagridis* infection in turkeys: I. Production losses. II. Feasibility of eradication. *Dissertation Abstracts International* 41B(2), 485.

Carpenter, T.E. (1983) A microeconomic evaluation of the impact of *Mycoplasma meleagridis* infection in turkey production. *Preventive Veterinary Medicine* 1(4), 289–301.

Carpenter, T. and Riemann, H. (1980) Benefit–cost analysis of a disease eradication program in the United States: a case study of *Mycoplasma meleagridis* in turkeys. In: *Proceedings of the Second International Symposium on Veterinary Epidemiology and Economics, 7–11 May 1979, Canberra, Australia*. ISVEE, Canberra, Australia, pp. 458–462.

Carpenter, T.E., Howitt, R., McCapes, R., Yamamoto, R. and Riemann, H.P. (1981a) Formulating a control program against *Mycoplasma meleagridis* using economic decision analysis. *Avian Diseases* 25(2), 260–271.

Carpenter, T.E., Edson, R.K. and Yamamoto, R. (1981b) Decreased hatchability of turkeys eggs caused by experimental infection with *Mycoplasma meleagridis*. *Avian Diseases* 25(1), 151–156.

Christiansen, K.H., Hird, D.W., Snipes, K.P., Danaye-Elmi, C., Palmer, C.W., McBride, M.D. and Utterback, W.W. (1996) California National Animal Health Monitoring System for meat turkey flocks – 1988–89 pilot study: management practices, flock health, and production. *Avian Diseases* 40(2), 278–284.

Copland, J.W., Ibrahim, A.L. and Spradbrow, P.B. (1988) A model for the epidemiological and economic evaluation of Newcastle disease of village poultry in South-east Asia and its control using heat tolerant V4 vaccine. *Acta Veterinaria Scandinavica* 84(Supplement), 405–407.

Ganesan, P.I., Rao, V.N.A. and Venugopal, K. (1993) Economic impact on production performance of layer poultry due to subclinical Ranikhet disease. *Indian Veterinary Journal* 70(6), 546–550.

Goren, E. (1979) Effect of *Mycoplasma synoviae* infection on the state of health and results of fattening of broiler chickens compared with the effects of various virus infections. A field study. [Dutch] Een praktijkonderzoek betreffende het effect van *Mycoplasma synoviae*-infectie ten opzichte van de invloed van diverse virus-infecties op de gezondheidstoestand en de mestresultaten van slachtkuikens. *Tijdschrift voor Diergeneeskunde* 104(9), 369–379.

Hafi, A., Reynolds, R. and Oliver, M. (1997) *Economic Impact of Newcastle Disease on the Australian Poultry Industry*. ABARE Research Report No. 94.7. Australian Bureau of Agricultural and Resource Economics, Canberra, Australia, vii + 70 pp.

Harada, Y. (1986) Field trial of oxytetracycline and doxycycline for preventing *Mycoplasma gallisepticum* and *M. synoviae* infections. [Japanese] *Journal of the Japan Veterinary Medical Association* 39(3), 175–179.

Heinze, E.M. (1984) Cost benefit analysis of the immunization of fowls against Marek's disease. [German] *Nutzen-Kosten-Analyse der Schutzimpfung gegen die Mareksche Krankheit der Huhner*. Tierarztliche Fakultat der Ludwig-Maximilians-Universitat, Munich, 103 pp.

Johnston, J. (1990) *Health and Productivity of Village Poultry in Southeast Asia. Economic Impact of Developing Techniques to Vaccinate Birds Orally Against Newcastle Disease*. ACIAR Working Paper No. 31. Australian Centre for International Agricultural Research, Canberra, Australia, 62 pp.

Johnston, J. (1993) Estimating the benefits of research to control Newcastle disease in smallholder village poultry. *Agricultural Systems and Information Technology Newsletter* 5(1), 39–40.

Johnston, J., Fontanilla, B. and Silvano, F. (1992) The economic impact of vaccinating village fowls: a case study from the Philippines. In: Spradbrow, P.B. (ed.) *Newcastle Disease in Village Chickens*. Australian Centre for International Agricultural Research, Canberra, Australia, pp. 62–71.

Jorgensen, P.H., Otte, L., Nielsen, O.L. and Bisgaard, M. (1995) Influence of subclinical virus infections and other factors on broiler flock performance. *British Poultry Science* 36(3), 455–463.

Kapetanov, R., Pejin, I., Tesic, M., Palic, T. and Kapetanov, M. (1998) Deterioration of natural productivity parameters in broilers from cooperative production. [Serbian] Retardacija naturalnih pokazatelja u kooperativnoj proizvodnji brojlerskih pilica. *Zivinarstvo* 33(1), 15–19.

Kvarnfors, E., Cerenius, F., Bjornerot, L., Engstrom, B., Engvall, A. and Renstrom, L. (1997) Newcastle disease outbreak in Skane in 1995. [Swedish] *Newcastleutbrottet i Skane 1995*. Svensk Veterinartidning, No. SUPP27. Svensk Veterinartidning, Stockholm, Sweden, 24 pp.

Landgraf, H. and Vielitz, E. (1983) Latent infections in flocks of laying hens; experimental infections in hens from flocks with several age groups. (Mycoplasma). [German] Latente Infektionen in Legehennenbestanden; Infektionsversuche mit Tieren aus Bestanden mit mehreren Altersgruppen. *Deutsche Tierarztliche Wochenschrift* 90(6) 219–221.

Lee, K. (1980) Long term effects of Marek's disease vaccination with cell-free herpesvirus of turkey and age at debeaking on performance and mortality of White Leghorns. *Poultry Science* 59(9), 2002–2007.

Lee, K. and Reid, I.S. (1977) The effect of Marek's disease vaccination and day-old debeaking on the performance of growing pullets and laying hens. *Poultry Science* 56(3), 736–740.

Leslie, J. (2000) Newcastle disease: outbreak losses and control policy costs. *Veterinary Record* 146(21), 603–606.

McIlroy, S.G. (1994) The epidemiology and control of economically important diseases of broiler and broiler breeder production. In: *Proceedings, Belfast, 13–15 April 1994*. Society for Veterinary Epidemiology and Preventive Medicine, Edinburgh, UK, pp. 114–127.

McIlroy, S.G., Goodall, E.A. and McCracken, R.M. (1989) Economic effects of subclinical infectious bursal disease on broiler production. *Avian Pathology* 18(3), 465–473, 475–480.

McIlroy, S.G., Goodall, E.A., Rice, D.A., McNulty, M.S. and Kennedy, D.G. (1993) Improved performance in commercial broiler flocks with subclinical infectious bursal disease when fed diets containing increased concentrations of vitamin E. *Avian Pathology* 22(1), 81–94.

Mohammed, H.O., Carpenter, T.E. and Yamamoto, R. (1987) Economic impact of *Mycoplasma gallisepticum* and *M. synoviae* in commercial layer flocks. *Avian Diseases* 31(3), 477–482.

Nawathe, D.R. and Lamorde, A.G. (1982) The impact of viral diseases on the Nigerian livestock economy and some suggestions on the control of rabies in Nigeria. *Bulletin of Animal Health and Production in Africa* 30(4), 309–314.

Omohundro, R.E. and Walker, J.W. (1973) A report on the exotic Newcastle disease situation in the United States. In: *Proceedings 77th Annual Meeting of the United States Animal Health Association, 1973*. United States Animal Health Association, St Joseph, Missouri, pp. 235–241.

Palic, T., Orlic, D., Miljkovic, B., Stojiljkovic, Lj., Rasic, Z., Nikolovski, J., Sekler, M., Ignjatovic, R. and Dekic, J. (1998) Analysis of poultry health in Serbia between 1989 and 1998. [Serbian] Analiza zdravstvene problematike u zivinarstvu Srbije za protekli period. *Zivinarstvo* 33(4/5), 81–90.

Permin, A. (1997) A study of the disease situation of rural scavenging poultry in the Morogoro Region of Tanzania. In: Dolberg, F. and Petersen, P.H. (eds) *Integrated Farming in Human Development*. Proceedings of a Workshop Tune, Landboskole, Denmark, 25–29 March 1996. DSR-Forlag, Frederiksberg, Denmark, pp. 135–140.

Powell, P.C. (1986) Marek's disease – a world poultry problem. *Worlds Poultry Science Journal* 42(3), 205–218.

Purchase, H.G. and Schultz, E.F. Jr (1978) The economics of Marek's disease control in the United States. *Worlds Poultry Science Journal* 34(4), 198–204.

Ring, C., Heinze, E.M. and Mayr, A. (1985) Cost benefit analysis of the immunization of fowls against Marek's disease. [German] Okonomische Bewertung der Schutzimpfung gegen die Mareksche Krankheit der Huhner mittels Nutzen-Kosten-Analyse. *Zentralblatt für Veterinarmedizin*, A 32(2), 143–148.

Ring, C., Mayr, A., Kandler, J. and Weinberg, E. (1988) Cost benefit analysis of vaccination of poultry against Newcastle disease. [German] Zur okonomischen Bewertung (NKA) der Schutzimpfung gegen die Newcastle Disease beim Nutzgeflugel. *Journal of Veterinary Medicine, B (Infectious Diseases, Immunology, Food Hygiene, Veterinary Public Health)* 35(3), 214–217.

Seré, S. and Steinfeld, H. (1995) *World Livestock Production Systems – Current Status, Issues and Trends.* FAO Animal Production and Health Paper No. 127. FAO, Rome, Italy.

Spradbrow, P.B. (1990) Village poultry and preventive veterinary medicine. *Preventive Veterinary Medicine* 8(4), 305–307.

Spradbrow, P.B. (1993) Newcastle disease in village chickens. *Poultry Science Review* 5(1993/4), 57–96.

Tadic, V. and Bidin, Z. (1988) Losses due to Marek's disease in hybrids of heavy breeds of fowl in Yugoslavia. *Acta Veterinaria Scandinavica* 84(Supplement), 155–157.

Voigtlander, B., Wolf, E. and Thom, B. (1991) Economic results of vaccinating broiler flocks against Marek's disease. [German] Okonomische Ergebnisse einer Vakzinierung gegen die Mareksche Krankheit in einem Broilermastbetrieb. *Monatshefte für Veterinarmedizin* 46(6), 213–215.

Werner, P., Werner, O., Schmidt, U., Hahnefeld, H., Pick, H. and Tesmer, S. (1987) Riems Marek's disease vaccine – a significant contribution to improving the efficiency of intensive poultry production. [German] Die Riemser Marekvakzine-Ein wesentlicher Beitrag zur Sicherung der industriemassigen Geflugelproduktion. *Archiv für Experimentelle Veterinarmedizin* 41(5), 635–639.

Index